Pediatric Disorders: Practical Imaging Guidelines and Recommendations

Editor

EDWARD Y. LEE

RADIOLOGIC CLINICS OF NORTH AMERICA

www.radiologic.theclinics.com

Consulting Editor
FRANK H. MILLER

January 2022 • Volume 60 • Number 1

ELSEVIER

1600 John F. Kennedy Boulevard • Suite 1800 • Philadelphia, Pennsylvania, 19103-2899

http://www.theclinics.com

RADIOLOGIC CLINICS OF NORTH AMERICA Volume 60, Number 1
January 2022 ISSN 0033-8389, ISBN 13: 978-0-323-84860-2

Editor: John Vassallo (j.vassallo@elsevier.com)
Developmental Editor: Karen Solomon

Radiologic Clinics of North America (ISSN 0033-8389) is published bimonthly by Elsevier Inc., 360 Park Avenue South, New York, NY 10010-1710. Months of issue are January, March, May, July, September, and November. Periodicals postage paid at New York, NY and additional mailing offices. Subscription prices are USD 529 per year for US individuals, USD 1335 per year for US institutions, USD 100 per year for US students and residents, USD 624 per year for Canadian individuals, USD 1362 per year for Canadian institutions, USD 717 per year for international individuals, USD 1362 per year for international institutions, USD 100 per year for Canadian students/residents, and USD 315 per year for international students/residents. To receive student and resident rate, orders must be accompanied by name of affiliated institution, date of term and the signature of program/residency coordinatior on institution letterhead. Orders will be billed at individual rate until proof of status is received. Foreign air speed delivery is included in all *Clinics* subscription prices. All prices are subject to change without notice. **POSTMASTER:** Send address changes to *Radiologic Clinics of North America*, Elsevier Health Sciences Division, Subscription Customer Service, 3251 Riverport Lane, Maryland Heights, MO63043. **Customer Service: Telephone: 1-800-654-2452** (U.S. and Canada); **1-314-447-8871** (outside U.S. and Canada). **Fax: 1-314-447-8029. E-mail: journalscustomerservice-usa@elsevier.com (for print support); journalsonlinesupport-usa@elsevier.com (for online support).**

Reprints. For copies of 100 or more of articles in this publication, please contact the Commercial Reprints Department, Elsevier Inc., 360 Park Avenue South, New York, New York 10010-1710. Tel.: +1-212-633-3874; Fax: +1-212-633-3820; E-mail: reprints@elsevier.com.

Radiologic Clinics of North America also published in Greek Paschalidis Medical Publications, Athens, Greece.

Radiologic Clinics of North America is covered in *MEDLINE/PubMed (Index Medicus), EMBASE/Excerpta Medica, Current Contents/Life Sciences, Current Contents/Clinical Medicine, RSNA Index to Imaging Literature, BIOSIS, Science Citation Index,* and *ISI/BIOMED.*

Contributors

CONSULTING EDITOR

FRANK H. MILLER, MD, FACR
Lee F. Rogers MD Professor of Medical Education, Chief, Body Imaging Section and Fellowship Program, Medical Director, MRI, Department of Radiology, Northwestern Memorial Hospital, Northwestern University, Feinberg School of Medicine, Chicago, Illinois, USA

EDITOR

EDWARD Y. LEE, MD, MPH
Associate Professor, Department of Radiology, Boston Children's Hospital, Harvard Medical School, Boston, Massachusetts, USA

AUTHORS

FREDERICK E. BUTT, MD
Department of Radiology, Dartmouth-Hitchcock Medical Center, One Medical Center Drive, Lebanon, New Hampshire, USA

APEKSHA CHATURVEDI, MD
Department of Imaging Sciences, University of Rochester Medical Center, School of Medicine and Dentistry, Rochester, New York, USA

NATHAN DAVID P. CONCEPCION, MD
Head, Section of Pediatric Radiology, Institute of Radiology, St. Luke's Medical Center-Global City, Philippines

SPENCER G. DEGERSTEDT, MD
Department of Radiology, Beth Israel Deaconess Medical Center, Harvard Medical School, Boston, Massachusetts, USA

MONICA EPELMAN, MD
Department of Radiology, Nemours Children's Health System/Nemours Children's Hospital, Orlando, Florida, USA

PILAR GARCIA-PEÑA, MD
Autonomous University of Barcelona (AUB), University Hospital Materno-Infantil Vall d'Hebron, Barcelona, Spain

JARED R. GREEN, MD
Chief of Pediatric Interventional Radiology, Joe DiMaggio Children's Hospital, Envision Radiology Associates of Hollywood, Pembroke Pines, Florida, USA

MAI-LAN HO, MD
Associate Professor, Director of Research, Department of Radiology, Director, Advanced Neuroimaging Core, Chair, Asian Pacific American Network, Secretary, Association for Staff and Faculty Women, Nationwide Children's Hospital, The Ohio State University, Columbus, Ohio, USA

NATHAN C. HULL, MD
Assistant Professor, Department of Radiology, Mayo Clinic, Rochester, Minnesota, USA

LINA KAROUT, MD
Research Fellow, Department of Radiology, Massachusetts General Hospital, Boston, Massachusetts, USA

HELEN H.R. KIM, MD
Assistant Professor, Department of Radiology, Seattle Children's Hospital and University of Washington, Seattle, Washington, USA

SUPIKA KRITSANEEPAIBOON, MD
Head, Section of Pediatric Imaging, Division of Diagnostic Radiology, Department of Radiology, Faculty of Medicine, Prince of Songkla University, Hat Yai, Thailand

BERNARD F. LAYA, MD, DO
Head, Section of Pediatric Radiology, Institute of Radiology, St. Luke's Medical Center-Quezon City, Quezon City, Philippines

EDWARD Y. LEE, MD, MPH
Associate Professor, Department of Radiology, Boston Children's Hospital, Harvard Medical School, Boston, Massachusetts, USA

TERESA I. LIANG, MD, FRCPC
Assistant Clinical Professor, Department of Radiology & Diagnostic Imaging, Stollery Children's Hospital and University of Alberta, Edmonton, Canada

LENA NAFFAA, MD
Radiology Department, Associate Professor of Radiology, University of Central Florida, Nemours Children's Hospital, Orlando, Florida, USA

JAISHREE NAIDOO, MD
Director, Paeds Diagnostic Imaging and Envisionit Deep AI, Johannesburg, South Africa

GRACE S. PHILLIPS, MD
Professor, Department of Radiology, Seattle Children's Hospital and University of Washington, Seattle, Washington, USA

SHANKAR RAJESWARAN, MD
Assistant Professor of Radiology, Ann and Robert H. Lurie Children's Hospital of Chicago, Northwestern University Feinberg School of Medicine, Chicago, Illinois, USA

RICARDO RESTREPO, MD
Professor of Radiology, Department of Interventional Radiology and Body Imaging, Nicklaus Children's Hospital, Miami, Florida, USA

JONATHAN D. SAMET, MD
Associate Professor of Radiology, Ann and Robert H. Lurie Children's Hospital of Chicago, Northwestern University Feinberg School of Medicine, Chicago, Illinois, USA

THOMAS SEMPLE, MDres, FRCR, MBBS, BSc
Department of Radiology, The Royal Brompton Hospital, London and Centre for Paediatrics and Child Health, Imperial College London, London, UK

PATRICK TIVNAN, MD
Department of Radiology, Boston Medical Center, Boston, Massachusetts, USA

ABBEY J. WINANT, MD
Department of Radiology, Boston Children's Hospital, Harvard Medical School, Boston, Massachusetts, USA

Contents

> Neck masses commonly present in children and several potential diagnostic and management pathways exist, though with a paucity of evidence-based recommendations. The purpose of this article is to evaluate the current literature and utilization of various diagnostic imaging modalities, with a review of imaging features and management pearls for pediatric neck masses. A comprehensive understanding and practical imaging workflow will guide optimal patient workup and management.

> Lower respiratory tract infection (LRTI) remains a major cause of morbidity and mortality in children. Various organisms cause LRTI, including viruses, bacteria, fungi, and parasites, among others. Infections caused by 2 or more organisms also occur, sometimes enhancing the severity of the infection. Medical imaging helps confirm a diagnosis but also plays a role in the evaluation of acute and chronic sequelae. Medical imaging tests help evaluate underlying pathology in pediatric patients with recurrent or long-standing symptoms as well as the immunocompromised.

> Congenital lung malformations are a spectrum of developmental anomalies comprised of malformations of the lung parenchyma, airways, and vasculature. Imaging assessment plays a pivotal role in the initial diagnosis, management, and follow-up evaluation of congenital lung malformations in the pediatric population. However, there is currently a lack of practical imaging guidelines and recommendations for the diagnostic imaging assessment of congenital lung malformations in infants and children. This article reviews the current evidence regarding the imaging evaluation of congenital lung malformations and provides up-to-date imaging recommendations for pediatric congenital lung malformations.

> Incidental pulmonary nodules are not infrequently identified on computed tomography imaging in the pediatric population and can be a challenge in suggesting appropriate follow-up recommendations. An evidence-based and practical imaging approach for diagnosis and appropriate directed management is essential for optimal patient care. This article provides an up-to-date review of the pediatric pulmonary nodule literature and suggests a practical algorithm to manage pulmonary nodules in the pediatric population.

In contrast with the algorithms and screening criteria available for adults with suspected pulmonary embolism, there is a paucity of guidance on the diagnostic approach for children. The incidence of pulmonary embolism in the pediatric population and young adults is higher than thought, and there is an urgent need for updated guidelines for the imaging approach to diagnosis in the pediatric population. This article presents an up-to-date review of imaging techniques, characteristic radiologic findings, and an evidence-based algorithm for the detection of pediatric pulmonary embolism to improve the care of pediatric patients with suspected pulmonary embolism.

Childhood interstitial lung disease (ChILD) is an umbrella term encompassing a diverse group of diffuse lung diseases affecting infants and children. Although the timely and accurate diagnosis of ChILD is often challenging, it is optimally achieved through the multidisciplinary integration of imaging findings with clinical data, genetics, and potentially lung biopsy. This article reviews the definition and classification of ChILD; the role of imaging, pathology, and genetics in ChILD diagnosis; treatment options; and future goals. In addition, a practical approach to ChILD imaging based on the latest available research and the characteristic imaging appearance of ChILD entities are presented.

Pediatric abdominal masses are commonly encountered in the pediatric population, with a broad differential diagnosis that encompasses benign and malignant entities. The primary role of abdominal imaging in the setting of a suspected pediatric abdominal mass is to establish its presence, as nonneoplastic entities can mimic an abdominal mass, and to identify characteristic imaging features that narrow the differential diagnosis. In the setting of a neoplasm, various imaging modalities play an important role to characterize the mass, stage extent of disease, and assist in presurgical planning. The purpose of this article is to discuss a practical imaging algorithm for suspected pediatric abdominal masses and to describe typical radiological findings of the commonly encountered abdominal masses in neonates and children with emphasis on imaging guidelines and recommendations.

Pediatric bowel obstructions are one of the most common surgical emergencies in children, and imaging plays a vital role in the evaluation and diagnosis. An evidence-based and practical imaging approach to diagnosing and localizing pediatric bowel obstructions is essential for optimal pediatric patient care. This article discusses an up-to-date practical diagnostic imaging algorithm for pediatric bowel obstructions and presents the imaging spectrum of pediatric bowel obstructions and their underlying causes.

Lina Karout and Lena Naffaa

Hip disorders are a wide range of conditions commonly affecting patients in the pediatric age group. Reaching an accurate diagnosis of these conditions in children may be challenging. The optimal use of image modalities in the approach of a child with possible hip pathology is essential, which allows radiologists and clinicians to narrow the differential diagnosis and reach a definitive diagnosis, which can consequently result in early and appropriate interventions leading to improved outcomes. Therefore, this article aims to provide practicing radiologists and clinicians with up-to-date and evidence-based imaging spectrum guidelines and recommendations for common pediatric hip disorders.

Frederick E. Butt, Edward Y. Lee, and Apeksha Chaturvedi

Pediatric musculoskeletal infections often pose a diagnostic challenge due to their frequently vague and nonspecific clinical presentation. Imaging evaluation is a crucial component to diagnostic workup of these entities. Changed epidemiology of these infections over the past 2 decades has resulted in increases in both disease incidence and severity in the pediatric population. Prompt and accurate diagnosis is essential in order to reduce the risk of morbid sequelae, and to optimize patient management. In this article, the unique pathophysiology of musculoskeletal infections and characteristic imaging findings in children compared with adults are reviewed.

Jonathan D. Samet, Ricardo Restrepo, Shankar Rajeswaran, Edward Y. Lee and Jared R. Green

Vascular malformations are commonly encountered in the pediatric population. This article reviews the imaging appearances of simple and syndromic vascular malformations in infants and children that radiologists should know and provides imaging guidelines based on an evidence-based approach. Malformations are discussed within the framework of the International Society for the Study of Vascular Anomalies classification system.

PROGRAM OBJECTIVE
The objective of the Radiologic Clinics of North America is to keep practicing radiologists and radiology residents up to date with current clinical practice in radiology by providing timely articles reviewing the state of the art in patient care.

TARGET AUDIENCE
Practicing radiologists, radiology residents, and other healthcare professionals who provide patient care utilizing radiologic findings.

LEARNING OBJECTIVES
Upon completion of this activity, participants will be able to:
1. Describe various pediatric disorders and characteristic imaging findings.
2. Discuss practical guidelines and recommendations for pediatric imaging.
3. Recognize newer pediatric imaging techniques and applications.

ACCREDITATION
The Elsevier Office of Continuing Medical Education (EOCME) is accredited by the Accreditation Council for Continuing Medical Education (ACCME) to provide continuing medical education for physicians.

The EOCME designates this journal-based CME activity for a maximum of 11 *AMA PRA Category 1 Credit*(s)™. Physicians should claim only the credit commensurate with the extent of their participation in the activity.

All other healthcare professionals requesting continuing education credit for this enduring material will be issued a certificate of participation.

DISCLOSURE OF CONFLICTS OF INTEREST
The EOCME assesses conflict of interest with its instructors, faculty, planners, and other individuals who are in a position to control the content of CME activities. All relevant conflicts of interest that are identified are thoroughly vetted by EOCME for fair balance, scientific objectivity, and patient care recommendations. EOCME is committed to providing its learners with CME activities that promote improvements or quality in healthcare and not a specific proprietary business or a commercial interest.

The planning committee, staff, authors, and editors listed below have identified no financial relationships or relationships to products or devices they or their spouse/life partner have with commercial interest related to the content of this CME activity:

Frederick E. Butt, MD; Apeksha Chaturvedi, MD; Regina Chavous-Gibson, MSN, RN; Nathan David P. Concepcion, MD; Spencer G. Degerstedt, MD; Monica Epelman, MD; Pilar Garcia-Peña, MD; Jared R. Green, MD; Mai-Lan Ho, MD; Nathan C. Hull, MD; Lina Karout, MD; Helen H.R. Kim, MD; Supika Kritsaneepaiboon, MD; Pradeep Kuttysankaran; Bernard F. Laya, MD, DO; Edward Y. Lee, MD, MPH; Teresa I. Liang, MD, FRCPC; Lena Naffaa, MD; Jaishree Naidoo, MD; Grace S. Phillips, MD; Shankar Rajeswaran, MD; Ricardo Restrepo, MD; Jonathan D. Samet, MD; Patrick Tivnan, MD; Abbey J. Winant, MD

The planning committee, staff, authors, and editors listed below have identified financial relationships or relationships to products or devices they or their spouse/life partner have with commercial interest related to the content of this CME activity:

Thomas Semple, MDres, FRCR, MBBS, BSc: Consultant: Boehringer Ingelheim, Parexel Biotech; Speaker: Vertex Pharmaceuticals; Researcher: Chiesi Pharmaceuticals

UNAPPROVED/OFF-LABEL USE DISCLOSURE
The EOCME requires CME faculty to disclose to the participants:
1. When products or procedures being discussed are off-label, unlabelled, experimental, and/or investigational (not US Food and Drug Administration [FDA] approved); and
2. Any limitations on the information presented, such as data that are preliminary or that represent ongoing research, interim analyses, and/or unsupported opinions. Faculty may discuss information about pharmaceutical agents that is outside of FDA-approved labelling. This information is intended solely for CME and is not intended to promote off-label use of these medications. If you have any questions, contact the medical affairs department of the manufacturer for the most recent prescribing information.

TO ENROLL
To enroll in the *Radiologic Clinics of North America* Continuing Medical Education program, call customer service at 1-800-654-2452 or sign up online at http://www.theclinics.com/home/cme. The CME program is available to subscribers for an additional annual fee of USD 356.00.

METHOD OF PARTICIPATION
In order to claim credit, participants must complete the following:
1. Complete enrolment as indicated above.
2. Read the activity.

3. Complete the CME Test and Evaluation. Participants must achieve a score of 70% on the test. All CME Tests and Evaluations must be completed online.

CME INQUIRIES/SPECIAL NEEDS

For all CME inquiries or special needs, please contact elsevierCME@elsevier.com.

RADIOLOGIC CLINICS OF NORTH AMERICA

FORTHCOMING ISSUES

March 2022
Imaging of Bone and SoftTissueTumors and Mimickers
Hillary W. Garner, *Editor*

May 2022
Imaging of Thoracic Infections
Loren Ketai, *Editor*

July 2022
Imaging of the Older Population
Eric Chang and Christine B. Chung, *Editors*

RECENT ISSUES

November 2021
Artificial Intelligence in Radiology
Daniel L. Rubin, *Editor*

September 2021
PET Imaging
Jonathan McConathy and Samuel J. Galgano, *Editors*

July 2021
Update on Incidental Cross-sectional Imaging Findings
Douglas S. Katz and John J. Hines, *Editors*

RELATED SERIES

Advances in Clinical Radiology
Available at: https://www.advancesinclinicalradiology.com/
Magnetic Resonance Imaging Clinics
Available at: https://www.mri.theclinics.com/
Neuroimaging Clinics
Available at: www.neuroimaging.theclinics.com
PET Clinics
Available at: www.pet.theclinics.com

THE CLINICS ARE AVAILABLE ONLINE!
Access your subscription at:
www.theclinics.com

Preface
Pediatric Imaging Guidelines and Recommendations

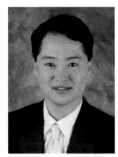

Edward Y. Lee, MD, MPH
Editor

Despite being the oldest radiologic subspecialty, pediatric imaging has traditionally been considered a clinical discipline with limited high-quality scientific investigation. Therefore, imaging evaluation often relies on anecdotal personal accounts rather than evidence-based research. However, practical and optimal imaging management requires imaging guidelines and recommendations based on scientific evidence. Thus, the focus of this issue of the *Radiologic Clinics of North America* is to provide the readers with written resources based on scientific evidence that can be used in managing pediatric patients with frequently encountered and clinically relevant pediatric disorders in their daily clinical practice.

As guest editor for this issue, I have selected topics that are considered to be of clinical importance in the pediatric body imaging in the neck, chest, abdomen, pelvis, and musculoskeletal system. Featured topics include pediatric neck masses, congenital lung malformations, lower respiratory tract infections, pulmonary nodules, interstitial lung disease, pulmonary embolism, bowel obstruction, abdominal masses, hip disorders, musculoskeletal infections, and vascular malformations. Articles in this issue focus on practical imaging guidelines and recommendations. In addition, up-to-date imaging techniques that can be easily employed and characteristic imaging findings of selected pediatric disorders for making an accurate diagnosis are highlighted. It is my hope that the readers of the articles included in this issue will recognize the currently limited available scientific evidence and become interested in future research that will continue to move forward the field of pediatric radiology.

It has been a great honor and privilege for me to work with both highly experienced and up-and-coming pediatric radiology rising stars in both academic and private practice settings. Their tremendous efforts and extraordinary expertise have undoubtedly helped create a resource of information that should facilitate understanding and management of various congenital and acquired pediatric disorders. First, I would like to thank the trainees and radiologists who have often requested written resources for the pediatric imaging guidelines and recommendations from me, which became an initial impetus and later became a motivation for me to take on this project. In addition, I would like to thank Frank H. Miller, MD, Consulting Editor of the *Radiologic Clinics of North America*, for the guidance in selecting topics; John Vassallo and his colleagues at Elsevier for their administrative and editorial assistance; and my family for their constant encouragement and support.

Edward Y. Lee, MD, MPH
Department of Radiology
Boston Children's Hospital
Harvard Medical School
300 Longwood Avenue
Boston, MA 02115, USA

E-mail address:
Edward.Lee@childrens.harvard.edu

Radiol Clin N Am 60 (2022) xi
https://doi.org/10.1016/j.rcl.2021.09.001
0033-8389/22/© 2021 Published by Elsevier Inc.

radiologic.theclinics.com

Pediatric Neck Masses
Imaging Guidelines and Recommendations

Mai-Lan Ho, MD

KEYWORDS

• Neck mass • Congenital • Acquired • Imaging • Infant • Child • Pediatric

KEY POINTS

- Evaluation of neck masses in children requires a practical synthesis of clinical information, laboratory testing, and imaging features.
- Major categories of pediatric neck masses include congenital, inflammatory, neoplastic, and vascular, each with distinct imaging features and management pathways.
- Diagnostic imaging workup typically begins with ultrasound for superficial lesions or computed tomography for rapid screening, followed by magnetic resonance imaging for detailed soft tissue evaluation.
- For potentially surgical lesions, interventional radiology can be consulted for percutaneous biopsy and minimally invasive therapeutic options.

INTRODUCTION

Neck masses commonly present in children and several possible diagnostic and management pathways exist, though with a paucity of evidence-based recommendations. The evaluation of neck masses in children requires practical synthesis of clinical information, laboratory testing, and imaging features. Imaging workup typically begins with ultrasound (US) for superficial lesions or computed tomography (CT) for rapid screening, followed by magnetic resonance (MR) for detailed soft tissue evaluation. Nuclear medicine (NM) has selected applications for functional assessment and staging of suspected neoplastic lesions. Following diagnostic imaging, interventional radiology (IR) can be consulted for minimally invasive alternatives to open surgery. Major categories of pediatric neck masses include congenital, inflammatory, neoplastic, and vascular, each with distinct imaging features and management pathways. The purpose of this article is to evaluate the current literature for pediatric neck masses, discuss utilization of various imaging modalities for diagnostic workup, and review characteristic imaging features and management pearls for pediatric neck masses typically encountered in daily clinical practice.

IMAGING MODALITIES

Five major imaging modalities for evaluating neck masses in pediatric patients include radiography, US, CT, MR, and NM.

1. US is recommended for initial evaluation of superficial neck masses following physical examination.
2. CT is used for rapid evaluation in acute clinical settings, including suspected infection, trauma, and/or airway compromise.
3. MR provides superior soft tissue evaluation of complex and deep neck masses in the nonurgent setting.
4. NM has selected applications for functional assessment and staging of suspected neoplastic lesions.

Department of Radiology, Nationwide Children's Hospital, The Ohio State University, 700 Children's Drive – ED4, Columbus, OH 43205, USA
E-mail address: mai-lan.ho@nationwidechildrens.org

Radiol Clin N Am 60 (2022) 1–14
https://doi.org/10.1016/j.rcl.2021.08.001

5. IR can be consulted for potentially surgical lesions amenable to percutaneous biopsy or minimally invasive therapy.

Radiography

Although radiography can detect sizable neck masses, it has limited utility in characterizing lesion composition, mass effect, and displacement of airway and vascular structures. When a neck mass is suspected to communicate with the airway, dynamic fluoroscopy can be performed during a swallow study or percutaneous contrast injection to evaluate for patent sinus tracts or fistulas.

Ultrasound

US is a useful screening tool for superficial neck masses in children. It is a readily available, inexpensive, and real-time imaging modality that does not involve potentially harmful ionizing radiation. US can characterize important imaging features, including the presence of solid and cystic components, as well as vascularity when Doppler imaging is used. The disadvantages of US include operator dependence with a limited acoustic window and depth penetration.[1,2]

Computed Tomography

CT is a fast and accessible cross-sectional imaging modality that involves ionizing radiation. CT is best used for rapid evaluation of suspected neck masses in acute clinical settings such as inflammation, infection, trauma, hemorrhage, and/or airway compromise. Although CT can distinguish different tissue densities such as calcium, fat, fluid, and blood, it is often limited for complex soft tissue evaluation, even with intravenous contrast administration.

Magnetic Resonance

MR is a more involved examination that uses nonionizing magnetic fields with multiple sequence weightings to enable superior soft tissue discrimination. Because the examination is longer and more detailed, infants and young children who cannot follow breathing instructions may require sedation or anesthesia. Nevertheless, MR imaging represents the current gold standard for evaluating pediatric neck masses, particularly congenital, neoplastic, and vascular lesions with complex anatomic involvement and multiple tissue components.

Nuclear Medicine

NM involves intravenous injection of various radiopharmaceuticals for single photon emission computed tomography (SPECT) and 18-fluoro-deoxyglucose for positron emission tomography (PET). NM is often used in oncologic evaluation. SPECT aids in the functional assessment of certain tumors, and PET is useful for whole body staging.

Interventional Radiology

Following diagnostic imaging, IR can be consulted for minimally invasive alternatives to open surgery. Interventional imaging options include angiography for evaluating vascular lesions, image-guided percutaneous tissue biopsy, and minimally invasive therapies such as sclerotherapy and ablation.[3–9]

EVIDENCE-BASED IMAGING ALGORITHM

Pediatric neck masses are common and invoke a wide range of diagnostic and management possibilities. Multivariate statistical analysis in large retrospective cohorts has demonstrated that no single clinical or radiologic feature can predict the final diagnosis.[6] Therefore, an ideal workflow for evaluation of pediatric neck masses should appropriately utilize and practically synthesize clinical features, laboratory testing, and imaging findings.

The clinical history should include the age and acuity of onset, recent history of infection or trauma, and any systemic symptoms including fever, night sweats, or weight loss. The physical examination should include location in the neck (medial or lateral, upper or lower, anterior or posterior), presence or absence of pain, mobile or fixed nature, signs of acute inflammation, and any findings outside the neck. Based on clinical assessment, various pertinent laboratory tests may be ordered, such as a complete blood cell count, metabolite concentrations, inflammatory markers, pathogen titers, hormone levels, and tumor markers.[10–16]

Diagnostic imaging can aid in the detection, localization, and characterization of pediatric neck masses. US is the preferred initial screening study following physical examination for most pediatric neck masses, particularly those that are superficially located. US helps to evaluate lesion location, size, and extent, as well as vascularity on color Doppler imaging.[1,2] For deep or complex neck lesions, cross-sectional imaging may be required for complete assessment. CT with iodinated contrast is recommended for rapid evaluation in urgent clinical settings, such as cellulitis, sialadenitis, abscess, and/or airway compromise. CT can also be used to evaluate acute trauma with suspicion for fractures and/or hemorrhage. In nonurgent settings, MR with gadolinium contrast is the current gold standard for evaluating complex soft tissue neck anatomy, including congenital, neoplastic, and vascular lesions. Because the examination is longer and more detailed, affected pediatric patients may require sedation or anesthesia.[3–9]

SPECTRUM OF PEDIATRIC NECK MASSES
Congenital Neck Disorders

Congenital neck anomalies are developmental malformations that are present at birth. Many of these lesions do not come to medical attention until later life, when they present with acute infection or inflammation. Acute inflammatory changes should be treated medically before any planned intervention to decrease the risk of iatrogenic neurovascular injury.[12–18] The current standard of care involves complete surgical excision to prevent lesion growth, repeat infection, and, in some cases, malignant transformation.[10–16] Some centers also offer minimally invasive percutaneous sclerotherapy and ablation approaches for benign congenital neck lesions.[17–19] Four common congenital neck lesions include branchial anomalies, cervical thymus, ectopic thyroid, and germ cell lesions.

Branchial anomalies

The branchial arches are 6 paired embryonic arches that form the structures of the head and neck. Branchial clefts form from ectoderm, branchial arches from mesoderm, and branchial pouches from endoderm. Incomplete obliteration of these embryonic precursors can result in the formation of a cyst, sinus (1 opening), or fistula (2 openings). Imaging helps to evaluate lesion location, size, superinfection, and abnormal communications with surrounding structures.

First branchial anomalies are located between the external ear and mandibular angle. Proposed classifications can be based on morphology (Arnot type I, parotid; II, anterior triangle) or tissue of origin (Work type I, ectoderm; II, ectoderm and mesoderm), but such systems do not correlate well with surgical risk or patient outcomes.[19,20] There may be communication with the periauricular soft tissues, parotid gland, parapharyngeal space, or anterior triangle of the neck.

Second branchial anomalies are the most common branchial apparatus anomalies and can be located in the anterior triangle of the neck, posterior to the submandibular gland, lateral to the carotid space, or anterior to the sternocleidomastoid muscle. Historic anatomic classifications exist, but are no longer commonly used in clinical practice (Bailey type I, anterior to sternocleidomastoid muscle; II, abutting internal carotid artery and internal jugular vein; III, between the internal and external carotid arteries; IV, pharyngeal mucosal space). Multiple or bilateral second branchial anomalies can be seen in the setting of brachio-oto-renal syndrome, along with deafness; auricular malformations; preauricular pits or tags; external, middle, and/or inner ear malformations; and renal anomalies.

Third branchial anomalies can be located in the upper posterior cervical space or lower anterior neck. Based on embryology, these lesions are often associated with the base of pyriform sinus, above the level of superior laryngeal and hypoglossal nerves and below the glossopharyngeal nerve. Fourth branchial anomalies are typically associated with the apex of the pyriform sinus and present with recurrent abscesses in the lower anterior neck, often in the thyroid gland or mediastinum. The clinical and radiologic features of third and fourth branchial anomalies can overlap greatly, with left lateralization more common owing to developmental asymmetries with persistence of the left thymopharyngeal duct, a remnant of the third pouch; and involution of the right ultimobranchial body, an outpocketing of the fourth pouch[17–26] (Fig. 1).

Cervical thymus

The thymus is a primary lymphoid organ derived from the third branchial pouch, which descends from the neck into the mediastinum during development. Cervical thymus refers to the presence of ectopic thymic remnants in the neck, which can present as a mass during childhood. Solid remnants can be located in the anterior triangle and deeper fascial layers, sometimes with a residual connection to the mediastinum. Cystic components can be present owing to congenital remnants of the thymopharyngeal duct, or from acquired inflammation or degeneration of thymic tissue. Thymic remnant lesions more commonly occur on the left, again related to persistence of the left thymopharyngeal duct component of the third branchial pouch [27,28] (Fig. 2).

Ectopic thyroid

The thyroid is an endocrine gland derived from the fourth branchial pouch. During development, the thyroid anlage migrates from the foramen cecum to the front of the trachea. Therefore, ectopic thyroid tissue can persist anywhere along this paramedian tract from the base of the tongue to mediastinum.[29] Owing to the presence of thyroglobulin, thyroid tissue is inherently hyperdense on CT and T1 hyperintense on MR. It is important to confirm the presence of a normal thyroid gland in the thyroid bed, prior to attempted excision of ectopic thyroid tissue.

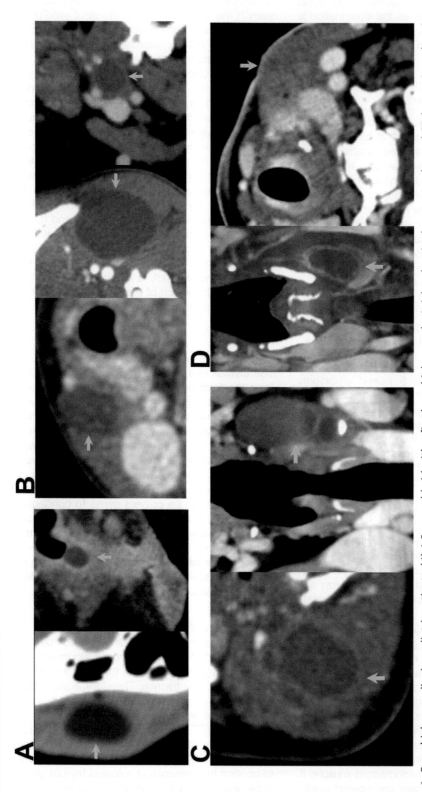

Fig. 1. Branchial anomalies in pediatric patients. (*A*) A 2-year-old girl with a first branchial anomaly. Axial and sagittal contrast-enhanced CT show a rim-enhancing cystic lesion (*arrows*) involving the right periauricular soft tissues and parotid gland. (*B*) Adolescent male patients with second branchial anomalies. Axial contrast-enhanced CT show well-circumscribed cystic lesions (*arrows*) located anterior to the right sternocleidomastoid muscle, lateral to left carotid space, and between the right internal and external carotid arteries. (*C*) Young boys with third branchial anomalies. Axial contrast-enhanced CT shows a complex rim-enhancing cystic lesion (*arrow*) located in the right upper posterior cervical space. Coronal contrast-enhanced CT demonstrates complex rim-enhancing cystic lesion (*arrow*) located adjacent to left piriform base. (*D*) A 6-year-old girl with a fourth branchial anomaly. Coronal and axial contrast-enhanced CT show a complex rim-enhancing cystic lesion involving the left piriform apex and thyroid lobe (*arrow*) with surrounding soft tissue edema and fistulization to the skin surface (*arrow*).

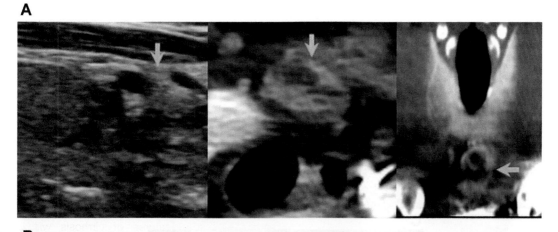

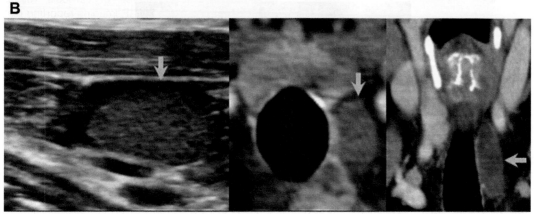

Fig. 2. Thymic variants in 2 pediatric patients. (*A*) A 9-year-old girl with cervical thymus. Longitudinal US and axial and coronal contrast-enhanced CT show solid and cystic thymic tissue (*arrows*) in the left inferior neck, contiguous with the mediastinum. (*B*) A 12-year-old boy with thymopharyngeal duct cyst. Longitudinal US and axial and coronal contrast-enhanced CT demonstrate thymopharyngeal duct cyst (*arrows*) in the left neck.

Thyroglossal duct cyst (TGDC) is the most common developmental cyst of the neck and can occur at the suprahyoid, hyoid, or infrahyoid levels. Suprahyoid TGDC is commonly located at the midline base of tongue (foramen cecum) or posterior floor of mouth. Hyoid TGDC is usually located anterior to the midline hyoid bone and may communicate with the airway. Infrahyoid TGDC is often paramedian and embedded in the thyroid strap muscles. Cystic lesions are at risk for malignant transformation to carcinoma, with suspicious imaging features including enhancement, nodularity, and coarse calcifications. Successful treatment involves a Sistrunk procedure with complete resection of the lesion and tract, along with the middle one-third of the hyoid bone[29–31] (Fig. 3).

Germ cell lesions

Germ cell lesions are classified based on their embryonic derivatives. The 3 main types are teratoma, dermoid cyst, and epidermoid cyst. Teratomas are true neoplasms containing tissues from all 3 germ cell layers and can be mature (well-differentiated), immature (incompletely differentiated), or malignant (poorly differentiated). The imaging appearance of germ cell lesions is heterogeneous with varying components of soft tissue, calcification, and bulk fat, which can produce substantial mass effect. Dermoid cysts are composed of both ectodermal and mesodermal components, including an epithelial lining and dermal substructure. Internal contents can include hair, macroscopic fat, and calcifications. Epidermoid cysts consist of purely ectodermal components, with a squamous epithelial lining and fluid contents. Both dermoid and epidermoid cysts can present as slowly expanding cystic masses, with recurrent infections when a fistulous tract is present. Internal contents and debris may be visible on US and CT, with restricted diffusion on MR[32,33] (Fig. 4).

Inflammatory Neck Disorders

Acute symptomatic pediatric neck conditions require urgent clinical and imaging workup, typically

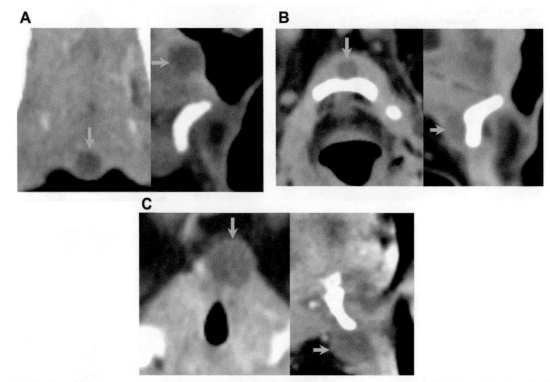

Fig. 3. Thyroglossal duct cyst (TGDC) in 3 pediatric patients. (*A*) A 14-year-old boy with TGDC. Axial and sagittal contrast-enhanced CT show suprahyoid TGDC (*arrows*) at the foramen cecum. (*B*) A 17-year-old girl with TGDC. Axial and sagittal contrast-enhanced CT demonstrate midline hyoid TGDC (*arrows*). (*C*) A 9-year-old boy with TGDC. Axial and sagittal contrast-enhanced CT show infrahyoid TGDC (*arrows*) embedded in strap muscles.

with contrast-enhanced CT. The major goals of imaging are to assess for any source of infection, drainable fluid collections, airway patency, and complications such as vascular thrombosis. In nonemergent cases, medical management can be instituted based on the presumed underlying etiology. Large fluid collections can be drained surgically or under imaging guidance. Critical airway cases may require intubation or tracheostomy.[34–37] Four common etiologies of pediatric neck inflammation include deep neck abscess, deep neck edema, lymphadenitis, and sialadenitis.

Deep neck abscess
Acute infections with deep neck involvement can produce suppurative collections in multiple spaces, most commonly the peritonsillar (parapharyngeal, masticator, and/or submandibular) and retropharyngeal spaces. Correct positioning for neck radiographs is important, because normal cervical spine ligamentous laxity and neck flexion can mimic the appearance of prevertebral soft tissue prominence and pseudosubluxation. Cross-sectional imaging with contrast can identify organized, rim-enhancing abscesses with mass effect

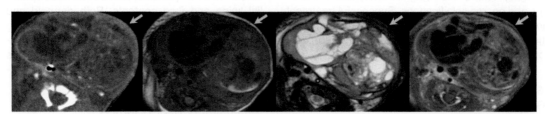

Fig. 4. Anterior neck teratoma in female newborn. Axial contrast-enhanced CT, T1-weighted, T2-weighted, and postcontrast T1-weighted MR with fat suppression show a large left anterior neck mass (*arrows*) with soft tissue, calcifications, and macroscopic fat, severely compressing the airway.

requiring drainage. With larger collections, there is a risk of dysphagia, airway obstruction, and atlantoaxial subluxation (Grisel syndrome), particularly in younger children with prominent lymphoid tissue. Severe infections may yield vascular complications, such as arterial pseudoaneurysm or septic thrombophlebitis (Lemierre syndrome)[34–38] (**Fig. 5**).

Deep neck edema

Reactive retropharyngeal edema can present similarly to retropharyngeal abscess on clinical examination. On imaging, retropharyngeal edema demonstrates a more symmetric appearance spanning the midline, with minimal rim enhancement or mass effect. The distinction is critical, because edema represents sterile fluid that arises secondary to an underlying infectious, inflammatory, or neoplastic condition, and resolves with treatment of the primary cause. Longus colli calcific tendinitis is an important mimicker in which calcium hydroxyapatite deposition in the longus colli tendon leads to inflammation and swelling of the prevertebral muscles.[39] The identification of linear prevertebral calcifications and symmetric retropharyngeal edema is diagnostic. Other clinically important conditions associated with retropharyngeal space edema include autoimmune conditions, bacterial and viral infections, head and neck carcinoma, and radiation therapy[40] (**Fig. 6**).

Lymphadenitis

Pediatric lymphadenitis is associated with a variety of infectious, inflammatory, and neoplastic etiologies.

For presumed infectious lymphadenopathy, empiric antibiotic therapy with observation can be instituted for up to 4 weeks. Features concerning for atypical or malignant lymphadenopathy include painless, firm or fixed, or matted nodes; supraclavicular location; diameter of more than 2 cm; enlargement on antibiotics; or persistence beyond 6 weeks.[13,41,42] Suspicious nodes should undergo fine needle aspiration and, if necessary, excisional biopsy for definitive pathologic diagnosis. Until malignancy has been excluded, corticosteroid therapy should be avoided unless absolutely necessary, since treatment can impact the accuracy of pathologic results.[13,41,42]

Benign reactive lymphadenopathy appears as nodal enlargement with preserved margins, ovoid morphology, and central fatty hila. Suppurative lymphadenitis can be seen with bacterial infection, beginning as inflammatory phlegmon and evolving to organized abscess. Associated findings may include cellulitis, myositis, and vascular complications, including extrinsic narrowing, vasospasm, or thrombosis. Tuberculosis (scrofula) presents with matted, thick, rim-enhancing, and centrally necrotic nodes. Atypical mycobacterial infections tend to manifest with cystic nodes and minimal surrounding inflammatory changes, complicated by fistulization to the skin surface over time. *Bartonella henselae* infection can occur after a cat scratch with fever, regional adenopathy, variable nodal necrosis, and calcified granulomas. Causes of inflammatory lymphadenitis include Kikuchi, Kimura, and Castleman diseases. Imaging findings are nonspecific, requiring laboratory testing and histologic confirmation for definitive diagnosis.

Malignant lymphadenopathy in the neck can arise in the setting of hematologic cancers and metastases from various primary tumors. Concerning imaging features include rounded nodal morphology, hyperenhancement, central necrosis,

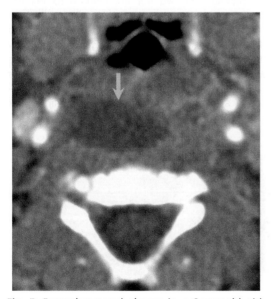

Fig. 5. Retropharyngeal abscess in a 6-year-old girl. Axial contrast-enhanced CT show expansile and rim-enhancing retropharyngeal fluid collection (*arrow*).

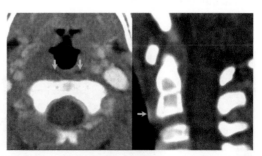

Fig. 6. Retropharyngeal edema in an 11-year-old boy with longus colli calcific tendinitis. Axial contrast-enhanced CT shows symmetric "bow-tie" edema (*arrows*) in the retropharyngeal space. Sagittal contrast-enhanced CT demonstrates linear calcification (*arrow*) of the longus colli tendon.

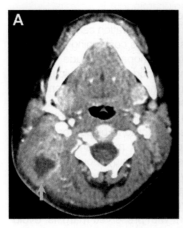
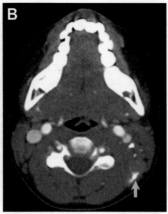

Fig. 7. Lymphadenopathy in 2 pediatric patients. (*A*) Bacterial lymphadenitis in a 5-year-old boy. Axial contrast-enhanced CT shows inflammatory phlegmon and abscess formation (*arrow*) in the right posterior neck. (*B*) Granulomatous lymphadenitis in a 12-year-old girl. An axial contrast-enhanced CT demonstrates enlarged lymph nodes with coarse calcifications (*arrow*) in the left posterior triangle.

microcalcification, replacement of fatty hila, and extranodal extension[41,42] (**Fig. 7**).

Sialadenitis

Sialadenitis refers to infection or inflammation of the salivary glands, most commonly the parotid or submandibular glands. Acute imaging findings typically include gland enlargement, hyperenhancement, inflammatory stranding, and abscess formation. When caused by an obstructing sialolith, imaging may be able to identify calcified stones along with proximal ductal dilation. Infectious causes of sialadenitis are usually viral or bacterial.[43] Chronic sialadenitis can present with gland atrophy and fatty replacement, ductal irregularity, and calcifications. Autoimmune etiologies of sialadenitis present with diffuse bilateral gland involvement and include immunoglobulin G4-related disease, Sjögren syndrome, and sarcoidosis. Malignant salivary gland neoplasms are rare in children, but should be considered in the setting of a focal mass that persists despite medical therapy[44] (**Fig. 8**).

Neoplastic Disorders

A wide variety of benign and malignant tumors can present in the pediatric neck. Imaging can help to identify lesion origin and extent, and provide a working differential diagnosis with regard to histology. Fine needle aspiration biopsy is a minimally invasive first-line approach that helps to assess tumor cytology. In some cases, a more invasive core or surgical biopsy is required to obtain a definitive tissue histology.[45–47] Five of the most commonly encountered pediatric neck neoplasms include nerve sheath tumor, neuroblastic tumor, paraganglioma, sarcoma, and thyroid cancer.

Nerve sheath tumors

Peripheral nerve sheath tumors include neurofibromas and schwannomas. Neurofibromas are seen in neurofibromatosis type 1. These lesions involve all nerve elements with an expansile and disorganized characteristic "target" morphology on CT and MR, consisting of a central fibrous and peripheral myxoid stroma. Plexiform lesions can involve multiple nerve branches with a transspatial appearance extending across multiple neck

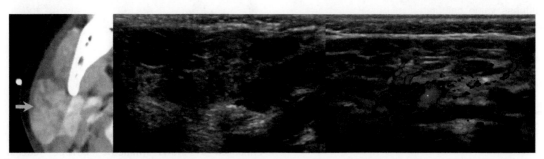

Fig. 8. Right parotitis in a 4-year-old girl. Axial contrast-enhanced CT and longitudinal view of US image show an enlarged heterogeneous parotid gland (*arrow*) with hyperenhancement and hypervascularity.

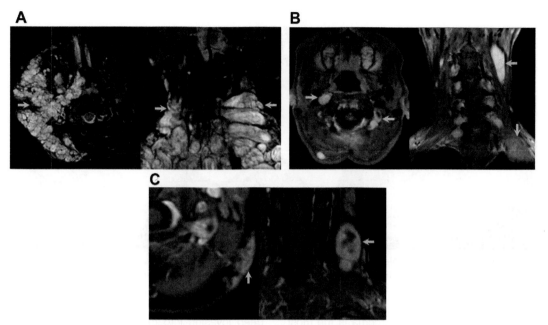

Fig. 9. Nerve sheath tumors in 3 pediatric patients. (*A*) A 9-year-old girl with neurofibromatosis type 1. Coronal and axial T2-weighted MR with fat suppression show multiple targetoid plexiform neurofibromas (*arrows*) of the right face, bilateral neck, and cervical spine. (*B*) A 15-year-old boy with neurofibromatosis type 2. Axial and coronal postcontrast T1-weighted MR with fat suppression show multiple cranial nerve and spinal schwannomas (*arrows*). (*C*) A 19-year-old man with neurofibromatosis type 3 (schwannomatosis). Axial and coronal postcontrast T1-weighted MR with fat suppression show multiple plexiform schwannomas (*arrows*) of the left posterior neck and brachial plexus.

spaces. Schwannomas are seen in neurofibromatosis types 2 and 3 (schwannomatosis). These encapsulated proliferations involve the Schwann cells that surround and myelinate peripheral nerve fibers, with a well-defined and elongated fusiform appearance. Plexiform lesions can involve multiple nerve branches with an interconnecting and multinodular appearance[48] (**Fig. 9**).

Neuroblastic tumors

Neuroblastic tumors arise from primitive sympathetic chain cells. The histologic classification, from most to least differentiated, includes ganglioneuroma, ganglioneuroblastoma, and neuroblastoma. Locations of neuroblastic tumors include the neck, mediastinum, adrenals, retroperitoneum, and pelvis.

In the neck, primary neuroblastoma typically arises in the posterior carotid space with mass effect on the carotid artery and internal jugular vein. Metastatic neuroblastoma can involve the lymph nodes, central nervous system, viscera, bones, and skin. Depending on the histology, nuclear medicine diagnosis and therapy can be performed using various radiolabeled somatostatin receptor analogs including octreotide, meta-iodobenzylguanidine, fluorodeoxyglucose, fluorodopa, and DOTA-conjugated peptides[49–51] (**Fig. 10**).

Paraganglioma

Glomus tumors are neuroendocrine tumors that typically arise from parasympathetic cell rests when arising in the head and neck. These tumors can be located in the middle ear (glomus tympanicum), jugular foramen (glomus jugulare), vagal nerve (glomus vagale), and carotid body (glomus caroticum). Lesions are hypervascular, with avid enhancement and permeative bone margins at the skull base. A "salt and pepper" appearance on MR can arise from the combination of intratumoral hemorrhage and flow-related signal voids. Hereditary paragangliomas are related to germline mutations in the succinate dehydrogenase (SDH) gene, responsible for oxygen sensing in mitochondrial complex II. There is also an association with syndromes such as multiple endocrine neoplasia and von Hippel–Lindau disease. Depending on the histology, nuclear medicine diagnosis and therapy can be performed using various radiolabeled somatostatin receptor analogs, including octreotide, meta-iodobenzylguanidine, fluorodeoxyglucose, fluorodopa, and DOTA-conjugated peptides[52–55] (**Fig. 11**).

Sarcoma

Sarcomas are heterogeneous malignancies of mesenchymal origin, which can arise from soft

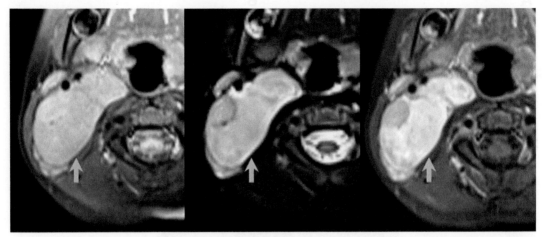

Fig. 10. Primary cervical neuroblastoma in a 2-year-old girl. Axial T1-weighted T2-weighted with fat suppression and postcontrast T1-weighted MR with fat suppression show a large mass (*arrows*) in the posterior cervical space.

tissue or bone. Rhabdomyosarcoma is the most common pediatric sarcoma and commonly involves the head and neck. Typical locations of involvement include orbital, parameningeal, and nonparameningeal, each with different prognostic implications.[56]

Thyroid cancer

Thyroid lesions in children can include diffuse lesions, such as goiter and thyroiditis, as well as focal masses including colloid cysts and various carcinomas. The American College of Radiology TI-RADS classification can help to stratify risk groups based on US appearance, with the caveat that pediatric thyroid lesions are more commonly malignant and invoke a lower threshold for fine needle aspiration.[57] Suspicious imaging features for thyroid masses include a solid appearance,

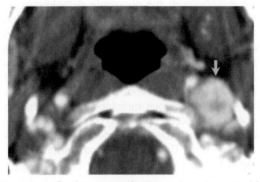

Fig. 11. Left glomus vagale tumor in a 12-year-old boy. Axial contrast-enhanced CT shows a hyperenhancing mass (*arrow*) in the left carotid space just inferior to the skull base.

deep invasion into the gland, irregular margins, extrathyroidal extension, peripheral or rim calcifications, and regional lymphadenopathy. Thyroid cancer histologies include papillary, follicular, medullary, and anaplastic thyroid carcinoma[57–59] (Fig. 12).

Vascular Anomalies

Vascular anomalies frequently occur in the pediatric head and neck. Vascular anomalies can be subclassified into vascular malformations, which are primary abnormalities of vascular morphology; and vascular tumors, which contain soft tissue with an increased endothelial turnover rate. US with Doppler is helpful for superficial lesion evaluation to identify vessel type and architecture, flow waveforms, soft tissue, fluid, and calcifications. Cross-sectional CT and MR with contrast can better evaluate the vascular supply and extent of deep lesions.[60]

High-flow vascular malformations include arteriovenous malformation (AVM) and arteriovenous fistula (AVF). AVMs have an abnormal tangle of vessels (nidus) connecting the arterial and venous systems. Associated syndromes include hereditary hemorrhagic telangiectasia, capillary malformation–arteriovenous malformation syndrome, Parkes–Weber syndrome, and Wyburn–Mason syndrome. AVFs have 1 or more direct connections between the arterial and venous systems.

Low-flow vascular malformations include venous, capillary, and lymphatic malformations. Venous malformations demonstrate gradual progressive "puddling" enhancement, often with calcified phleboliths due to slow flow. Associated syndromes

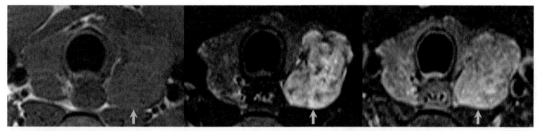

Fig. 12. Left papillary thyroid carcinoma in an 8-year-old boy. Axial T1-weighted, T2-weighted with fat suppression, and postcontrast T1-weighted MR with fat suppression show a large lobulated and heterogeneous mass (*arrows*) arising from the left thyroid lobe.

include multiple cutaneous and mucosal venous malformations, blue rubber bleb nevus syndrome, and Klippel–Trenaunay syndrome. Capillary malformations involve small, often superficial vessels that are difficult to characterize by imaging. A subtle reticulated blush is sometimes visible on contrast-enhanced CT or MR. Associated syndromes include macrocephaly–capillary malformation and other overgrowth syndromes. Lymphatic malformations demonstrate minimal flow with peripheral and septal enhancement. Macrocystic lesions can enlarge

rapidly after trauma or infection, with layering internal debris or hemorrhage. Microcystic lesions have tiny cysts that may be below the resolution of imaging, yielding a pseudo-solid, diffusely echogenic appearance on US and infiltrative enhancement on CT and MR. Multiple lymphatic malformations of the soft tissues, viscera, and bones can be seen in the setting of generalized lymphatic anomaly[60,61] (Fig. 13).

Vascular tumors can be benign, borderline, or malignant. Hemangiomas are the most common

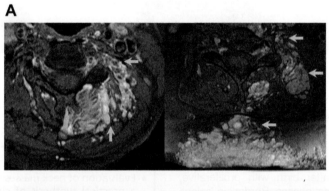

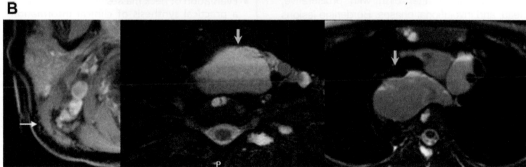

Fig. 13. Slow-flow vascular malformations in pediatric and young adult patients. (*A*) A 22-year-old man with blue rubber bleb nevus syndrome. Axial postcontrast T1-weighted MR with fat suppression shows multiple trans-spatial venous malformations (*arrows*) in the posterior neck and left paraspinal soft tissues. (*B*) A 3-year-old girl with generalized lymphatic anomaly. Axial postcontrast T1-weighted MR with fat suppression demonstrates microcystic lymphatic malformation in the right posterior neck (*thin white arrow*) (*left*). Axial T2-weighted MR with fat suppression shows trans-spatial macrocystic lymphatic malformations in the vertebral bodies, anterior neck, and mediastinum with layering fluid-debris levels (*thick yellow arrows*) (*middle and right*).

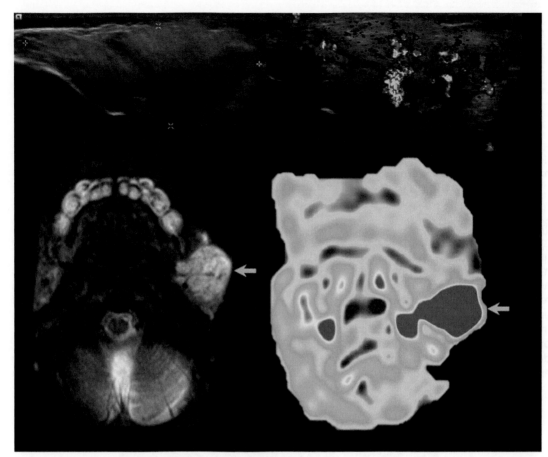

Fig. 14. A 6-month-old girl with left infantile parotid hemangioma in proliferative phase. Longitudinal US with Doppler shows hyperechogenic and hypervascular parotid mass. Axial T2-weighted MR shows a hyperintense left parotid mass (*arrow*) with elevated blood flow on arterial spin labeling (*arrow*).

benign vascular tumors seen in infants and young children. Congenital hemangiomas develop during fetal life and are present at birth, undergoing various degrees of involution after birth. Infantile hemangiomas arise shortly after birth with proliferative, plateau, and involutional phases. Borderline lesions have a locally aggressive or intermediate histology and can include tufted angioma, Kaposiform hemangioendothelioma, and juvenile nasopharyngeal angiofibroma[62] (**Fig. 14**).

SUMMARY

Initial evaluation of pediatric neck masses is based on clinical history and a detailed physical examination. Next, targeted imaging is used to refine the diagnosis and provide guidance for biopsy and therapy of potentially surgical lesions. A practical evidence-based imaging workflow with appropriate differential diagnostic considerations is key to optimal patient workup, subspecialty referral, and management.

CLINICS CARE POINTS

- Evaluation of neck masses in children requires a practical synthesis of clinical information, laboratory testing, and imaging features.
- Major categories of pediatric neck masses include congenital, inflammatory, neoplastic, and vascular, each with distinct imaging findings and management pathways.
- Diagnostic imaging workup typically begins with US for superficial lesions or CT for rapid screening, followed by MR for detailed soft tissue evaluation.
- For potentially surgical lesions, IR can be consulted for percutaneous biopsy and minimally invasive therapeutic options.

DISCLOSURE

The authors have no relevant disclosures.

REFERENCES

1. Bansal AG, Oudsema R, Masseaux JA, et al. US of pediatric superficial masses of the head and neck. Radiographics 2018;38(4):1239–63.
2. Rosenberg HK. Sonography of pediatric neck masses. Ultrasound Q 2009;25(3):111–27.
3. Meuwly JY, Lepori D, Theumann N, et al. Multimodality imaging evaluation of the pediatric neck: techniques and spectrum of findings. Radiographics 2005;25(4):931–48.
4. Brown RE, Harave S. Diagnostic imaging of benign and malignant neck masses in children-a pictorial review. Quant Imaging Med Surg 2016;6(5):591–604.
5. Stern JS, Ginat DT, Nicholas JL, et al. Imaging of pediatric head and neck masses. Otolaryngol Clin North Am 2015;48(1):225–46.
6. Riva G, Sensini M, Peradotto F, et al. Pediatric neck masses: how clinical and radiological features can drive diagnosis. Eur J Pediatr 2019;178(4):463–71.
7. Buch K, Reinshagen KL, Juliano AF. MR imaging evaluation of pediatric neck masses: review and update. Magn Reson Imaging Clin N Am 2019;27(2):173–99.
8. Ho ML, Courtier J, Glastonbury CM. The ABCs (Airway, Blood Vessels, and Compartments) of pediatric neck infections and masses. AJR Am J Roentgenol 2016;206(5):963–72.
9. Friedman ER, John SD. Imaging of pediatric neck masses. Radiol Clin North Am 2011;49(4):617–32.
10. Goins MR, Beasley MS. Pediatric neck masses. Oral Maxillofac Surg Clin North Am 2012;24(3):457–68.
11. Geddes G, Butterly MM, Patel SM, et al. Pediatric neck masses. Pediatr Rev 2013;34(3):115–24 [quiz 125].
12. Jackson DL. Evaluation and management of pediatric neck masses: an otolaryngology perspective. Physician Assist Clin 2018;3(2):245–69.
13. Meier JD, Grimmer JF. Evaluation and management of neck masses in children. Am Fam Physician 2014;89(5):353–8.
14. Curtis WJ, Edwards SP. Pediatric neck masses. Atlas Oral Maxillofac Surg Clin North Am 2015;23(1):15–20.
15. Shengwei H, Zhiyong W, Wei H, et al. The management of pediatric neck masses. J Craniofac Surg 2015;26(2):399–401.
16. Torsiglieri AJ Jr, Tom LW, Ross AJ 3rd, et al. Pediatric neck masses: guidelines for evaluation. Int J Pediatr Otorhinolaryngol 1988;16(3):199–210.
17. Quintanilla-Dieck L, Penn EB Jr. Congenital neck masses. Clin Perinatol 2018;45(4):769–85.
18. Erikci VS. Pediatric congenital neck masses: a review article. Clin Surg 2017;2:1791.
19. Al-Khateeb TH, Al Zoubi F. Congenital neck masses: a descriptive retrospective study of 252 cases. J Oral Maxillofac Surg 2007;65(11):2242–7.
20. LaRiviere CA, Waldhausen JH. Congenital cervical cysts, sinuses, and fistulae in pediatric surgery. Surg Clin North Am 2012;92(3):583–97, viii.
21. Koeller KK, Alamo L, Adair CF, et al. Congenital cystic masses of the neck: radiologic-pathologic correlation. Radiographics 1999;19(1):121–46 [quiz 152–3].
22. Vaughn JA. Imaging of pediatric congenital cystic neck masses. Oper Tech Otolaryngol Head Neck Surg 2017;28(3):143–50.
23. Bagchi A, Hira P, Mittal K, et al. Branchial cleft cysts: a pictorial review. Pol J Radiol 2018;83:e204–9.
24. Adams A, Mankad K, Offiah C, et al. Branchial cleft anomalies: a pictorial review of embryological development and spectrum of imaging findings. Insights Imaging 2016;7(1):69–76.
25. Thomas B, Shroff M, Forte V, et al. Revisiting imaging features and the embryologic basis of third and fourth branchial anomalies. AJNR Am J Neuroradiol 2010;31(4):755–60.
26. James A, Stewart C, Warrick P, et al. Branchial sinus of the piriform fossa: reappraisal of third and fourth branchial anomalies. Laryngoscope 2007;117:1920–4.
27. Kuperan AB, Quraishi HA, Shah AJ, et al. Thymopharyngeal duct cyst: a case presentation and literature review. Laryngoscope 2010;120(Suppl 4):S226.
28. Kaufman MR, Smith S, Rothschild MA, et al. Thymopharyngeal duct cyst: an unusual variant of cervical thymic anomalies. Arch Otolaryngol Head Neck Surg 2001;127(11):1357–60.
29. Oomen KP, Modi VK, Maddalozzo J. Thyroglossal duct cyst and ectopic thyroid: surgical management. Otolaryngol Clin North Am 2015;48(1):15–27.
30. Fujii NJ, Gibson TM, Satheesh KM, et al. Thyroglossal duct cyst: abbreviated review and case report. Compend Contin Educ Dent 2017;38(2):97–101 [quiz 102].
31. Rayess HM, Monk I, Svider PF, et al. Thyroglossal duct cyst carcinoma: a systematic review of clinical features and outcomes. Otolaryngol Head Neck Surg 2017;156(5):794–802.
32. Pupić-Bakrač J, Pupić-Bakrač A, Bačić I, et al. Epidermoid and dermoid cysts of the head and neck. J Craniofac Surg 2021;32(1):e25–7.
33. Smirniotopoulos JG, Chiechi MV. Teratomas, dermoids, and epidermoids of the head and neck. Radiographics 1995;15(6):1437–55.
34. Abudinen-Vasquez S, Marin MN. Management of pediatric head and neck infections in the emergency department. Pediatr Emerg Med Pract 2020;17(11):1–24.
35. Huang CM, Huang FL, Chien YL, et al. Deep neck infections in children. J Microbiol Immunol Infect 2017;50(5):627–33.
36. Maharaj S, Mungul S, Ahmed S. Deep neck space infections: changing trends in pediatric versus adult patients. J Oral Maxillofac Surg 2020;78(3):394–9.

37. Bochner RE, Gangar M, Belamarich PF. A clinical approach to tonsillitis, tonsillar hypertrophy, and peritonsillar and retropharyngeal abscesses. Pediatr Rev 2017;38(2):81–92.

38. Al-Sabah B, Bin Salleen H, Hagr A, et al. Retropharyngeal abscess in children: 10-year study. J Otolaryngol 2004;33(6):352–5.

39. Langner S, Ginzkey C, Mlynski R, et al. Differentiation of retropharyngeal calcific tendinitis and retropharyngeal abscess: a case series and review of the literature. Eur Arch Otorhinolaryngol 2020; 277(9):2631–6.

40. Hoang JK, Branstetter BF 4th, Eastwood JD, et al. Multiplanar CT and MRI of collections in the retropharyngeal space: is it an abscess? AJR Am J Roentgenol 2011;196(4):W426–32.

41. Weinstock MS, Patel NA, Smith LP. Pediatric cervical lymphadenopathy. Pediatr Rev 2018;39(9):433–43.

42. Rosenberg TL, Nolder AR. Pediatric cervical lymphadenopathy. Otolaryngol Clin North Am 2014;47(5): 721–31.

43. Francis CL, Larsen CG. Pediatric sialadenitis. Otolaryngol Clin North Am 2014;47(5):763–78.

44. Abdel Razek AAK, Mukherji S. Imaging of sialadenitis. Neuroradiol J 2017;30(3):205–15.

45. Qaisi M, Eid I. Pediatric head and neck malignancies. Oral Maxillofac Surg Clin North Am 2016; 28(1):11–9.

46. Lilja-Fischer JK, Schrøder H, Nielsen VE. Pediatric malignancies presenting in the head and neck. Int J Pediatr Otorhinolaryngol 2019;118:36–41.

47. Chadha NK, Forte V. Pediatric head and neck malignancies. Curr Opin Otolaryngol Head Neck Surg 2009;17(6):471–6.

48. Fisher MJ, Belzberg AJ, de Blank P, et al. 2016 Children's Tumor Foundation conference on neurofibromatosis type 1, neurofibromatosis type 2, and schwannomatosis. Am J Med Genet A 2018;176(5): 1258–69.

49. Lonergan GJ, Schwab CM, Suarez ES, et al. Neuroblastoma, ganglioneuroblastoma, and ganglioneuroma: radiologic-pathologic correlation. Radiographics 2002;22(4):911–34.

50. Bar-Sever Z, Biassoni L, Shulkin B, et al. Guidelines on nuclear medicine imaging in neuroblastoma. Eur J Nucl Med Mol Imaging 2018;45(11):2009–24.

51. Brisse HJ, McCarville MB, Granata C, et al, International Neuroblastoma Risk Group Project. Guidelines for imaging and staging of neuroblastic tumors: consensus report from the International Neuroblastoma Risk Group Project. Radiology 2011;261(1):243–57.

52. Persky M, Tran T. Acquired vascular tumors of the head and neck. Otolaryngol Clin North Am 2018; 51(1):255–74.

53. Fishbein L. Pheochromocytoma and paraganglioma: genetics, diagnosis, and treatment. Hematol Oncol Clin North Am 2016;30(1):135–50.

54. Tokgöz SA, Saylam G, Bayır Ö, et al. Glomus tumors of the head and neck: thirteen years' institutional experience and management. Acta Otolaryngol 2019;139(10):930–3.

55. Desai H, Borges-Neto S, Wong TZ. Molecular imaging and therapy for neuroendocrine tumors. Curr Treat Options Oncol 2019;20(10):78.

56. Huh WW, Fitzgerald N, Mahajan A, et al. Pediatric sarcomas and related tumors of the head and neck. Cancer Treat Rev 2011;37(6):431–9.

57. Richman DM, Benson CB, Doubilet PM, et al. Assessment of American College of Radiology Thyroid Imaging Reporting and Data System (TI-RADS) for pediatric thyroid nodules. Radiology 2020; 294(2):415–20.

58. Silva CT, Navarro OM. Pearls and pitfalls in pediatric thyroid imaging. Semin Ultrasound CT MR 2020; 41(5):421–32.

59. Uner C, Aydin S, Ucan B. Thyroid image reporting and data system categorization: effectiveness in pediatric thyroid nodule assessment. Ultrasound Q 2020;36(1):15–9.

60. Buckmiller LM, Richter GT, Suen JY. Diagnosis and management of hemangiomas and vascular malformations of the head and neck. Oral Dis 2010;16(5): 405–18.

61. Puttgen KB, Pearl M, Tekes A, et al. Update on pediatric extracranial vascular anomalies of the head and neck. Childs Nerv Syst 2010;26(10):1417–33.

62. Bouchard C, Peacock ZS, Troulis MJ. Pediatric vascular tumors of the head and neck. Oral Maxillofac Surg Clin North Am 2016;28(1):105–13.

Pediatric Lower Respiratory Tract Infections
Imaging Guidelines and Recommendations

Bernard F. Laya, MD, DO[a],*, Nathan David P. Concepcion, MD[a],
Pilar Garcia-Peña, MD[b], Jaishree Naidoo, MD[c],
Supika Kritsaneepaiboon, MD[d], Edward Y. Lee, MD, MPH[e]

KEYWORDS

- Lower respiratory tract infections • Pneumonia • Chest imaging • Radiologic imaging • Infant
- Children • Pediatric patients

KEY POINTS

- Lower respiratory tract infections (LRTIs), caused by various pathogens, either alone or in combination, remain a substantial cause of morbidity and mortality in children.
- Medical imaging can demonstrate both acute and chronic complications of LRTI in children.
- Chest radiograph is usually the initial imaging tool in the evaluation of LRTI in children. Other imaging modalities, including ultrasound, computed tomography, and magnetic resonance imaging, all play important roles, depending on the clinical condition. It is important to understand the appropriateness of each imaging modality for a particular indication to maximize its utility.
- Cross-sectional imaging is recommended for further evaluation of patients with recurrent or persistent chest radiographic abnormalities to exclude underlying congenital lung and airway malformations or other disorders.
- There is a wide spectrum of imaging manifestations of LRTI in children, and, although some demonstrate typical imaging features, it is often that these imaging features do overlap.

INTRODUCTION

Lower respiratory tract infection (LRTI) in children is a spectrum of illness that may affect the peripheral airways (bronchiolitis) or the alveoli (pneumonia),[1] but these can occur sequentially or simultaneously. There has been a considerable decrease in the incidence and mortality from LRTIs in the past 20 years; however, they remain the single largest cause of death in children worldwide.[2–5] Pneumonia can cause substantial morbidity in children, with potential development of various acute and chronic complications.[3] In 2017, approximately 15% of mortality among children below 5 years old was due to pneumonia.[2] The disease burden remains substantial in low-income and middle-income countries, where more than 90% of pneumonia deaths occur.[4]

Etiologies of LRTI include various organisms, such as viruses, bacteria, bacteria-like organisms, mycobacteria, fungi, and parasites. Mixed pathogens, however, also can occur. Among hospitalized children with pneumonia, approximately 26% to

[a] Section of Pediatric Radiology, Institute of Radiology, St. Luke's Medical Center-Quezon City, 279 E. Rodriguez Sr. Ave., Quezon City, 1112 Philippines; [b] Autonomous University of Barcelona (AUB), University Hospital Materno-Infantil Vall d'Hebron, Pso. Vall d'Hebron 119-129, 08035 Barcelona, Spain; [c] Paeds Diagnostic Imaging and Envisionit Deep AI, 2nd Floor, One-on Jameson Building, 1 Jameson Avenue, Melrose Estate, Johannesburg, 2196, South Africa; [d] Division of Diagnostic Radiology, Department of Radiology, Faculty of Medicine, Prince of Songkla University, Kanjanavanich Road, Hat Yai, 90110, Thailand; [e] Department of Radiology, Boston Children's Hospital, Harvard Medical School, 300 Longwood Avenue, Boston, MA 02115, USA
* Corresponding author.
E-mail address: bflaya@stlukes.com.ph

Radiol Clin N Am 60 (2022) 15–40
https://doi.org/10.1016/j.rcl.2021.08.003
0033-8389/22/© 2021 Elsevier Inc. All rights reserved.

radiologic.theclinics.com

35% had mixed pathogens of various combinations believed to function synergistically and likely enhancing the severity of the infection.[6–9]

Medical imaging has been used to confirm or exclude the presence of pneumonia, but it also is helpful in the evaluation of recurrent or persistent abnormalities, in assessment of acute or chronic complications, and to exclude other underlying pathologic processes.[9] This article aims to review the various imaging modalities utilized in the evaluation of LRTIs in children, present systematic and evidence-based diagnostic imaging recommendations and algorithms, and discuss the spectrum of acute and chronic imaging manifestations of these conditions.

EVIDENCE-BASED IMAGING RECOMMENDATIONS AND ALGORITHM

An extensive search of the medical literature, which includes peer-reviewed systematic reviews/meta-analysis, review articles, evidence-based guidelines, and consensus statements, was performed. In addition to American College of Radiology Appropriateness Criteria for pneumonia in the immunocompetent child,[10] Appropriateness Criteria for acute respiratory illness in the immunocompromised patients,[11] and Appropriateness Criteria for fever without source or unknown origin–child,[12] many other references were utilized in order to generate various clinical scenarios in pediatric patients with LRTI along with corresponding recommended imaging tests (Table 1). To analyze the strength of the references used, strength of recommendation (SORT) was utilized. The SORT category levels are the following: (A) recommendation is based on consistent and good quality patient-oriented evidence; (B) recommendation is based on inconsistent or limited quality patient-oriented evidence; and (C) recommendation is based on consensus, usual practice, opinion, disease-oriented evidence, or case series for studies of diagnosis, treatment, prevention, or screening.[32] The SORT level of the references used in developing the recommendations falls under category C. After a careful synthesis of all the available information reviewed, which includes various clinical scenarios and recommended imaging tests, an evidence-based algorithm for children with LRTIs was developed (Fig. 1).

PRACTICAL IMAGING APPROACH TO LOWER RESPIRATORY TRACT INFECTIONS IN CHILDREN
Radiography

The chest radiograph (chest x-ray) is widely available and the imaging examination performed most frequently not only in adults but also in children. This imaging modality can serve as a screening tool for the detection of lung parenchymal opacities or as a monitoring tool to evaluate response to therapy.[33,34] Prior to a radiologist's interpretation of the radiograph, several parameters, including proper patient positioning, adequate inspiratory effort, and acceptable radiograph exposure, initially must be assessed and satisfied to determine the diagnostic quality of the films or images.[33]

A frontal projection of the chest, either in anteroposterior or posteroanterior view, may be sufficient to demonstrate presence of lung opacities, but a lateral view also is recommended in children to better detect other associated findings, such as lymphadenopathy and minimal pleural effusion, among others.[18,33,35] A lateral decubitus view, right or left, depending on the perceived abnormality on the frontal chest radiograph, also may be obtained in some cases: (1) to assess presence of minimal free pleural fluid in situations where the lateral costophrenic sulcus is blunted or (2) to differentiate a loculated from a nonloculated pleural effusion. The low specificity of the imaging findings, however, makes the evaluation of pediatric patients with suspected pulmonary infections challenging because of various potential causes that have similar radiographic characteristics. For example, a chest radiograph cannot accurately differentiate between viral and bacterial pneumonia.[16,18,26,34]

Ultrasound

Ultrasound (US) is used primarily in the evaluation of pleural fluid, better characterizing the nature, type, presence of septations, and volume of pleural effusion.[33,36–40] In a radiographically opaque hemithorax, US also can differentiate pleural effusion from consolidation.[19] Recent technological advancements in US also have improved the spatial resolution, tissue penetration, and characterization of the lung parenchyma. Moreover, the chest of infants and young children has less subcutaneous fat than adults with partially or unossified ribs and sternum, making it easier to perform transosseous scanning.[33,40–43]

Chest radiographs are less sensitive in the detection of small pleural fluid, but US is able to detect even less than 10 mL of pleural fluid, especially when a patient is in an upright position.[19,40,41,44–47] US has other various advantages over the other imaging modalities, including its portability and real-time scanning, without a need for sedation or exposure to ionizing radiation.

US may demonstrate lung consolidation as heterogeneous, low echogenicity similar to the liver,

Table 1
Clinical condition and appropriateness of chest imaging tool based on American College of Radiology appropriateness criteria and other references

Imaging Recommendations	References	Comments
Chest radiograph is the initial imaging tool in the neonate, infant or child up to 36 mo with fever of unknown source and respiratory symptoms.	12	May disclose an occult pneumonia
Imaging is not recommended in immunocompetent children with suspected uncomplicated community acquired pneumonia who does not require hospitalization.	10,13–16	Imaging does not change the management of these pediatric patients.
Chest radiograph is the initial imaging tool in immunocompetent children with community acquired-pneumonia that does not respond to initial outpatient treatment or requires hospitalization.	10,16–18	US may be appropriate.[10,19–23]
Chest radiograph is the initial imaging tool recommended in immunocompetent with suspected hospital acquired pneumonia.	10	US may be appropriate.[10,19–21]
Chest radiograph is the initial imaging tool in immunocompromised children with cough, dyspnea, chest pain, or fever.	11	Chest CT without or with contrast may be appropriate.[11]
Chest radiograph is the initial imaging tool for a child when TB is suspected.	18,24	
US usually is appropriate in immunocompetent children with pneumonia complicated with moderate or large effusion on chest radiograph.	10	A decubitus view chest radiograph or a chest CT with IV contrast also may be appropriate.[10]
Chest CT with IV contrast is an appropriate imaging tool for immunocompetent children with pneumonia complicated by suspected bronchopleural fistula seen on chest radiograph.	10,18,25,26	Chest CT without IV contrast may be appropriate.[10]
Chest CT with IV contrast is an appropriate imaging tool in immunocompetent children with pneumonia complicated by suspected lung abscess seen on chest radiograph.	1,10,18,25,26	US of the chest[10] or chest MRI with IV contrast[10,27–29] may be appropriate.
Chest CT without IV contrast is appropriate in immunocompetent children with nonlocalized recurrent pneumonia seen on chest radiograph.	1,10,30	To evaluate underlying pulmonary disease. such as bronchiectasis and interstitial or diffuse lung disorders, HRCT is appropriate.
Chest CT with IV contrast or chest CTA is appropriate studies for immunocompetent children with localized recurrent pneumonia seen on chest radiograph.	1,10,30	Causes of recurrent localized infections include congenital bronchopulmonary malformations or possible foreign body aspiration.
Chest CT is appropriate in immunocompromised children when chest radiographs are equivocal.	1,11,17,26,31	Chest CT without IV contrast usually is appropriate, but IV contrast can be given depending on the clinical indication, which includes suspected TB.

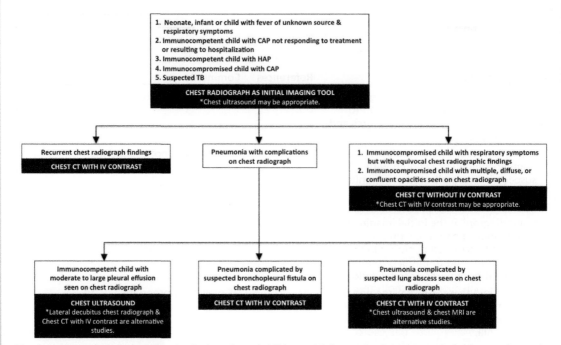

1. Neonate, infant or child with fever of unknown source & respiratory symptoms
2. Immunocompetent child with CAP not responding to treatment or resulting to hospitalization
3. Immunocompetent child with HAP
4. Immunocompromised child with CAP
5. Suspected TB

CHEST RADIOGRAPH AS INITIAL IMAGING TOOL
*Chest ultrasound may be appropriate.

Recurrent chest radiograph findings
CHEST CT WITH IV CONTRAST

Pneumonia with complications on chest radiograph

1. Immunocompromised child with respiratory symptoms but with equivocal chest radiographic findings
2. Immunocompromised child with multiple, diffuse, or confluent opacities seen on chest radiograph

CHEST CT WITHOUT IV CONTRAST
*Chest CT with IV contrast may be appropriate.

Immunocompetent child with moderate to large pleural effusion seen on chest radiograph
CHEST ULTRASOUND
*Lateral decubitus chest radiograph & Chest CT with IV contrast are alternative studies.

Pneumonia complicated by suspected bronchopleural fistula on chest radiograph
CHEST CT WITH IV CONTRAST

Pneumonia complicated by suspected lung abscess seen on chest radiograph
CHEST CT WITH IV CONTRAST
*Chest ultrasound & chest MRI are alternative studies.

Fig. 1. Evidence-based algorithm in the imaging of children with lower respiratory tract infection. * Alternative imaging study that may be appropriate. CAP, community acquired pneumonia; CT, computed tomography; HAP, hospital acquired pneumonia; IV, intravenous contrast; TB, tuberculosis.

also known as lung hepatization. Bronchograms within the solid-appearing lung may be seen either as multiple, linear, branching bright dots within the lung (sonographic air bronchograms) or as hypoechoic branching structures filled with entrapped fluid or mucoid material within bronchi (sonographic fluid bronchograms) in pediatric patients with necrotizing or postobstructive pneumonias.[33] Complications in pneumonia, such as abscess and empyema, also are readily visualized in US. Color Doppler imaging also may be helpful in detecting necrotizing pneumonia even without the use of intravenous (IV) contrast media.

Computed Tomography

Computed tomography (CT) is a highly useful imaging tool in the evaluation of the thorax, including the lungs, mediastinum, and chest wall in infants and children. Multidetector CT and dual-energy CT technologies with advanced multiplanar and 3-dimensional (3-D) reconstructions as well as artificial intelligence software currently are available, not only increasing image quality and lesion detection but also decreasing the sedation rates, scanning time, and radiation dose, which are of particular importance in infants and young children.

CT is considered an adjunct to conventional radiography[34,48] and often used in the evaluation of nonresponding pulmonary infection as well as its complications.[18,33] Unlike chest radiography, where

there is superimposition of anatomic structures, CT provides cross-sectional images where pattern and distribution of pulmonary diseases are better visualized than chest radiography.[34,49] Various scanning protocols are available for different clinical indications, such as high-resolution CT (HRCT) or CT angiography (CTA) but usually are not appropriate for evaluation of acute respiratory illnesses.

Iodinated contrast agents may be administered IV and greatly improve the image quality by enhancing the differentiation of various tissues in the body, which could help radiologists distinguish normal structures from abnormal findings.

Magnetic Resonance Imaging

Magnetic resonance imaging (MRI) is an imaging modality that has no ionizing radiation. It uses strong magnetic fields and gradients as well as computer-generated radio waves to produce multiplanar images of various parts of the body. MRI, however, is less sensitive compared with CT in the evaluation of the lung parenchyma due to the lung's inherent low proton density, high loss of signal due to susceptibility, and substantial cardiac and respiratory motion artifacts.[33,50,51] Scan times also are longer, increasing the need for sedation in infants and young children as well as those pediatric patients with claustrophobia.

Even with disadvantages, pathologic processes with high fluid or proton content, such as pneumonia, pulmonary edema, and pleural and pericardial effusion, are readily depicted on MRI. In addition, various technological advances in the imaging protocols with electrocardiograph and respiratory gating as well as motion correction, the lungs now can be examined better than before.[27,33,52] Gadolinium-based IV contrast media may be administered, similar to CT, for better detection of acute complications, such as necrotizing pneumonia, lung abscess, and empyema.

SPECTRUM OF LOWER RESPIRATORY TRACT INFECTIONS IN CHILDREN
Viral Infections

Demographics and clinical symptoms
Viruses are common causes of respiratory tract infection among children and are substantial causes of morbidity and mortality.[5,9] It often is difficult to determine the underlying etiology of pneumonia in a child, but a patient's age can be helpful.[3,4,53–56] Viral pneumonia is rare in neonates because of maternal antibody protection, but viruses are the most frequent cause of community-acquired pneumonia (CAP) in infants older than 4 months and in preschool-aged children (95%).[17] For school-aged children, viral infections also are common but the incidence of bacterial infection increases.[10,18,25,57] In developed countries, infants and preschool-aged children experience a mean of 6 to 10 viral infections annually, and school-aged children and adolescents experience 3 to 5 illnesses annually.[58] In hospitalized children with pneumonia, viral pathogens were detected in 73% of patients, and bacteria were seen in 15%.[7]

The clinical signs and symptoms of viral pneumonia are highly variable, usually are nonspecific, and depend on the infectious agent, patient age, and state of immunity.[18,25] Affected pediatric patients typically present with cough, coryza, and wheezing, although severe respiratory distress that requires hospitalization also may occur.

Following inhalation of the viral agent in the nasopharynx and upper respiratory tract, the virus migrates inferiorly to small airways and alveoli.[9,25] There is resultant inflammation and necrosis of the ciliated epithelial cells, goblet cells, and bronchial mucous glands that lead to bronchial and bronchiolar edema, often with involvement of the peribronchial tissue and interlobular lung septa. The affected small airway reacts with bronchoconstriction and increased mucous secretion, which narrows the already small airways causing peripheral atelectasis and hyperaeration[31] (Fig. 2). Both small airways and lung parenchymal changes do occur.[33,34,59] Coinfection with 2 or more microbial agents can happen and a majority of mixed infections are viral-bacterial infections, but viral-viral coinfections also are seen.[7,8]

DNA viruses Adenovirus is an important cause of acute respiratory illness in children, accounting for 5% to 17% of all respiratory infections, and can occur endemically or in epidemics.[34,60–62] The peak incidence of infection in children is 6 months to 5 years. They can cause necrotizing bronchitis, bronchiolitis, bronchopneumonia, and severe respiratory disease in up to 20% of children, with fatality rates from 5% to 12%.[34,60–64] LRTI from DNA viruses can develop frequent sequela (22%–30%) as postinfectious bronchiolitis obliterans (PIBO), bronchiectasis, and Swyer-James-McLeod syndrome.[61,62,65,66] Varicella zoster virus is the etiologic agent of varicella or chickenpox and belongs to the herpesvirus family. The virus becomes latent in the neural tissue and can be reactivated later, causing herpes zoster.[67] Infection generally is mild, but there is risk of complications in neonates and immunocompromised pediatric patients.[67,68] Varicella pneumonia is a serious complication, with an incidence from 5.6% to 30.3%.[68–70] Cytomegalovirus (CMV) is the largest and most complex member of the herpes virus family, and can remain latent and with potential for reactivation. It is a major cause of morbidity and mortality in the immunocompromised pediatric patients.[34,61,71–73]

RNA viruses Respiratory syncytial virus (RSV) is a common pathogen in children younger than 5 years old,[4,34,55,57,74] and there is great risk of infection in premature infants and children with chronic lung disease and heart disease.[75–77] Infection includes upper respiratory infection, bronchiolitis, pneumonia, and respiratory failure.[61,74–78] Measles is a contagious worldwide infectious disease transmitted by direct contact that causes substantial mortality in children.[34,79,80] Typical symptoms with characteristic maculopapular skin rash and Koplik spots develop 10 days to 12 days after the exposure and last 7 days to 10 days. It may involve the airways, leading to bronchitis, bronchiolitis, and pneumonia (6%–15%).[34,79] RNA viruses also cause neurologic complications (encephalitis) and can suppress the immune system, which predisposes a child to other infections.[66,81,82] Rhinovirus is a common etiology of childhood viral upper respiratory tract infections worldwide (18%–27%) but affects the lower respiratory tract less commonly, leading to bronchiolitis and pneumonia.[61,83,84]

There are 3 groups of influenza virus, types A, B, and C. Type A and occasionally type B can cause viral pneumonia.[34,61] One of the most severe outbreaks of this infection was the pandemic of 1918, Spanish influenza, resulting in approximately

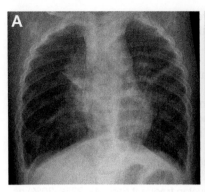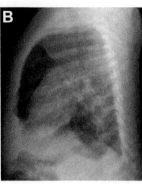

Fig. 2. Respiratory syncytial virus (RSV) infection in a 10-month-old boy who presented with cough, runny nose, low-grade fever, and wheezing. (*A*) Frontal and (*B*) lateral view chest radiographs show flattened diaphragm and increased anteroposterior thoracic diameter compatible with hyperaeration. There is increased interstitial markings particularly in the perihilar regions, with areas of linear and wedge-shaped opacities compatible with subsegmental atelectasis.

50 million deaths.[34] Influenza A can be classified in subtypes. Influenza A virus subtype H1N1 is a zoonotic virus of swine origin. It was discovered in Mexico and was known as the cause of the swine flu pandemic of 2009. Infection usually presents with nonspecific symptoms, but pneumonia and severe pulmonary complications as acute respiratory distress syndrome (ARDS) can occur, due to an exaggerated inflammatory response.[34,76,85,86] Influenza virus A subtype H5N1 is the causative agent of avian flu. Infection occurs after close contact with infected birds or their products. It first was isolated in Hong Kong in 1997 and later spread to other countries. The symptoms are fever, cough, diarrhea, shortness of breath, lymphocytopenia, and thrombocytopenia. Fatal and rapid progression to ARDS resulting in death could exceed 60%.[34,76]

Coronaviruses (CoVs) have an approximately spherical shape with prominent spike projections resembling a crown.[85] They can infect birds, humans, and others vertebrates.[78] CoVs can cause mild to moderate upper respiratory tract infection in healthy individuals, but they also can infect lower respiratory tract, causing severe or fatal pneumonia and even ARDS.[87,88] The most highly pathogenic are, severe acute respiratory syndrome CoV (SARS-CoV), Middle East respiratory syndrome CoV (MERS-CoV), and SARS–CoV-2.

The SARS-CoV was detected in Guangdong province, China, in 2002. Chinese ferret-badgers, raccoon dogs, and masked palm civets are the animal hosts for this virus. During 2002 and 2003, the infection spread to 29 countries, with 8098 infected individuals and 916 deaths.[86] The transmission was via respiratory droplets, and the infected patients presented with flulike symptoms. Affected pediatric patients can develop pneumonia and lymphocytopenia. Children, especially under the age of 10 years, have a mild clinical course, but adults can develop severe complications (ARDS).[34,61,76,89] The MERS-CoV was detected in Saudi Arabia, where camels and bats are reservoirs. It spread across the world,

but 80% of cases occurred in Middle East Asia. A total of 2254 individuals were infected, and 800 deaths occurred between 2012 and 2018.[85] In the literature, there are few MERS-CoV infections in children, and 42% are asymptomatic.[88] In adults, the infection can progress to pneumonia, ARDS, multiorgan failure, and death.[61,76,85] The SARS–CoV-2 was detected in Wuhan, China, in December 2019, and on March 11, 2020, the World Health Organization (WHO) declared this infection as a pandemic.[90–92] The transmission is via respiratory droplets and fomites, with an incubation period of 5 days to 6 days. Children are affected less severely than adults, and most cases are asymptomatic or with mild moderate disease.[85,93,94] General hospitalization is approximately 4% in children.[95] Typical symptoms are fever, diarrhea, rash, conjunctivitis, and, in severe illness, edema, shock, myocardial dysfunction, and neurologic findings. Multisystem inflammatory syndrome also was reported in children.[96,97]

Human immunodeficiency virus (HIV) causes acquired immunodeficiency syndrome.[98–100] Children represent 2% of the HIV reported cases.[18] Most children are infected after vertical transmission from their mothers, but there are other causes, such as sexual transmission, illicit drug use, and blood transfusions.[18,98] HIV damages or destroys vital cells in the human immune system; therefore, pulmonary infections are a highly important cause of morbidity and mortality.[14,33,101–104] These pediatric patients are highly susceptible to viral, bacterial, fungal, protozoal, and opportunistic infections.[33,98,101,105–109] Lymphocytic interstitial pneumonia can occur in these pediatric patients.[101,110] Imaging findings of lymphocytic interstitial pneumonia are diffuse, symmetric, reticular, or round opacities, which can coalesce and form pulmonary opacifications.[102,105,107,111] These imaging findings should be distinguished from TB infection.[33,103,105,109]

Imaging of viral lower respiratory tract infections

Chest radiograph remains the mainstay of pneumonia imaging, supplemented with US and CT for specific indications.[14,19,112–114] It can be normal in children with mild disease, but peribronchial inflammation manifests as symmetric and bilateral peribronchial interstitial opacities radiating from the hila and extending peripherally, with segmental and subsegmental areas of atelectasis.[33] There also is hyperaeration due to the narrowing of the distal airway lumen due to bronchial wall edema, and mucous plugging, resulting in air trapping and subsequent hyperinflation. This is shown well on the chest radiographs as hyperlucency, increased transverse and anteroposterior chest diameter, and flattening of the diaphragms[31,57,115] (see Fig. 2). The radiographic pattern of viral pneumonia, however, can be diverse and nonspecific because it can be seen in nonviral LRTIs as bacterial pneumonia and other diseases, such as asthma.[6,61,116] Viral infection also can mimic the radiological findings of bacterial infection, with bilateral areas of consolidation.[31,115–117] This can occur in pandemic virus infections, such as influenza A H1N1, influenza A H5N1, and CoVs, in which initially it can appear as focal or diffuse interstitial opacities but rapidly progress to bilateral areas of consolidation[25,86] (Figs. 3–5). In varicella and CMV infection, the imaging findings are ground-glass opacities (GGOs) or diffuse nodular opacities that may progress to large segmental areas of patchy airspace disease. Total clearing is expected but punctate calcifications could be seen after a varicella pneumonia. So, viral pneumonia can have a diverse imaging appearance on chest radiograph depending on the infecting agent, and the host response that depends on age, immune status, and presence of underlying comorbidity. The chest radiograph alone is a poor indicator of specific causative agent of pneumonia, but, with inclusion of clinical and laboratory data, sensitivity can increase.[115,117,118]

CT is a useful adjunct to chest radiograph in selected cases, and HRCT is the modality of choice to evaluate lung parenchyma.[33,34,113,119–121] The wide spectrum of CT findings of viral LRTIs includes patchy mosaic perfusion pattern, GGOs, consolidation, micronodules and tree-in-bud opacities, interlobular septal thickening, and bronchial and bronchiolar wall thickening with areas of hyperaeration and atelectasis.[59,61] GGOs with or without consolidation is the predominant finding in viral pneumonia[92,93,98,122] (see Figs. 3 and 4). The halo sign, which is seen as a focal consolidation with a rim of GGO, may be found in 50% of SARS–CoV-2 infection[92,93] (Fig. 5).

Complication of viral lower respiratory tract infections

The most frequent acute complication of viral pneumonia in children is a superimposed bacterial infection[25] and immune reconstitution inflammatory syndrome (IRIS) in HIV.[25,105,113,123] The most common chronic complications of viral pneumonia are bronchiectasis, PIBO, or Swyer-James-MacLeod syndrome. The radiological findings for bronchiectasis could be subtle on chest radiograph, but they are well shown on CT, where the bronchus is dilated and larger than its accompanying pulmonary artery. Chronic bronchiectasis commonly is seen with adenovirus infection (Fig. 6).

PIBO is an irreversible, chronic, and obstructive complication of viral pneumonia and can be seen as sequela of adenovirus, RSV, parainfluenza, measles, and CMV.[25,31,124,125] Radiographic findings of PIBO usually are nonspecific and even can appear normal but also can show hyperlucent lung, atelectasis, confluent densities, peribronchial thickening, and bronchiectasis.[25,125,126] CT is the best radiological examination to analyze PIBO findings, demonstrating mosaic perfusion pattern, peribronchial thickening, bronchiectasis, atelectasis, and reduced vessels size in low-attenuation areas, indicating diminished perfusion,

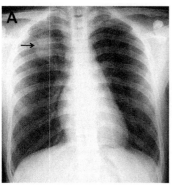
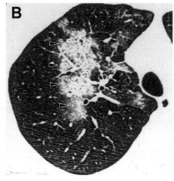

Fig. 3. Severe Acute Respiratory Syndrome-CoV (SARS-CoV) infection in a 10-year-old boy who presented with fever, cough, and myalgia. (A) Frontal chest radiograph shows airspace opacity (arrow) in the right upper lobe. (B) Axial lung window HRCT image demonstrates a large area of mixed ground-glass opacity with interlobular septal thickening, crazy paving (arrowheads), along with other areas of airspace consolidation in the right upper lobe.

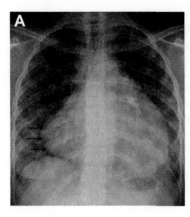
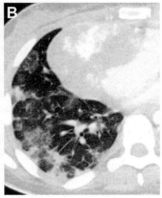

Fig. 4. Middle East Respiratory Syndrome-CoV (MERS-CoV) infection in a 17-year-old boy with a cardiac tumor (angiosarcoma) who presented with increasing cough and shortness of breath. (*A*) Frontal chest radiograph shows cardiomegaly with a prominent right cardiac border (*arrows*) due to the cardiac mass. There also are multifocal lung consolidations in both lower lobes. (*B*) Axial lung window CT image demonstrates multiple peripheral areas of ground-glass opacities and consolidations in the right lung.

air trapping, and sometimes lung volume reduction[25,34,56,125,127] (see **Fig. 6**). Swyer-James-MacLeod syndrome is a form of PIBO, where the lung involvement typically is unilateral, affecting the entire lung or lobe, although it also can affect both lungs. Characteristic findings on chest radiographs are hyperlucency due to pulmonary hypoperfusion, small pulmonary artery with small hilum, reduced volume of the affected lung or lobe, and air trapping. CT shows these findings in more detail and precision.[25,31,128] Expiratory CT imaging could be useful to better demonstrate the air trapping and hyperlucencies, especially in detecting bilateral lung involvement (30%)[65,129] (**Fig. 7**).

Bacterial Infection

Demographic and clinical symptoms
Viral infections are encountered more commonly than pyogenic bacteria in CAP. Even after the new conjugate vaccines have become more widely available, however, bacterial infections still result in severe and/or complicated pneumonia that sometimes requires hospitalization and even mortality.[3,7,130,131] In addition, viral-bacterial coinfections (7%–34.6%) of RSV and potentially pathogenic bacteria augment the disease severity.[3,7,8,58,132] Co-

mmon bacterial agents causing pneumonia in immunocompetent hosts vary by age, whereas in immunocompromised hosts bacterial agents also may vary depending on the types of immunologic defects as well.[1,33,133–137] Children without fever or respiratory tract symptoms are unlikely to have pneumonia. Nonspecific and nonrespiratory signs and symptoms, such as irritability, malaise, pleuritic chest pain, abdominal pain, or stiff neck, are not uncommon, especially in infants and smaller children.[17,18,33,130,134,137,138]

Imaging of bacterial lower respiratory tract infections
Bacterial pneumonia tends to have unilateral, segmental or lobar airspace opacification.[1,25,33,137,139,140] This alveolar pattern or endpoint consolidation, categorized by the WHO as radiographic definition for identifying pneumonia, has a high sensitivity (93%) and high negative predictive value (92%) in diagnosing bacterial pneumonia and high agreement in imaging interpretation[17,141–143] (**Fig. 8**). Expansile pneumonia can be found in *Klebsiella pneumoniae* and *Staphylococcus aureus* infections.[26] The chest radiographs, however, are not able to differentiate causative agent and interstitial (or nonendpoint)

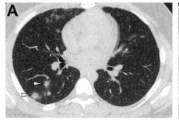
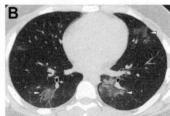

Fig. 5. Severe Acute Respiratory Syndrome-CoV-2 (SARS-CoV-2) infection in a 14-year-old boy who presented with fever, cough, shortness of breath, and myalgia. (*A*) Axial lung window CT image shows multifocal small round consolidations surrounded by a rim of ground–glass opacity (GGO) referred to as the halo sign (*arrowheads*) in right lower lobe, along with areas of GGO in middle lobe. (*B*) Axial lung window CT image shows bilateral multifocal areas of GGO (*arrowheads*) in the lower lobes and lingula.

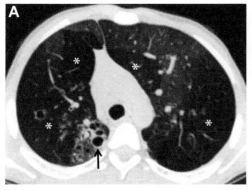
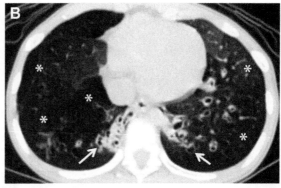

Fig. 6. Bronchiectasis and bronchiolitis obliterans as chronic sequelae of adenovirus infection in a 9-year-old boy who presented with persistent cough and wheezing. (A) and (B) Axial lung window CT images show multiple areas of hyperlucent lung with low attenuation and reduced vessels size (asterisks), peribronchial thickening, and multiple bronchiectasis (arrows) in both lower lobes and in right upper lobe.

opacities seen in both viral and bacterial pneumonia.[6,18,138] Round pneumonia, a unique pattern seen in children less than 8 years of age, can mimic tumor or developmental pulmonary malformations[25,144,145] (Fig. 9). The chest radiograph is not recommended in a child who appears well and can be treated as outpatient. Follow-up chest radiographs at 2 weeks to 4 weeks should be reserved for those with persistent or recurrent symptoms or patients with immuno-deficiency.[10,17,137,146]

Complication of bacterial lower respiratory tract infections

Complicated bacterial pneumonia is considered in healthy children who do not respond to treatment or in children with underlying comorbidities.[147] Acute complications can be categorized as lung parenchymal complications (cavitary

necrosis, lung abscess, pneumatocele, pulmonary gangrene, and bronchopleural fistula) and pleural complications (parapneumonic effusion and empyema)[1,25,26,137,140] (Figs. 10–12). Rare mycotic pulmonary arterial aneurysm may occur either as direct extension from necrotizing pneumonia or secondary septic emboli[148] (Fig. 13). Pneumatocele is caused most frequently by Staphylococcus aureus as the offending organism.[25,149,150] Chronic complications of bacterial pneumonia include bronchiectasis and pulmonary fibrosis.[1] US is appropriate in determining the echogenicity, presence of loculation, and septation of parapneumonic effusions.[1,10,114,137] Contrast-enhanced CT is helpful to evaluate lung parenchymal complications and plan for surgical treatments or interventions when appropriate.[10,25,114,137] Although MRI can characterize

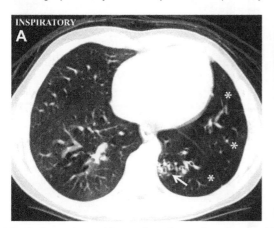
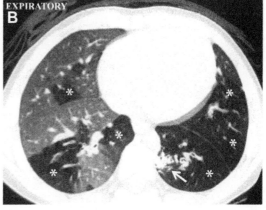

Fig. 7. Swyer-James-MacLeod syndrome in a 5-year-old boy who presented with a previous severe adenovirus lung infection. (A) Axial inspiratory phase lung window CT image shows a generalized hyperlucent small left lung (asterisks) with focal area of atelectasis and associated bronchiectasis in the left lower lobe (arrow). (B) Axial expiratory phase lung window CT image reveals more pronounced hyperlucency and decreased vessel caliber in the left lung (asterisks). There also are multifocal areas of hyperlucency in the right lung (asterisks), which were not evident in the inspiratory phase. Bronchiectasis (arrow) is again seen in the left lower lobe.

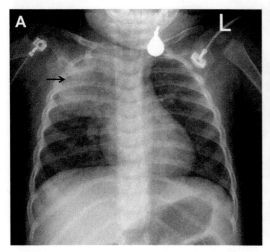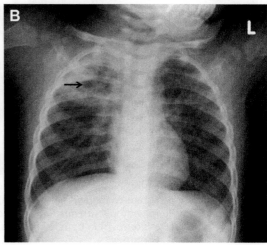

Fig. 8. Alveolar pattern, or endpoint consolidation, in a 6-year-old boy who presented with fever, chest pain, and respiratory distress. (*A*) Frontal chest radiograph shows a patchy opacity at the right upper lobe with faint internal air density (*arrow*). (*B*) Follow-up frontal chest radiograph obtained after 3 days reveals multiple cysts (*arrow*) in the consolidated lung, compatible with necrotizing pneumonia.

complicated pneumonia, it is advocated only for children with substantial radiation exposure from repeated CT scans.[1,27,29,146,151]

Atypical Pneumonia

Demographic and clinical symptoms
Mycoplasma pneumoniae, *Chlamydia pneumoniae*, and *Legionella* spp are the common causative pathogens in atypical pneumonia.[25,152] *M pneum-*

oniae and *C pneumoniae* often are found in school-aged children, frequently presenting with nonspecific clinical symptoms, for example, fever, myalgia, and gradually worsening cough, which is self-limiting.[130,137,152,153] *M pneumonia* may cause extrapulmonary symptoms, such as myocarditis, arthritis, meningoencephalitis, and skin/rash manifestation.[1,17,130,154–156] Legionella pneumonia is rare in children and the risk factors include immunodeficiency, organ transplantation, underlying

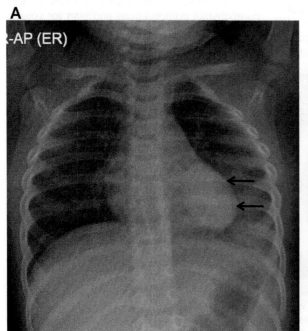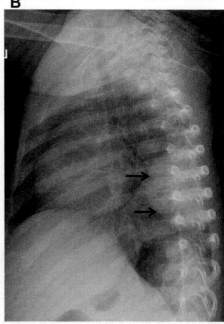

Fig. 9. Round pneumonia in a 3-year-old boy who presented with fever and cough. (*A*) Frontal and (*B*) lateral chest radiographs show a well-defined, rounded opacity (*arrows*) that resembles a mass in the left lower lobe.

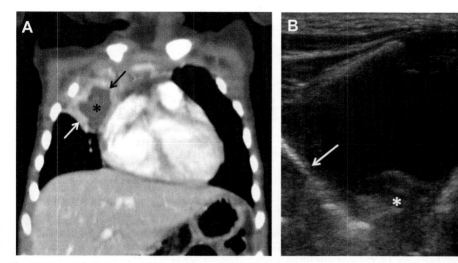

Fig. 10. Lung abscess in an 8-year-old boy after a 3-week treatment of bacterial pneumonia. (*A*) Coronal soft tissue window contrast-enhanced CT image shows a well-defined irregular and thick rim-enhancing lesion (*asterisk*) in the consolidated lung (*arrows*). (*B*) Corresponding ultrasound (US) image reveals presence of proteinaceous debris within the fluid. A percutaneous US-guided aspiration was performed showing the needle (*arrow*) and layering proteinaceous debris (*asterisk*).

chronic pulmonary disease, corticosteroid use, neonatal age, prematurity, and inhalation of contaminated aerosolized water.[152,157] Clinical presentation ranges from mild symptoms to multiple organ failure, with 23% to 41% mortality rate in the pediatric age.[157,158]

Imaging of atypical pneumonia

Radiographic findings of atypical pneumonia are nonspecific, including minimal patchy opacity or segmental/subsegmental airspace and usually more than 1 single dense consolidation. It also can present as reticulonodular opacities, atelectasis, bilobar reticular pattern, and bilateral parahilar peribronchial opacities, mimicking viral pneumonia[1,25,156,159–162] (**Fig. 14**A–B). Centrilobular nodules and thickening of bronchovascular bundles also may be seen from CT study.[161] Hilar adenopathy and pleural and pericardial effusions can occur in *M pneumoniae* pneumonia (MPP) and lobar or unilateral shadow and atelectasis are high risks for refractory MPP, leading to difficult treatment[152,163,164] (see **Fig. 14**C–D). Round pneumonia has also been reported in *C pneumoniae* infections.[165] Clinical, laboratory, and radiographic findings cannot distinguish between MPP and *C pneumoniae* pneumonia.[166] Legionella pneumonia may present with unilateral or bilateral nodular opacities, pleural effusion, and, albeit rarely, cavitation.[167]

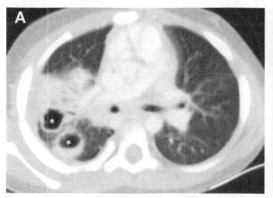
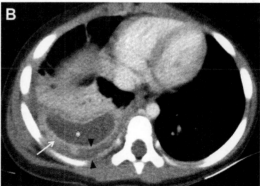

Fig. 11. Pneumatoceles and empyema thoracis in a 2-year-old boy with prior history of pneumonia. (*A*) Axial lung window CT image shows 2 thin-walled cysts (*asterisks*) with internal fluid level and adjacent consolidated lung. (*B*) Axial soft tissue window contrast-enhanced CT image demonstrates loculated pleural effusion (*asterisk*) with thickened parietal pleura (*arrow*), and increased attenuation of the extrapleural space (*arrowheads*) suggestive of empyema thoracis. The patient subsequently underwent thoracostomy and decortication.

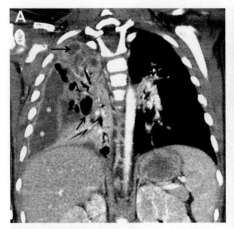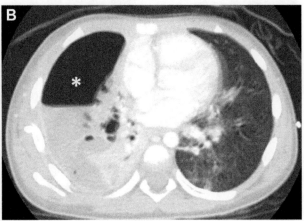

Fig. 12. Complicated pneumonia with cavitary necrosis and bronchopleural fistula in a 1-year-old girl who presented with fever and chest pain. (*A*) Coronal soft tissue window contrast-enhanced CT image shows consolidated right lung with multiloculated cysts (*arrows*) and adjacent pleural fluid collection (*asterisks*). (*B*) Axial lung window CT image demonstrates a large amount of air (*asterisk*) in the pleural space compatible with bronchopleural fistula subsequently developed from the peripherally located, fluid-filled cavitary lung necrosis.

Complication of atypical pneumonia

Although the commonly observed patterns usually are interstitial or bronchopneumonia patterns, acute and chronic complications of complicated pneumonia, including parapneumonic effusion and necrotizing pneumonia, bronchiolitis obliterans, Swyer-James-McLeod syndrome, pulmonary fibrosis, ARDS, and thrombosis in any part of the body have been reported in severe MPP.[152,156,168] Lung abscess, empyema, and rhabdomyolysis are common complications in Legionella pneumonia.[152,167]

Tuberculosis

Demographic and clinical symptoms

Tuberculosis (TB), an airborne infectious disease caused by species in the *Mycobacterium tuberculosis* complex is an important public health concern because it is a major cause of morbidity and mortality in children worldwide. In 2019, 1.2 million children fell ill with TB globally with Africa and Southeast Asia found to have the highest number of children infected.[169] Infection begins when the inhaled infected droplets are deposited in the terminal airway, followed by a localized parenchymal inflammation called the primary (Ghon) focus. The inflammation spreads via the draining lymphatic vessels, usually to the ipsilateral central or regional lymph nodes that enlarge in response. The parenchymal primary focus and the enlarged lymph nodes are called the primary (Ranke or Ghon) complex.[170,171]

If a child is immunocompetent, these lesions become dormant while still causing continuous

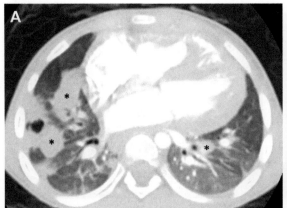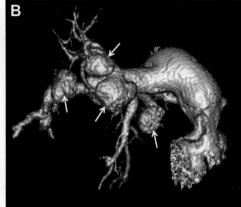

Fig. 13. Mycotic aneurysms in a 3-year-old boy with underlying tetralogy of Fallot and infective endocarditis from *Streptococcus viridans*. (*A*) Axial lung window CT image shows multiple small fluid-filled cavities (*asterisks*) are compatible with septic emboli. (*B*) A 3-D volume-rendered CT image demonstrates multiple mycotic aneurysms (*arrows*) involving lobar branches of right and left pulmonary arteries.

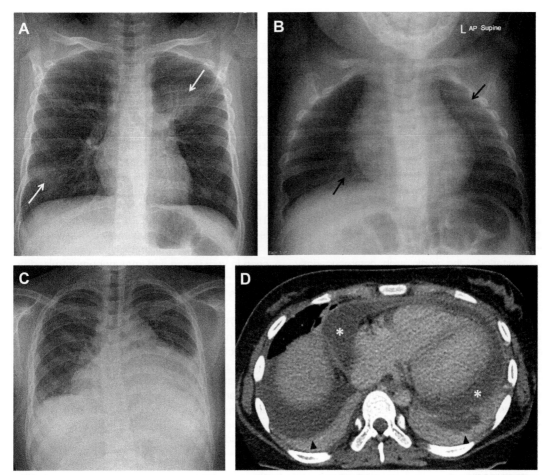

Fig. 14. Spectrum of abnormalities in atypical pneumonia in 3 different pediatric patients. (*A*) Frontal chest radiograph of a 10-year-old boy with *M pneumonia* shows segmental airspace opacities (*arrows*) in the right lower lobe and left upper lobe. (*B*) Frontal chest radiograph of a 4-month-old boy who presented with fever, cough, and conjunctivitis and was diagnosed with *C pneumonia* shows patchy opacities (*arrows*) at right lower lobe and left upper lobe. (*C*) Frontal chest radiograph of a 13-year-old boy with severe *M pneumonia* demonstrates cardiomegaly and airspace densities at both lower lungs. (*D*) Axial soft tissue window contrast-enhanced CT image corresponding to (*C*) shows pericardial effusion (*asterisks*), bilateral pleural effusion (*arrowheads*), and atelectatic lungs.

antigenic stimulation for maintenance of hypersensitivity to TB antigen. This has been referred to as latent TB infection. The caseating necrosis within the Ghon focus and infected lymph node frequently calcifies.[170] If the host is unable to contain the infection and disease progression occurs, this results in primary progressive TB disease.[33] Progression of primary pulmonary TB can manifest in the lungs, lymph nodes, pleural space, or adjacent thoracic structures; however, hematogenous dissemination can occur that can lead to involvement of the distant organs.[33,172]

TB is confirmed when the culture from a specimen representative of intrathoracic disease (eg, sputum, nasopharyngeal/gastric aspirate, or pleural fluid) is positive. The Xpert MTB/RIF is a rapid test to detect

M tuberculosis as well as in detecting resistance to rifampicin from any specimen.[170,173,174] Affected children often display nonspecific clinical signs and symptoms and it can be difficult in obtaining microbiological confirmation.

Imaging of tuberculosis

Imaging of TB, therefore, can play a critical role in the initial diagnosis and evaluation of children suspected of having active TB. A chest radiograph generally is the initial investigation at the time of diagnosis[24,33] with US, CT, and MRI providing additional and more detailed evaluation of the lymph nodes, parenchymal disease, and the associated complications.[33] In many settings, however, the use of chest radiography in screening and triage for TB disease is limited by the unavailability of radiologists to interpret radiographic images. In recent years, computer-aided detection software has been developed to augment and automate the interpretation of digital chest radiography in screening for TB. The WHO has updated its recommendations for TB screening to include the use of computer-aided detection.[24]

Mediastinal and hilar lymphadenopathy is the most common radiologic manifestation of primary TB and is seen in 83% to 96% of cases.[175,176] Due to the normal pattern of lymphatic circulation, a right-sided predominance of lymphadenopathy is seen.[33] On lateral chest radiography, these enlarged lymph nodes demonstrate the classic doughnut sign, which is formed by the normal right main pulmonary arteries anteriorly, left main pulmonary artery posteriorly, the aortic arch anterosuperiorly, and the hilar and subcarinal lymphadenopathy inferiorly[176] (Fig. 15). These nodes may calcify in 15% of cases.[33,170]

Contrast-enhanced CT or MRI can demonstrate the enlarged tuberculous lymph nodes having the characteristic rim sign with an enhancing rim secondary to peripheral granulomatous inflammation and a central low density due to caseous necrosis.[33,170,172,176] TB lymphadenopathy on MRI may have a low signal on T2-weighted short tau inversion recovery imaging, probably related to the free radicals, which are paramagnetic and associated with caseous necrosis[176] (Fig. 16). Airway involvement commonly is seen in children with primary TB. The extrinsic compression of adjacent bronchi by the enlarged lymph nodes may cause symptoms related to airway compression or postobstructive pneumonia.[33,170,172]

Lung parenchymal disease manifests most frequently as consolidation depicted as an area of opacity with a strong lobar predilection in primary TB.[175,177] The radiologic features of the parenchymal disease often appear similar to bacterial pneumonia; however, the presence of lymphadenopathy can be a clue that points toward primary TB. Cavitation rarely occurs in patients with primary TB (29%) in 1 series; and when cavitation occurs, it is known as progressive primary disease.[175]

Hematogenous (miliary) dissemination, usually seen in very young and immunocompromised pediatric patients, manifests radiographically in the lung as nodular interstitial granulomas, usually 1 mm to 2 mm in size, throughout both lungs; however, CT is more sensitive in demonstrating these miliary nodules.[33,172] (Fig. 17). Caseating necrosis, liquefaction, or calcifications can be seen within the consolidation and can progress into extensive lung damage.[33] Fibrosis and destruction of the lung parenchyma result in traction bronchiectasis and formation of cavities, which is known as progressive Ghon focus.[170,178] Bronchopneumonic consolidation may result from the intrabronchial

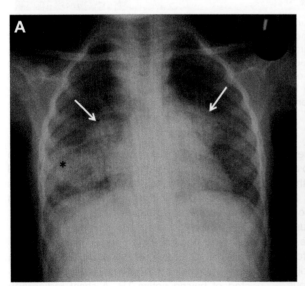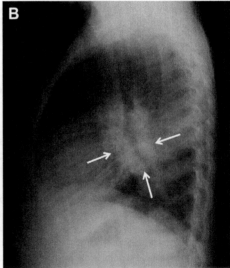

Fig. 15. Mediastinal and hilar lymphadenopathy in a 3-year-old boy with primary tuberculosis who presented with progressively worsening cough and chest pain. (A) Frontal chest radiograph demonstrates dense mass-like structures in the hilar and subcarinal regions compatible with lymphadenopathy (arrows). Right lower lobe consolidation (asterisk) is also seen. (B) Lateral chest radiograph demonstrates the typical doughnut sign (arrows), which is formed by the normal right main pulmonary artery anteriorly, left main pulmonary artery posteriorly, the aortic arch anterosuperiorly, and the hilar and subcarinal lymphadenopathy inferiorly. The radiolucent center is formed by the trachea and upper lobe bronchi.

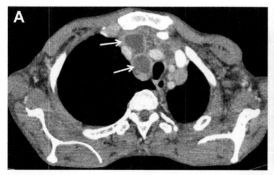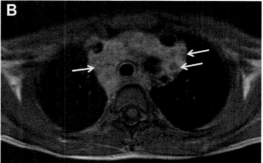

Fig. 16. Characteristic cross-sectional imaging appearance of tuberculosis (TB) lymphadenopathy in a 17-year-old boy who presented with weight loss, low grade fever, chest pain, and cough. (A) Axial soft tissue window contrast-enhanced CT image of the chest demonstrates multiple enlarged lymph nodes with central low attenuation and enhancing periphery compatible with typical rim sign of TB lymphadenopathy (arrows). (B) Corresponding axial contrast-enhanced T1-weighted MRI shows enlarged heterogeneously enhancing mediastinal lymph nodes also showing areas of necrosis with enhancing rim (arrows).

spread of the parenchymal cavity or after eruption of a caseated lymph node into the bronchial tree. Radiography depicts irregular patchy infiltration, usually involving more than 1 lobe of a single lung. CT may show poorly defined nodules or rosettes of nodules, 2 mm to 10 mm in diameter, and the centrilobular or branching centrilobular opacities seen in approximately 95% of cases with a tree-in-bud appearance.[33,175]

Tuberculous pleural effusions usually result from hypersensitivity to the tuberculous protein. Effusions are uncommon in infants and young children with pulmonary TB and may appear in only 6% to 11% of pediatric cases, with increasing prevalence with age. US of the chest is an alternative to chest radiograph in characterizing the pleural effusion and identifying lymph nodes and diagnosing pulmonary TB, especially in a resource-limited setting. Tuberculous empyemas typically are loculated and associated with pleural thickening and enhancement on CT imaging[33,170,171] (Fig. 18).

Postprimary TB, also known as reactivation TB disease or adult-type TB disease, often is seen in children over 10 years of age and adults. The typical radiographic pattern is bilateral ill-defined parenchymal densities mainly involving the apical segments of the upper lobes. It usually is associated with nodular and linear fibrosis. There could be associated distortion of the adjacent mediastinal and bronchovascular structures. Cavitation with air–fluid levels, pleural effusions, bronchiectasis, and even colonization of the cavities with Aspergillus species also can be seen.[33]

The immune response to mycobacteria has important implications for the clinical and imaging appearance of TB, particularly in immunocompromised patients.[175]

Tuberculosis and human immunodeficiency virus coinfection in children

Progressive immune dysfunction caused by HIV infection increases the susceptibility to TB infection as well as progression from latent infection to active TB disease. When HIV and TB coinfected individuals are treated with antiretroviral drugs against HIV, they may develop an IRIS, where the recovering immune system starts to react to the bacterial infection, resulting in increased morbidity.[176] The most common manifestations of TB-associated IRIS in the lungs include worsening or new hilar or mediastinal lymphadenopathy with or without tracheobronchial compression, worsening or new airspace consolidation, and pleural effusions. The radiographic manifestations of HIV-associated TB depends on the level of immunosuppression. HIV-infected pediatric patients with a CD4 T-lymphocyte count of less than 200/mm have had a higher prevalence of hilar or mediastinal adenopathy, extrapulmonary involvement, and lower prevalence of cavitation in the lungs. Miliary or dis

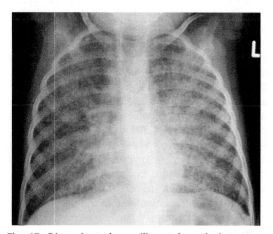

Fig. 17. Disseminated or miliary tuberculosis pattern in a 1-year-old girl who presented with low grade fever and cough. Frontal chest radiograph demonstrates minute (2–3 mm) nodules diffusely throughout both lungs.

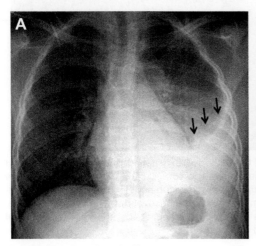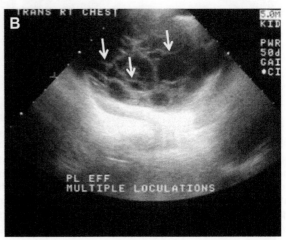

Fig. 18. Complex pleural effusion in a 3-year-old boy with pulmonary tuberculosis. (*A*) Frontal chest radiograph shows an opacity in the left hemithorax with meniscus (*arrows*), obscuring the left hemidiaphragm and left heart margin. (*B*) Corresponding US examination of the chest reveals a complex pleural fluid collection with multiple loculations (*arrows*).

seminated disease has been associated with severe immunosuppression.[176,179]

Fungal and Opportunistic Infections

Fungal infections of the lungs are relatively common and a potentially life-threatening condition, especially in immunocompromised children. Other populations at risk include those who live in areas where mycoses, such as coccidioidomycosis, blastomycosis, and histoplasmosis, are persistently endemic, premature neonates and those who are critically ill or have medically placed catheters or prostheses.[180,181] Five relatively common and clinically important fungal and opportunistic infections in the pediatric population include aspergillosis, histoplasmosis, coccidioidomycosis, candidiasis, and pneumocystis pneumonia, which are discussed in the following sections.

Aspergillosis

The sinopulmonary tract is the most common portal of entry via inhalation of the spores of *Aspergillus* conidia into the respiratory tract, but other routes include the gastrointestinal tract and skin.[33,180,182] Due to the host-impaired immune response, the conidia germinate into hyphae, then invade the pulmonary arteries and cause pulmonary arterial thrombosis, hemorrhage, lung necrosis, and thereafter systemic dissemination.

The respiratory tract can be involved in 3 main forms and depends on the host immune response[180]: (1) aspergilloma by colonization of preexisting space from various conditions[181]; (2) allergic bronchopulmonary aspergillosis due to saprophytic infestation in the body of the host[182]; and (3) invasive pulmonary aspergillosis, which usually is acute and

rapidly progressive disease.[33,182,183] Aspergilloma or mycetoma is a fungus ball, which represents a colonization of intertwined fungal hyphae growing in a space, such as an ectatic bronchus or a postpneumonic cavity. The typical appearance on radiographs or CT is a rounded soft tissue mass within a cavity forming an air crescent sign and represents the separation of necrotic lung tissue from the neighboring pulmonary parenchyma.[180,184] Any cavity within the lung can facilitate the development of an aspergilloma, which moves within the cavity according to a patient's position[180] (**Fig. 19**).

Allergic bronchopulmonary aspergillosis is caused by a hypersensitivity reaction to *Aspergillus* antigens and usually develops in children with chronic respiratory diseases, such as cystic fibrosis or asthma. The fungi are trapped in the tenacious secretions and this results in an immune response, which further exacerbates their respiratory symptoms.[33,180,182,185] Due to the chronic mucoid impaction of the ectatic proximal bronchi, the typical imaging finding is the pulmonary airspace consolidation and finger-in-glove appearance on radiographs, which frequently leads to a postobstructive lobar atelectasis. These imaging features usually involve the middle or upper lobes and can be transient or permanent.[180] HRCT is more sensitive than radiography and demonstrates the mucoid impaction of the central airways and the bronchiectasis of the segmental or subsegmental airways.[33,180]

Invasive pulmonary aspergillosis occurs predominantly in pediatric patients with a hematologic malignancy or aplastic anemia or in those who are undergoing corticosteroid or other immunosuppressive therapy.[186] The characteristic CT findings

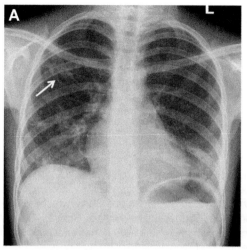
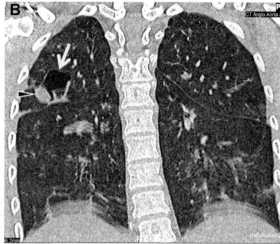

Fig. 19. Aspergilloma in a 4-year-old boy who presented with fever, cough and chest pain. (*A*) Frontal chest radiograph shows a suspicious cystic lesion (*arrow*) in the right upper lobe. There also are linear streaky opacities in the right lower lobe and airspace consolidation in the left lower lobe. (*B*) Corresponding coronal lung window CT image confirms the cystic lesion (*arrow*) with a round intracavitary mass (*arrowhead*) that moved within the cavity as the child's position changed.

of acute angioinvasive aspergillosis consist of a nodule or nodules surrounded by a halo of ground-glass attenuation (halo sign) or pleura-based wedge-shaped areas of consolidation.[180] These nodules are composed of infected hemorrhagic and infarcted lung tissue. The air crescent sign, that can be seen on CT imaging, is due to the peripheral reabsorption of the necrotic tissue, which causes the retraction of the infarcted center with air filling the space in-between. This usually occurs 2 weeks to 3 weeks after the onset of treatment when a patient mounts an immune response[183] (**Fig. 20**).

Histoplasmosis

Histoplasmosis is caused by the dimorphic fungus *Histoplasma capsulatum* that is found in soil contaminated with avian or bat droppings and is endemic in Central America, Northern South America, and some parts of Asia.[1] Histoplasmosis is acquired mainly through the respiratory tract by inhalation of the spores, which germinate and infiltrate within the alveoli and thereby incites an interstitial inflammation characterized by granulomas, which may calcify.[33,182] This infection also spreads to the hilar and mediastinal nodes. Children with a competent immune system usually do not manifest the disease, because histoplasmosis predominantly is a disease of the immunocompromised, the very young, and the very old.[1,33,187] There is a wide range of clinical forms of histoplasmosis from the very mild, self-limiting cases that respond favorably to therapy to the more chronic form, appearing similar radiographically to postprimary

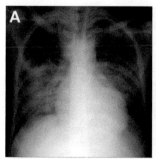
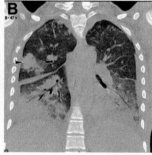
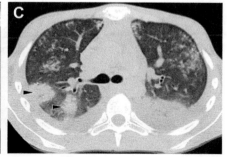

Fig. 20. Angioinvasive aspergillosis in a 15-year-old boy with acute lymphoblastic leukemia who presented with fever and worsening respiratory distress. (*A*) Frontal chest radiograph with corresponding (*B*) coronal and (*C*) axial lung window CT images demonstrate multiple nodules throughout both lungs. The large nodules in the right upper lobe are surrounded by ground-glass opacity compatible with halo sign (*arrowheads*). Airspace consolidations with air bronchograms are also noted in both lower lobes.

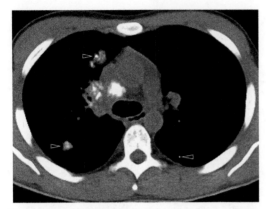

Fig. 21. Histoplasmosis infection in a 7-year-old boy who presented with low-grade fever, chills, dry cough, and headache. Axial soft tissue window noncontrast CT image shows calcified mediastinal lymphadenopathy and calcified pulmonary nodules (*arrowheads*).

TB and paralleling the clinical phase of the disease, to the most extreme acute and disseminated form that is fatal.

Radiologic manifestations are dependent on the stage of the disease and immune state of the patient. Acute histoplasmosis usually manifests as focal parenchymal consolidation with or without ipsilateral hilar or mediastinal adenopathy, which resolves over weeks or months. Pulmonary nodules representing a histoplasmoma may develop and may show central or dystrophic calcification after a few months (**Fig. 21**). Pleural effusion (<5%), mediastinal granuloma, mediastinal fibrosis, and pericarditis are rare and are late complications.[33,180,188] Chronic histoplasmosis, which is more common in adults, manifests radiographically as an upper lobe fibrocavitary disease similar to

postprimary TB.[33,180] Disseminated histoplasmosis commonly manifests with small, single or multiple, nodular opacities that are less than 3 mm in diameter, depicting a miliary or diffuse reticulonodular pattern that could progress to diffuse airspace opacification.[33,188] Mediastinal histoplasmosis may complicate the pulmonary disease and can lead to mediastinal fibrosis, causing vascular compromise as well as esophageal and bronchial stenosis, best demonstrated on CT imaging of the chest.[187]

Coccidioidomycosis

Coccidioidomycosis is caused by *Coccidioides immitis* and *Coccidioides posadasii*, which are endemic in southwestern United States, Central America, South America, and the arid regions of Mexico and also is known as valley fever.[189,190] The spores are inhaled and manifest clinically most commonly as a mild, self-limiting respiratory illness to a CAP in older children and adults. The 3 forms of coccidioidomycosis identified based on the clinical and imaging findings are (1) acute, (2) disseminated, and (3) chronic. The degree of exposure and a patient's immune status could determine the severity and extent of the disease.[189,190]

Radiographs and CT of affected pediatric patients may show pulmonary nodules or consolidation with associated enlargement of mediastinal or hilar lymph nodes, which usually resolve in 6 weeks[189,190] (**Fig. 22**). The parenchymal consolidation may resolve at 1 site and migrate to another area as so-called phantom infiltrates.[191] Pulmonary nodules, thin-walled cavitations, and small pleural effusions may occur in a small fraction of the pediatric patients. Chronic disease is characterized by the presence of clinical or imaging findings beyond 6 weeks. Imaging features include residual pulmonary abnormalities, including fibrosis,

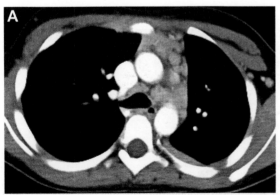
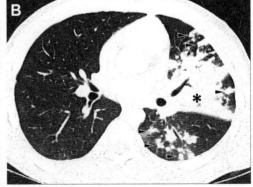

Fig. 22. Coccidioidomycosis infection in a 16-year-old boy with travel history to South America who presented with fever, cough, chills, and chest pain. (*A*) Axial soft tissue window contrast-enhanced CT image shows multiple enlarged mediastinal lymph nodes. (*B*) Axial lung window CT image demonstrates consolidation (*asterisk*) and multiple pulmonary nodues (*arrowheads*).

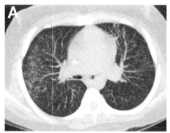
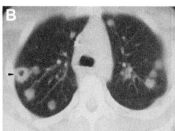

Fig. 23. Pulmonary candidiasis in 2 different pediatric patients. (*A*) A 10-year-old girl with acute lymphocytic leukemia undergoing hematopoietic stem cell transplantation developed *Candida krusei* sepsis. Axial lung window CT image demonstrates innumerable 3 mm to 5 mm interstitial nodules on both lungs compatible with miliary pattern of pulmonary Candidiasis. (*B*) Axial lung window CT image of a 14-year-old girl with leukemia undergoing chemotherapy shows multiple bilateral lung nodules, some exhibiting cavitation (*arrowhead*).

cavity formations, lymphadenopathy, pleural effusion, or uncommonly mycetoma, abscess formation, and bronchopleural fistula.[189] On CT, the residual pulmonary nodule, called coccidioidoma, can have a smooth, spiculated, or lobulated margin surrounded by GGOs and, rarely, calcify.[189] Disseminated infection, which may involve any organ of the body, is seen in minority of affected children, especially those with impaired immune status. The presence of miliary nodules is the classic pulmonary finding in disseminated coccidioidomycosis and is secondary to hematogenous spread leading to ARDS in immunocompromised pediatric patients.

Candidiasis

Candida is the most common cause of fungal infections worldwide, especially when the immune system is compromised as in those patients undergoing steroid therapy, prolonged antibiotic treatment, and in patients with indwelling catheters. *Candida albicans* is the most commonly isolated species.[33,182,192] Pulmonary candidiasis can enter the lungs hematogenously, from other sites of infection or, less commonly, from the aspiration of contaminated oropharyngeal secretions.

In the early stage of the disease, chest imaging findings may be normal and diagnosis may be difficult because there is no specific clinical or radiologic presentation. Pediatric patients with *Candida*

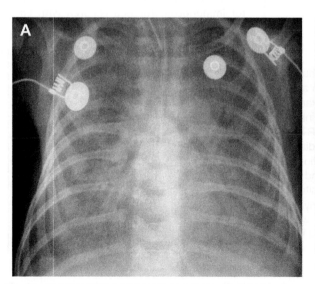
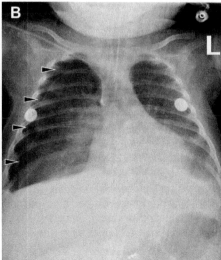

Fig. 24. Pneumocystis pneumonia in a 3-month-old girl who presented with fever and hypoxia. (*A*) Frontal chest radiograph demonstrates diffuse bilateral ground-glass opacity in both lungs. (*B*) Subsequent frontal chest radiograph reveals a large right-sided pneumothorax (*arrowheads*).

pneumonia may present with bilateral interstitial or multifocal alveolar patchy opacifications on chest radiograph. A miliary pattern is common in hematogenous *Candida* pneumonia and cystic or cavitary masses and exudative pleural effusions also have been described. CT findings are nonspecific and may include miliary nodules ranging from 3 mm to 30 mm in diameter, associated with other parenchymal findings, such as airspace consolidation, tree-in-bud changes, or GGOs[33,193] (**Fig. 23**).

Pneumocystis pneumonia

Pneumocystis pneumonia, caused *by Pneumocystis jirovecii*, an atypical fungus transmitted mainly via respiratory secretions, is the most common opportunistic infection in the immunocompromised, particularly in HIV-infected infants, occurring in up to 50%.[33,182] The imaging appearance is variable and may be normal in pediatric patients with early or mild disease, but a majority of infected children have abnormal chest radiographs.[33] Coinfection with CMV in HIV-infected infants is common and results in a more rapid disease progression.[105]

The typical radiographic findings include diffuse bilateral interstitial or nodular opacification extending from the perihilar region and progression to widespread alveolar opacities with air bronchograms. Cavitary nodules and cysts also can be seen, with common complications including pneumothorax, pneumomediastinum, and interstitial emphysema (**Fig. 24**). Pleural effusions, lymphadenopathy, and nodules rarely are seen in children. Typical HRCT findings include patchy or diffuse ground-glass attenuation with a background of interlobular septal thickening, known as crazy paving pattern.[33,106,122]

SUMMARY

LRTI is a common disease entity in children, but it can have a diverse spectrum of manifestation and complications. Clinical history and physical examination remain the most important tools in the initial evaluation of a child suspected of having LRTIs. Medical imaging plays a role in confirming diagnosis, characterization, evaluation of complications, and as a guide for treatment and intervention and for assessment of long-term sequelae. In some situations, medical imaging demonstrates an underlying abnormality particularly in pediatric patients with long-standing and recurrent infections. Various imaging tools and its appropriate indications are presented in this review. These recommendations and algorithm are intended to guide radiologists and clinicians in making decisions regarding radiologic studies. The severity of a patient's condition, the availability of imaging equipment, and expertise of the imaging physician or radiologist, however, would have to be considered carefully.

CLINICS CARE POINTS

- Chest imaging may not be needed in children with noncomplicated CAP responding to therapy.
- Chest radiograph is the initial imaging tool recommended for the following: a neonate or child with fever of unknown source and respiratory symptoms; an immunocompetent child with CAP not responding to treatment or resulting to hospitalization; an immunocompetent child with hospital-acquired pneumonia (HAP); immunocompromised child with CAP; and a child with suspected TB.
- There is some evidence for the use of US detection of pneumonia in children and it may be used as an alternative imaging tool although future studies confirming the initial results currently are needed. US also can be used to evaluate moderate to large pleural effusion and suspected lung abscess seen on the initial chest radiograph. Training and expertise are required in the performance of this test.
- Chest CT without or with IV contrast can be used for further evaluation of immunocompromised children with multiple, diffuse, or confluent chest radiographic findings and for immunocompromised children with equivocal chest radiographic results.
- Chest CT with IV contrast is recommended for children with recurrent pneumonia, pneumonia with complicated lung parenchymal disease (eg, abscess and necrotizing pneumonia), or pneumonia with complicated pleural disease (eg, empyema, bronchopleural fistula, and moderate to large effusion).
- Evidence is available for the use of MRI in complicated pneumonia particularly in abscess formation. MRI also is utilized to evaluate mediastinal lymphadenopathy, especially in children with thoracic TB.
- A majority of the available literature for childhood LRTIs and chest imaging are focused on imaging detection and characterization of abnormalities. It is recommended further that more studies be conducted with regard to the utility of various imaging studies and patient-centered outcomes for these indications.

DISCLOSURE

The authors have nothing to disclose.

REFERENCES

1. Eslamy HK, Newman B. Pneumonia in normal and immunocompromised children: an overview and update. Radiol Clin North Am 2011;49:895–920.
2. WHO fact sheet on Pneumonia. 2019. Available at: https://www.who.int/news-room/fact-sheets/detail/pneumonia.pdf. Accessed March 15, 2021.
3. le Roux DM, Zar HJ. Community-acquired pneumonia in children – a changing spectrum of disease. Pediatr Radiol 2017;47:1392–8.
4. Rudan I, O'Brien KL, Nair H, et al. Epidemiology and etiology of childhood pneumonia in 2010: estimates of incidence, severe morbidity, mortality, underlying risk factors and causative pathogens for 192 countries. J Glob Health 2013;3:10401.
5. McAllister DA, Liu L, Shi T, et al. Global, regional, and national estimates of pneumonia morbidity and mortality in children younger than 5 years between 2000 and 2015: a systematic analysis. Lancet Glob Health 2019;7(1):e47–57.
6. Virkki R, Juven T, Rikalainene H, et al. Differentiation of bacterial and viral pneumonia in children. Thorax 2002;57:438–41.
7. Jain S, Williams DJ, Arnold SR, et al. Community-acquired pneumonia requiring hospitalization among U.S. children. N Engl J Med 2015;372(9):835–45.
8. Jiang W, Wu M, Zhou J, et al. Etiologic spectrum and occurrence of co-infections in children hospitalized with community-acquired pneumonia. BMC Infect Dis 2017;17:787.
9. Ruuskanen O, Lahti E, Jennings LC, et al. Viral pneumonia. Lancet 2011;377:1264–75.
10. Chan SS, Kotecha MK, Rigsby CK, et al. ACR appropriateness criteria pneumonia in the immunocompetent child. J Am Coll Radiol 2020;17:S215–25.
11. Lee C, Colletti PM, Chung JH, et al. ACR appropriateness criteria acute respiratory illness in immunocompromised patients. J Am Coll Radiol 2019;16(11):S331–9.
12. Westra SJ, Karmazyn BK, Alazraki AL, et al. ACR appropriateness criteria fever without source or unknown origin – child. J Am Coll Radiol 2016;13(8):922–30.
13. Ambroggio L, Mangeot C, Kurowski EM, et al. Guideline adoption for community-acquired pneumonia in the outpatient setting. Pediatrics 2018;142(4):e20180331.
14. O'Grady KA, Torzillo PJ, Frawlwy K, et al. The radiological diagnosis of pneumonia in children. Pneumonia 2014;5:38–51.
15. Harris M, Clark J, Coote N, et al. British Thoracic Society guidelines for management of community acquired pneumonia in children: update 2011. Thorax 2011;66(Suppl2):ii1–23.
16. Bradley JS, Byington CL, Shah SS, et al. Executive summary: the management of community-acquired pneumonia in infants and children older than 3 months of age: clinical practice guidelines by the pediatric infectious diseases society and the infectious diseases society of America. Clin Infect Dis 2011;53(7):617–30.
17. Donnelly LF. Maximizing the usefulness of imaging in children with community-acquired pneumonia. AJR Am J Roentgenol 1999;172:505–12.
18. Zar HJ, Moore DP, Andronikou A, et al. Diagnosis and management of community-acquired pneumonia in children: South African Thoracic Society guidelines. South Afr Med J 2020;110(7):588–93.
19. Cox M, Soudack M, Podberesky DJ, et al. Pediatric chest ultrasound: a practical approach. Pediatr Radiol 2017;47:1058–68.
20. Xin H, Li J, Hu HY. Is lung ultrasound useful for diagnosing pneumonia in children? a meta-analysis and systematic review. Ultrasound Q 2018;34(1):3–10.
21. Pereda MA, Chavez MA, Hooper-Miele CC, et al. Lung ultrasound for the diagnosis of pneumonia in children: a meta-analysis. Pediatrics 2015;135(4):714–22.
22. Urbankowska E, Krenke K, Drobczyński Ł, et al. Lung ultrasound in the diagnosis and monitoring of community acquired pneumonia in children. Respir Med 2015;109(9):1207–12.
23. Ho MC, Ker CR, Hsu JH, et al. Usefulness of lung ultrasound in the diagnosis of community-acquired pneumonia in children. Pediatr Neonatol 2015;56(1):40–5.
24. WHO consolidated guidelines on tuberculosis. Module 2: screening – systematic screening for tuberculosis disease. Geneva: World Health Organization; 2021. Licence: CC BY-NC-SA 3.0 IGO.
25. Daltro P, Santos EN, Gasparetto TD, et al. Pulmonary infections. Pediatr Radiol 2011;41(Suppl 1):S69–82.
26. Andronikou S, Lambert E, Halton J, et al. Guidelines for the use of chest radiographs in community-acquired pneumonia in children and adolescents. Pediatr Radiol 2017;47(11):1405–11.
27. Yikilmaz A, Koc A, Coskun A, et al. Evaluation of pneumonia in children: comparison of MRI with fast imaging sequences at 1.5 T with chest radiographs. Acta Radiol 2011;52(8):914–9.
28. Liszewski MC, Görkem S, Sodhi KS, et al. Lung magnetic resonance imaging for pneumonia in children. Pediatr Radiol 2017;47:1420–30.
29. Konietzke P, Mueller J, Wuennemann F, et al. The value of chest magnetic resonance imaging compared to chest radiographs with and without additional lung ultrasound in children with complicated pneumonia. PLoS One 2020;15(3):e0230252.

30. Montella S, Corcione A, Santamaria F. Recurrent pneumonia in children: a reasoned diagnostic approach and a single centre experience. Int J Mol Sci 2017;18(2):298.

31. Donnelly LF. Practical issues concerning imaging of pulmonary infection in children. J Thorac Imaging 2001;16(4):238–50.

32. Ebell MH, Siwek J, Weiss BD, et al. Strength of Recommendation Taxonomy (SORT): a patient-centered approach to grading evidence in the medical literature. Am Fam Physician 2004;69:548–56.

33. Laya BF, Amini B, Zucker EJ, et al. Chapter 6: lung. In: Lee EY, editor. Pediatric radiology: practical imaging evaluation of infants and children. Philadelphia: Wolters Kluwer; 2018. p. 358–458.

34. Franquet T. Imaging of pneumonia: trends and algorithms. Eur Respir J 2001;18:196–208.

35. Feigin DS. Lateral chest radiograph: a systematic approach. Acad Radiol 2010;17:1560–6.

36. Ayyala RS, Nosaka S, Khashoggi K, et al. Chapter 7: pleura. In: Lee EY, editor. Pediatric radiology: practical imaging evaluation of infants and children. Philadelphia: Wolters Kluwer; 2018.

37. Mercer RM, Psallidas I, Rahman NM. Ultrasound in the management of pleural disease. Expert Rev Respir Med 2017;11:323–31.

38. Hassan M, Rizk R, Essam H, et al. Validation of equations for pleural effusion volume estimation by ultrasonography. J Ultrasound 2017;20(4):267–71.

39. Aboudara M, Maldonado F. Update in the management of pleural effusions. Med Clin North Am 2019; 103(3):475–85.

40. Coley BD. Chest sonography in children: current indications, techniques, and imaging findings. Radiol Clin North Am 2011;49(5):825–46.

41. Goh Y, Kapur J. Sonography of the pediatric chest. J Ultrasound Med 2016;35(5):1067–80.

42. Shah CC, Greenberg SB. The pediatric chest. In: Rumack C, Levine D, editors. Diagnostic ultrasound. 5th edition. Philadelphia: Elsevier; 2018.

43. Joshi P, Vasishta A, Gupta M. Ultrasound of the pediatric chest. Br J Radiol 2019;92:20190058.

44. Ferreiro L, Toubes ME, Valdés L. The utility of ultrasonography in diseases of the pleura. Arch Bronconeumol 2017;53(12):659–60.

45. Soni NJ, Franco R, Velez MI, et al. Ultrasound in the diagnosis and management of pleural effusions. J Hosp Med 2015;10(12):811–6.

46. Marchetti G, Arondi S, Baglivo F, et al. New insights in the use of pleural ultrasonography for diagnosis and treatment of pleural disease. Clin Respir J 2018;12(6):1993–2005.

47. Rea G, Sperandeo M, Di Serafino M, et al. Neonatal and pediatric thoracic ultrasonography. J Ultrasound 2019;22(2):121–30.

48. Tomiyama N, Muller NL, Johkoh T, et al. Acute parenchymal lung disease in immunocompetent patients: diagnostic accuracy of high-resolution CT. AJR Am J Roentgenol 2000;174:1745–50.

49. Gruden JF, Huang L, Turner J, et al. High-resolution CT in the evaluation of clinically suspected Pneumocystis carinii pneumonia in AIDS patients with normal, equivocal, or non-specific radiographic findings. AJR Am J Roentgenol 1997;169:967–75.

50. Wielpütz M, Kauczor HU. MRI of the lung: state of the art. Diagn Interv Radiol 2012;18:344–53.

51. Hirsch W, Sorgea I, Krohmera S, et al. MRI of the lungs in children. Eur J Radiol 2008;68:278–88.

52. Sodhi KS, Khandelwal N, Saxena AK, et al. Rapid lung MRI: paradigm shift of febrile neutropenia in children with leukemia: a pilot study. Leuk Lymphoma 2015;57(1):70–5.

53. Kusel MM, de Klerk NH, Holt PG, et al. Role of respiratory viruses in acute upper and lower respiratory tract illness in the first year of life: a birth cohort study. Pediatr Infect Dis J 2006;25(8):680–6.

54. Nair H, Simooes EA, Rudan I, et al. Global and regional burden of hospital admissions for severe acute lower respiratory infections in young children in 2010: a systematic analysis. Lancet 2013; 381(9875):1380–90.

55. Zar HJ. Bacterial and viral pneumonia: new insights from the drakenstein child health study. Paediatr Respir Rev 2017. https://doi.org/10.1016/j.prrv.2017.06.009.

56. Virkki R, Juven T, Mertsola J, et al. Radiographic follow-up of pneumonia in children. Pediatr Pulmonol 2005;40:223–7.

57. Winant AJ, Schooler GR, Concepcion NDP, et al. Current updates on pediatric pulmonary infections. Semin Roentgenol 2017;52(1):35–42.

58. Korppi M, Heiskanen-Kosma T, Jalonen E, et al. Aetiology of community-acquired pneumonia in children treated in hospital. Eur J Pediatr 1993;152:24–30.

59. Yoo JK, Kim TS, Hufford MW, et al. Viral infection of the lung: host response and sequelae. J Allergy Clin Immunol 2013;132:1263–76.

60. Kwon HJ, Rhie YJ, Seo WH, et al. Clinical manifestations of respiratory adenoviral infection among hospitalized children in Korea. Pediatr Int 2013;55:450–4.

61. Koo HJ, Lim S, Choe J, et al. Radiographic and CT features of viral pneumonia. Radiographics 2018;38: 719–39.

62. Lim LM, Woo YY, de Bruyne JA, et al. Epidemiology, clinical presentation and respiratory sequelae of adenovirus pneumonia in children in Kuala Lumpur, Malaysia. PLoS One 2018;13(10):e0205795.

63. Hong JY, Lee HJ, Piedra PA, et al. Lower respiratory tract infections due to adenovirus in hospitalized Korean children: epidemiology, clinical features, and prognosis. Clin Infect Dis 2001;32:1423–9.

64. Lee N, Qureshi ST. Other viral pneumonia. coronavirus, respiratory syncytial virus, adenovirus, hantavirus. Crit Care Clin 2013;29(4):1045–68.

65. Lucaya J, Gartner S, Garcia-Peña P, et al. Spectrum of manifestations of Swyer-James-MacLeod syndrome. J Comput Assist Tomogr 1998;22: 592–7.

66. Posfay-Barbe KM. Infections in paediatrics: old and new diseases. Swiss Med Wkly 2012;142: w13654.

67. Diniz LMO, Maia MMM, de Oliveira YV, et al. Study of complications of Varicella-Zoster Virus infection in hospitalized children at a reference hospital for infectious disease treatment. Hosp Pediatr 2018; 8:419–25.

68. Bozzola E, Gattinara GC, Bozzola M, et al. Varicella associated pneumonia in a pediatric population. Ital J Pediatr 2017;43:49.

69. Kim JS, Ryu CW, Lee SI, et al. High resolution CT findings of varicella zoster pneumonia. AJR Am J Roentgenol 1999;172:113–6.

70. Cameron JC, Allan G, Johnson F, et al. Severe complications of chickenpox in hospitalized children in the UK and Ireland. Arch Dis Child 2007; 92:1062–6.

71. Moon JH, Kim EA, Lee KS, et al. Cytomegalovirus pneumonia: high resolution CT findings in ten non-AIDS immunocompromised patients. Korean J Radiol 2000;1:73–8.

72. Restrepo-Gualteros SM, Jaramillo-Barberi LE, Gonzales-Santos M, et al. Characterization of cytomegalovirus lung infection in non-HIV infected children. Viruses 2014;6:2038–51.

73. Gasparetto EL, Ono SE, Escuissato D, et al. Cytomegalovirus pneumonia after bone marrow transplantation: high resolution CT findings. Br J Radiol 2004;77:724–7.

74. Mejias A, Chavez-Bueno S, Ramilo O. Respiratory syncytial virus pneumonia: mechanisms of inflammation and prolonged airway hyperresponsiveness. Curr Opin Infect Dis 2005;18:199–204.

75. Dawson-Caswell M, Muncie HL. Respiratory syncytial virus in children. Am Fam Physician 2011;83: 141–6.

76. Nye S, Whitley RJ, Kong M. Viral infection in the development and progression of pediatric acute respiratory distress syndrome. Front Pediatr 2016; 4:128.

77. Weisman LE. Populations at risk for developing respiratory syncytial virus and risk factors for respiratory syncytial virus severity: infants with predisposing conditions. Pediatr Infect Dis J 2003;22:S33–7.

78. Sloots TP, Whiley DM, Lambert SB, et al. Emerging respiratory agents: new viruses for old diseases. J Clin Virol 2008;42:233–43.

79. Orenstein WA, Perry RT, Halsey NA. The clinical significance of measles: a review. J Infect 2004; 189:S4–16.

80. Rota PA, Moss WJ, Takeda M, et al. Measles. Nat Rev 2016;2:16049.

81. Quiambao BP, Gatchalian SR, Halonen P, et al. Co-infection is common in measles-associated pneumonia. Pediatr Infect Dis J 1998;17:89–93.

82. Peltola H, Heinonen OP, Valle M, et al. The elimination of indigenous measles, mumps, and rubella from Finland by a 12-year, two-dose vaccination program. N Engl J Med 1994;331:1397–402.

83. Chu HY, Englund JA, Strelitz B, et al. Rhinovirus disease in children seeking care in a tertiary pediatric emergency department. J Pediatr Inf Dis Soc 2016;5:29–38.

84. Drysdale SB, Mejias A, Ramilo O. Rhinovirus-not just the common cold. J Infect 2017;74:S41–6.

85. Foust AM, Winant AJ, Chu WC, et al. Pediatric SARS, H1N1, MERS, EVALI, and Now Coronavirus Disease (COVID-19) Pneumonia: what radiologists need to know. Am J Radiol AJR 2020;215:1–9.

86. Lee EY, McAdam A, Chaudry G, et al. Swine-origin influenza A (H1N1) viral infection in children: initial chest radiographic findings. Radiology 2010;254: 934–41.

87. Ye Q, Wang B, Mao J. The pathogenesis and treatment of the 'Cytokine Storm' in COVID-19. J Infect 2020;80:607–13.

88. Zimmerman P, Curtis N. Coronavirus infections in children including COVID-19. an overview of the epidemiology, clinical features, diagnosis, treatment and prevention options in children. Pediatr Infect Dis J 2020;39:355–68.

89. Babyn PS, Chu Winnie CW, Tsou IYY. Severe acute respiratory syndrome (SARS) chest radiographic features in children. Pediatr Radiol 2004;34:47–58.

90. Gulati A, Pomeranz C, Qamar Z, et al. A Comprehensive review of manifestations of novel coronaviruses in the context of deadly COVID-19 global pandemic. AM J Med Sci 2020. https://doi.org/10.1016/j.amjms.2020.05.006.

91. Jin Y, Yang H, Ji W, et al. Virology, epidemiology, pathogenesis, and control of COVID-19. Viruses 2020;12:372.

92. Foust AM, Phillips GS, Chu WC, et al. International expert consensus statement on chest imaging in pediatric Covid-19 patient management: imaging findings, imaging study reporting, and imaging study recommendations. Radiol Cardiothorac Imaging 2020;2(2):e200214.

93. Foust AM, McAdam AJ, Chu WC, et al. practical guide for pediatric pulmonologist on imaging management of pediatric patients with COVID-19. Pediatr Pulmonol 2020;55:2213–24.

94. Kanne JP, Little BP, Chung JH, et al. Essentials for radiologists on COVID-19: an update-radiology scientific expert panel. Radiology 2020;296(2):E113–4.

95. Garazzino S, Montagnani C, Dona D, et al. Multicentre Italian study of SARS-CoV-2 infection in children and adolescents, preliminary data as at 10 April 2020. Euro Surveill 2020;25(18):2000600.

96. Chiotos K, Bassiri H, Behrens EM, et al. Multi-system inflammatory syndrome in children during the coronavirus 2019 pandemic: a case series. J Pediatr Infect Dis Soc 2020;9:393–8.

97. Hameed S, Elbaaly H, Reid CEL, et al. Spectrum of Imaging Findings on Chest Radiographs, US, CT, and MRI Images in Multisystem Inflammatory Syndrome in Children Associated with COVID-19. Radiology 2020;298(1):E1–10. https://doi.org/10.1148/radiol.2020202543.

98. Marks MJ, Haney PJ, McDermott MP, et al. Thoracic diseases in children with AIDS. Radiographics 1996;16:139–1362.

99. Maartens G, Celum C, Lewin SR. HIV infection: epidemiology, pathogenesis, treatment and prevention. Lancet 2014;384:258–71.

100. Holland DV, Guillerman RP, Brody AS. Thoracic manifestations of systemic diseases. In: Garcia-Peña P, Guillerman RP, editors. Pediatric chest imaging. 3rd edition. Springer-Verlag Berlin Heidelberg; 2014. p. 395–429.

101. Pitcher RD, Lombard C, Cotton MF, et al. Clinical and immunological correlates of chest X-ray abnormalities in HIV-infected South African children with limited access to anti-retroviral therapy. Pediatr Pulmonol 2014;49:581–8.

102. Theron S, Andronikou S, George R, et al. Non-infective pulmonary disease in HIV-positive children. Pediatr Radiol 2009;39:555–64.

103. Oldham SA, Castillo M, Jacobson FL, et al. HIV-associated lymphocytic interstitial pneumonia: Radiologic manifestations and pathologic correlation. Radiology 1989;170:83–7.

104. Mahomed N, van Ginneken B, Philipsen RHHM, et al. Computer-aided diagnosis for World Health Organization-defined chest radiograph primary-endpoint pneumonia in children. Pediatr Radiol 2020;50:482–91.

105. Kilborn T, Chu WCW, Das KM, et al. Current updates on HIV-related pulmonary disease in children: what do radiologists and clinicians need to know? S Afr J Rad 2015;19:928–33.

106. Jeanes AC, Owens CM. Chest imaging in the immunocompromised child. Pediatr Respir Rev 2002;3:59–69.

107. Graham SM. Impact of HIV on childhood respiratory illness: Differences between developing and developed countries. Pediatr Pulmonol 2003;36:462–8.

108. Zar HJ. Chronic lung disease in human immunodeficiency virus (HIV) infected children. Pediatr Pulmonol 2008;43:1–10.

109. George R, Andronikou S, Theron S, et al. Pulmonary infections in HIV-positive children. Pediatr Radiol 2009;39:545–54.

110. Dufour V, Wislez M, Burgot E, et al. Improvement of symptomatic human immunodeficiency virus-related lymphoid interstitial pneumonia in patients receiving highly active antiretroviral therapy. Clin Infec Dis 2003;36:e127–30.

111. Becciolini V, Gudinchet F, Cheseaux JJ, et al. Lymphocytic interstitial pneumonia in children with AIDS: high-resolution CT findings. Eur Radiol 2001;11:1015–20.

112. Rigsby CK, Strife JL, Johnson ND, et al. Is the frontal radiograph alone sufficient to evaluate for pneumonia in children? Pediatr Radiol 2004;34:379–83.

113. Zampoli M, Kilborn T, Eley B. Tuberculosis during early antiretroviral-induced immune reconstitution in HIV-infected children. Int J Tuberc Lung Dis 2007;11:417–23.

114. Andronikou S, Goussard P, Sorantin E. Computed tomography in children with community-acquired pneumonia. Pediatr Radiol 2017;47:1431–40.

115. Guo W, Wang J, Sheng M, et al. Radiological findings in 210 paediatric patients with viral pneumonia: a retrospective case study. Br J Radiol 2012;85:1385–9.

116. Swingler GH. Radiologic differentiation between bacterial and viral lower respiratory infection in children: a systemic literature review. Clin Pediatr 2000;39:627–33.

117. Don M, Valent F, Korppi M, et al. Differentiation of bacterial and viral community-acquired pneumonia in children. Pediatr Int 2009;51:91–6.

118. Wahlgren H, Mortensson W, Eriksson, et al. Radiographic patterns and viral studies in childhood pneumonia at various ages. Pediatir Radiol 1995;25:627–30.

119. Reittner P, Ward S, Heyneman L, et al. Pneumonia: high-resolution CT findings in 114 patients. Eur Radiol 2003;13:515–21.

120. Lucaya J, Coma A. High-resolution CT of the lung in children: technique, indications, anatomy, and features of lung disease. In: Garcia-Peña P, Guillerman RP, editors. Pediatric chest imaging. 3rd edition. Berlin Heidelberg: Springer-Verlag; 2014. p. 111–34.

121. le Pointe HD. High-resolution CT of the lung in children: clinical applications. In: Garcia-Peña P, Guillerman RP, editors. Pediatric chest imaging. 3rd edition. Berlin Heidelberg: Springer-Verlag; 2014. p. 135–55.

122. Collingsworth CL. Thoracic disorders in the immunocompromised. Radiol Clin North Am 2005;43:435–47.

123. Mahomed N, Reubenson G. Immune Reconstitution Inflammatory Syndrome in children. S Afr J Rad 2017;21(2):a1257.

124. Li YN, Liu L, Qiao HM, et al. Post-infectious bronchiolitis obliterans in children: a review of 42 cases. BMC Pediatr 2014;14:238.

125. Kim J, Kim MJ, So IS, et al. Quantitative CT and pulmonary function in children with post-infectious bronchiolitis obliterans. PLoS One 2019;14(4):e0214647.

126. Chang AB, Masel JP, Masters B. Post-infectious bronchiolitis obliterans: clinical, radiological and pulmonary function sequelae. Pediatr Radiol 1998;28:23–9.

127. Fischer GB, Sarria EE, Mattiello R, et al. Post-infectious bronchiolitis obliterans in children. Paediatr Respir Rev 2010;11:233–9.

128. Yikilmaz A, Güleç M, Tuna IS, et al. Swyer-James syndrome with pulmonary vein hypoplasia detected by multislice CT. Eur J Radiol Extra 2005;56:79–81.

129. Garcia-Peña P, Lucaya J. HRCT in children: technique and indications. Eur Radiol 2004;14:L13–30.

130. Boyd K. Back to the basics: community-acquired pneumonia in children. Pediatr Ann 2017;46(7):e257–61.

131. Yun KW, Wallihan R, Juergensen A, et al. Community-acquired pneumonia in children: myths and facts. Am J Perinatol 2019;36(S02):S54–7.

132. Gavrieli H, Dagan R, Givon-Lavi N, et al. Unique features of hospitalized children with alveolar pneumonia suggest frequent viral-bacterial co-infections. Am Fam Physician 2004;70:899–908.

133. Sandora TJ, Harper MB. Pneumonia in hospitalized children. Pediatr Clin North Am 2005;52:1059–81.

134. McIntosh K. Community-acquired pneumonia in children. N Engl J Med 2002;346:429–37.

135. Bénet T, Sánchez Picot V, Messaoudi M, et al. Microorganisms associated with pneumonia in children <5 years of age in developing and emerging countries: the GABRIEL pneumonia multicenter, prospective, case-control study. Clin Infect Dis 2017;65:604–12.

136. Peck KR, Kim TJ, Lee MA, et al. Pneumonia in immunocompromised patients: updates in clinical and imaging features. Precision Future Med 2018;2:95–108.

137. Donnelly LF. Imaging in immunocompetent children who have Pneumonia. Radiol Clin N Am 2005,43.253–65.

138. Ostapchuk M, Roberts DM, Haddy R. Community-acquired pneumonia in infants and children. Am Fam Physician 2004;70:899–908.

139. Reynolds JH, McDonald G, Alton H, et al. Pneumonia in the immunocompetent patient. Br J Radiol 2010;83:998–1009.

140. Reynolds JH, Banerjee AK. Imaging pneumonia in immunocompetent and immunocompromised individuals. Curr Opin Pulm Med 2012;18:194–201.

141. Nascimento-Carvalho CM, Araújo-Neto CA, Ruuskanen O. Association between bacterial infection and radiologically confirmed pneumonia among children. Pediatr Infect Dis J 2015;34:490–3.

142. Ben Shimol S, Dagan R, Givon-Lavi N, et al. Evaluation of the World Health Organization criteria for chest radiographs for pneumonia diagnosis in children. Eur J Pediatr 2012;171:369–74.

143. Cherian T, Mulholland EK, Carlin JB, et al. Standardized interpretation of paediatric chest radiographs for the diagnosis of pneumonia in epidemiological studies. Bull World Health Organ 2005;83:353–9.

144. Kim YW, Donnelly LF. Round pneumonia: imaging findings in a large series of children. Pediatr Radiol 2007;37:1235–40.

145. Restrepo R, Palani R, Matapathi UM, et al. Imaging of round pneumonia and mimics in children. Pediatr Radiol 2010;40:1931–40.

146. Zar HJ, Andronikou S, Nicol MP. Advances in the diagnosis of pneumonia in children. BMJ 2017;358:j2739.

147. Tracy MC, Mathew R. Complicated pneumonia: current concepts and state of the art. Curr Opin Pediatr 2018;30:384–92.

148. Ahmed B, Ageeli M, Abdali H, et al. Mycotic aneurysms of pulmonary artery in a young girl with sickle cell disease: a case report. Curr Pediatr Res 2019;23:17–20.

149. Goel A, Bamford L, Hanslo D, et al. Primary staphylococcal pneumonia in young children: a review of 100 cases. J Trop Pediatr 1999;45:233–6.

150. Highman JH. Staphylococcal pneumonia and empyema in childhood. Am J Roentgenol Radium Ther Nucl Med 1969;106:103–8.

151. Sodhi KS, Khandelwal N, Saxena AK, et al. Rapid lung MRI in children with pulmonary infections: time to change our diagnostic algorithms. J Magn Reson Imaging 2016;43:1196–206.

152. Shim JY. Current perspectives on atypical pneumonia in children. Clin Exp Pediatr 2020;63(12):469–76.

153. Hammerschlag MR. Pneumonia due to Chlamydia pneumoniae in children: epidemiology, diagnosis, and treatment. Pediatr Pulmonol 2003;36:384–90.

154. Søndergaard MJ, Friis MB, Hansen DS, et al. Clinical manifestations in infants and children with Mycoplasma pneumoniae infection. PLoS One 2018;13:e0195288.

155. Krafft C, Christy C. Mycoplasma pneumonia in children and adolescents. Pediatr Rev 2020;41:12–9.

156. John SD, Ramanathan J, Swischuk LE. Spectrum of clinical and radiographic findings in pediatric mycoplasma pneumonia. Radiographics 2001;21:121–31.

157. Moscatelli A, Buratti S, Castagnola E, et al. Severe neonatal legionella pneumonia: full recovery after extracorporeal life support. Pediatrics 2015;136:e1043–6.

158. Greenberg D, Chiou CC, Famigilleti R, et al. Problem pathogens: paediatric legionellosis—implications for improved diagnosis. Lancet Infect Dis 2006;6:529–35.

159. Ma YJ, Wang SM, Cho YH, et al. Clinical and epidemiological characteristics in children with community-acquired mycoplasma pneumonia in Taiwan: a nationwide surveillance. J Microbiol Immunol Infect 2015;48:632–8.

160. Hsieh SC, Kuo YT, Chern MS, et al. Mycoplasma pneumonia: clinical and radiographic features in 39 children. Pediatr Int 2007;49:363–7.

161. Reittner P, Müller NL, Heyneman L, et al. Mycoplasma pneumoniae pneumonia: radiographic and high-resolution CT features in 28 patients. AJR Am J Roentgenol 2000;174:37–41.

162. Radkowski MA, Kranzler JK, Beem MO, et al. Chlamydia pneumonia in infants: radiography in 125 cases. AJR Am J Roentgenol 1981;137:703–6.

163. Cho YJ, Han MS, Kim WS, et al. Correlation between chest radiographic findings and clinical features in hospitalized children with Mycoplasma pneumoniae pneumonia. PLoS One 2019;14: e0219463.

164. Zhai YY, Wu SZ, Yang Y, et al. An analysis of 20 clinical cases of refractory mycoplasma pneumonia in children. Ann Palliat Med 2020;9:2592–9.

165. Koinuma G, Shinjoh M, Kageyama T, et al. Round pneumonia due to Chlamydia pneumoniae in a child. Radiol Case Rep 2019;14:436–8.

166. Esposito S, Blasi F, Bellini F, et al. Mycoplasma pneumoniae and Chlamydia pneumoniae infections in children with pneumonia. Mowgli Study Group. Eur Respir J 2001;17:241–5.

167. Quagliano PV, Das Narla L. Legionella pneumonia causing multiple cavitating pulmonary nodules in a 7-month-old infant. AJR Am J Roentgenol 1993; 161:367–8.

168. Liu J, He R, Wu R, et al. Mycoplasma pneumoniae pneumonia associated thrombosis at Beijing Children's hospital. BMC Infect Dis 2020;20:51.

169. Global tuberculosis report 2019. Geneva: World Health Organization; 2019. Licence: CC BY-NC-SA 3.0 IGO. Available at: https://tbsouthafrica.org.za/resources/who-global-tuberculosis-report-2019.

170. Concepcion ND, Laya BF, Andronikou S, et al. Standardized radiographic interpretation of thoracic tuberculosis in children. Pediatr Radiol 2017;47:1237–48.

171. Van Dyck J, Vanhoenacker FM, Van den Brande P, et al. Imaging of pulmonary tuberculosis. Eur Radiol 2003;13:1771–85.

172. Nelson LJ, Wells CD. Global epidemiology of childhood TB. Int J Tuberc Lung Dis 2004;8(5):536–647.

173. Wang XW, Pappoe F, Huang Y, et al. Xpert MTB/RIF assay for pulmonary tuberculosis and rifampicin resistance in children: a meta-analysis. Clin Lab 2015;61:1775–85.

174. Ardizzoni E, Fajardo E, Saranchuk P, et al. Implementing the Xpert1MTB/RIF diagnostic test for tuberculosis and rifampicin resistance: outcomes and lessons learned in 18 countries. PLoS One 2015;10:e0144656.

175. Nacgiappan AC, Rahbar K, Shi X, et al. Pulmonary tuberculosis: role of Radiology in diagnosis and management. Radiographics 2017;37:52–72.

176. Naidoo J, Mahomed N, Moodley H. A systemic review of tuberculosis with HIV co-infection in children. Mini-symposium: Imaging of Childhood Tuberculosis. Paediatr Radiol 2017;47:1269–76.

177. Woodring JH, Vandiviere HM, Fried AM, et al. Update: the radiographic features of pulmonary tuberculosis. AJR Am J Roentgenol 1986;146(3):497–506.

178. Perez-Velez CM, Marais BJ. Tuberculosis in children. Nengl J Med 2012;367:348–61.

179. Murray JF, Mills J. Pulmonary infectious complications of human immunodeficiency virus infection. Part I. Am Rev Respir Dis 1990;141:1356–72.

180. Katragkou A, Fisher BT, Groll AH, et al. Diagnostic imaging and invasive fungal diseases in children. J Pediatr Infect Dis Soc 2017;6(S1):S22–31.

181. Steinbach WJ. Epidemiology of invasive fungal infections in neonates and children. Clin Microbiol Infect 2010;16:1321–7.

182. Liszewski MC, Laya BF, Zucker EJ, et al. Section 1: lung. In: Lee EY, editor. Pediatric thoracic imaging. Philadelphia, PA: Wolters Kluwer; 2019.

183. Aquino SL, Kee ST, Warnock ML, et al. Pulmonary aspergillosis: imaging findings with pathologic correlation. AJR Am J Roentgenol 1994;163:811–5.

184. Tragiannidis A, Roilides E, Walsh TJ, et al. Invasive aspergillosis in children with acquired immunodeficiencies. Clin Infect Dis 2012;54:258–67.

185. Laya BF. Chapter 13: Infections. In: Kim IO, editor. Radiology illustrated: pediatric radiology. Springer, Verlag Berlin Heidelberg; 2014.

186. Hatziagorou E, Walsh TJ, Tsanakas JN, et al. Aspergillus and the paediatric lung. Paediatr Respir Rev 2009;10:178–85.

187. Houston S. Histoplasmosis and pulmonary involvement in the tropics. Thorax 1994;49:598–601.

188. Fischer GB, Mocelin H, Severo CB, et al. Histoplasmosis in children. Paediatr Respir Rev 2009;10(4):172–7.

189. Wheat LJ, Conces D, Allen SD, et al. Pulmonary histoplasmosis syndromes: recognition, diagnosis, and management. Semin Respir Crit Care Med 2004;25(2):129–214.

190. Jude CM, Nayak NB, Patel MK, et al. Pulmonary coccidioidomycosis: pictorial review of chest radiographic and CT findings. Radiographics 2014; 34(4):912–25.

191. McCarty JM, Demetral LC, Dabrawski L, et al. Pediatric coccidioidomycosis in central California: a retrospective case series. Clin Infect Dis 2013; 56(11):1579–85.

192. Orlowski HL, McWilliams S, Mellnick VM, et al. Imaging spectrum of invasive fungal and fungal-like infections. Radiographics 2017;37(4):1119–34.

193. Kassner EG, Kauffman SL, Yoon JJ, et al. Pulmonary candidiasis in infants: clinical, radiologic, and pathologic features. AJR Am J Roentgenol 1981;137:707–16.

Pediatric Congenital Lung Malformations
Imaging Guidelines and Recommendations

Patrick Tivnan, MD[a],*, Abbey J. Winant, MD[b], Monica Epelman, MD[c],
Edward Y. Lee, MD, MPH[b]

KEYWORDS

- Congenital lung malformations • Children • Imaging evaluation • Radiography • Ultrasound
- Computed tomography • MR imaging • Imaging guidelines

KEY POINTS

- Pediatric congenital lung malformations (CLMs) comprise a spectrum of developmental anomalies of the lung parenchyma, airways, and vasculature. CLMs are increasingly diagnosed prenatally, but remain best characterized by postnatal cross-sectional imaging.
- Management of CLMs, including imaging, in infants and young children depends on associated symptoms and institutional standards.
- Chest CT angiography (CTA) performed not before 4 weeks of age is usually the most appropriate initial postnatal imaging modality for assessing prenatally diagnosed or clinically suspected CLMs in asymptomatic infants and children.
- Chest magnetic resonance (MR) imaging / magnetic resonance angiography (MRA) may be considered as a complementary, problem-solving, or follow-up imaging modality for evaluation of CLMs.

INTRODUCTION

Congenital lung malformations (CLMs) comprise a spectrum of developmental anomalies including malformations of the lung parenchyma, airways, and vasculature.[1] Although the historical incidence of CLMs is 1 in 10,000 to 35,000,[2,3] CLMs are being increasingly detected, especially prenatally, with an apparently increasing incidence, recently as frequent as 4 in 10,000 births.[4] This apparent increase in the incidence of CLMs is at least partially caused by recent improvements in and increased use of fetal ultrasound and fetal magnetic resonance (MR) imaging. Over the past three decades, this increased incidence and detec-tion of CLMs has aided the understanding of the imaging features of various types of CLMs, their potential etiologies, and the natural history of these anomalies.[5–7]

Diagnostic imaging evaluation plays a pivotal role in the initial diagnosis, preoperative planning, and follow-up evaluation of CLMs in the pediatric population. Unfortunately, there is currently a paucity of practical imaging guidelines and recommendations for the imaging assessment of CLMs in infants and children. Therefore, the purpose of this article is to review the current imaging modalities and techniques for evaluating CLMs postnatally, and provide up-to-date imaging guidelines and recommendations for practicing radiologists and clinicians managing pediatric patients with CLMs.

EVIDENCE-BASED IMAGING ALGORITHM

Table 1 provides a brief summary of the findings of selected previously published articles, comparing the currently available imaging modalities for evaluating CLMs postnatally.

[a] Department of Radiology, Boston Medical Center, One Boston Medical Center Place, Boston, MA 02118, USA;
[b] Department of Radiology, Boston Children's Hospital, Harvard Medical School, 300 Longwood Avenue, Boston, MA 02115, USA; [c] Department of Radiology, Nemours Children's Health System/Nemours Children's Hospital, 6535 Nemours Parkway, Orlando, FL 32827, USA
* Corresponding author.
E-mail address: Patrick.Tivnan@bmc.org

Radiol Clin N Am 60 (2022) 41–54
https://doi.org/10.1016/j.rcl.2021.08.002

Table 1
Comparison of currently available postnatal imaging modalities for detecting congenital lung malformations in infants and children

Imaging Modality	Sensitivity	Specificity	Pathology Concordance	Advantages	Disadvantages	References
Radiography	50%–61%	N/A	N/A	Wide availability Low cost	Low sensitivity Limited characterization Radiation (low)	16,17
Ultrasound	N/A	N/A	N/A	Wide availability Less costly No radiation	Operator dependent	76-79
Chest CTA with contrast	85%–100%	75%–100%	83.5%	Best spatial resolution Best lung parenchyma evaluation Best feeding vessel evaluation Wide availability	Radiation Limited in patients with suboptimal renal function and allergy to contrast More expensive than radiography and ultrasound Possible small risk from iodinated contrast use	8,12,15,78,79
Chest MR imaging without contrast	57%	100%	96%	Best soft tissue characterization No radiation	Longer examination often requiring sedation Susceptibility artifact from air cant limit evaluation of lung parenchyma Costly	10,14,15
Chest MR imaging/MR angiography with contrast			96%	Best soft tissue characterization No radiation Able to delineate feeding vessel	Longer examination requiring sedation Susceptibility artifact from air limits evaluation of lung parenchyma Costly Possible small risks from gadolinium use	13

Abbreviations: CTA, computed tomography angiography; N/A, nonapplicable.

In the prenatal period, fetal ultrasound and fetal MR imaging have high sensitivity for detecting CLMs; however, imaging characterization of CLMs with fetal ultrasound and fetal MR imaging is often incomplete, especially for solid lung parenchymal CLMs. For example, Mon and colleagues[8] found that prenatal ultrasound had an accuracy of 72% and fetal MR imaging had slightly higher accuracy of 80% for correctly identifying an aberrant systemic vessel in a series of 103 parenchymal CLMs that were found be 25% pulmonary sequestration, 44% congenital pulmonary airway malformation (CPAM), and 21% CPAM/sequestration hybrid lesions at the time of surgical excision. In this same study, postnatal chest computed tomography angiography (CTA) had a superior accuracy of 90% for identifying the systemic feeding vessel in these CLMs. The presence of a systemic feeding vessel is an important diagnostic feature for distinguishing CLMs, especially when differentiating CPAM from pulmonary sequestration. In this study, approximately 25% of CLMs diagnosed by prenatal ultrasound were found to have a different pathology at the time of surgical excision, likely at least partially caused by missing the systemic feeding vessel.[8] Of note, the opposite finding was noted by Beydon and colleagues[9] who found that fetal ultrasound had higher systemic vessel detection than fetal MR imaging, although this was a smaller study (n = 23). Lastly, prenatal imaging has reduced sensitivity for lesions whose predominant imaging features relate to aeration of the lung, such as congenital lobar overinflation (CLO). Collectively, these studies and others continue to demonstrate that prenatal ultrasound and fetal MR imaging can provide important information early, but have reduced sensitivity and specificity for accurately diagnosing CLMs compared with postnatal chest CTA.[8–11]

Although the use of chest CTA for assessing CLMs has been investigated more thoroughly, MR imaging of the chest is now being evaluated as a possible postnatal imaging alternative to chest CTA. Historically, MR imaging of the chest had a specific complementary role in assessing vascular CLMs, allowing for assessment of cardiac blood flow and shunt vascularity. More recently, MR imaging of the chest has been used to assess parenchymal CLMs. For example, in a series of 23 cases, Zirpoli and colleagues[12] compared chest MR imaging without contrast with chest CTA and found comparable sensitivity and specificity between the two modalities except in regards to aberrant vessel detection. In addition, Kellenberger and colleagues[13] recently found that postnatal chest MR imaging with contrast correctly diagnosed 96% of abnormalities (n = 46), including aberrant vessel detection, when compared with surgical pathology or other gold standard imaging modalities, such as echocardiogram and computed tomography (CT). Although direct comparison between postnatal CT and postnatal MR imaging was only available in 33% (n = 13) of these cases, 100% concordance was noted in these 13 cases. All of the CLMs in the study demonstrated reduced perfusion compared with normal lung parenchyma at peak pulmonary enhancement, a sensitive imaging feature on MR imaging that is not assessed by CTA.[13] Newman[14] recently described typical scenarios where MR imaging is being used in place of CTA for CLMs, including: (1) follow-up of a known CLM, defined previously either by prenatal MR imaging or prior CTA, if repeat radiation exposure is of concern; (2) to define a mass that might not initially be suspected to be a CLM if present in a less common location, such as paraspinal, mediastinal, or intra-abdominal; (3) as a supplemental imaging modality if there is incomplete characterization of the CLM by CTA, often in the case of complex lesions; and (4) incidentally noted CLMs on an MR imaging obtained for other reasons, such as cardiac or abdominal pathology.

Despite these early optimistic findings demonstrating the utility of chest MR imaging for postnatal CLM evaluation, CTA remains the first choice for characterizing CLM for several reasons. First, CTA is more readily available and a less expensive modality than MR imaging. Second, although sedation can sometimes be avoided in infants obtaining MR imaging (using feed and wrap protocol) and occasionally is needed for CTA, of the two examinations, CTA can more often be performed without sedation. Additionally, if sedation is to be used, it often is quicker and with lesser anesthetic depth for chest CTA than with chest MR imaging. A recently published study showed that sedation can often be avoided in the assessment of CLMs in infants and young children (≤6 years old) using the newer dual-source CT imaging without compromise of the diagnostic quality.[15] Avoiding sedation in young children is important because animal studies have indicated there is a possible small risk of neurotoxicity with the use of anesthetics in neonatal and young pediatric patients.[16] For this reason, the Food and Drug administration has placed warning labels on several sedative medications, such as propofol, ketamine, and lorazepam, stating that "exposure to these agents for lengthy periods of time or over multiple procedures may negatively affect brain development in children younger than 3 years."[17]

Third, the contrast agents used for both examinations have slightly different risks associated with them. Iodinated contrast agents are generally well tolerated with the main concern being a potential small risk of contrast-induced nephropathy, which has been previously reported to occur most commonly in a small percentage of adults with risk factors, such as underlying renal dysfunction, although this remains controversial. In the pediatric population, this association is even less well-delineated with a recent study by Gilligan and colleagues[18] finding no evidence of contrast-induced nephropathy in hospitalized pediatric patients with stable renal function (glomerular filtration rate->60). Another recent study by McGaha and colleagues[19] found no occurrence of contrast-induced nephropathy in injured pediatric patients undergoing CT scan for trauma assessment.

Gadolinium-based MR imaging contrast agents also have good safety profiles, with the main reported association being a small risk of nephrogenic systemic fibrosis, which most often occurs in the setting of renal dysfunction.[20] Although there are reported cases of nephrogenic systemic fibrosis in the pediatric population, the rate of nephrogenic systemic fibrosis has significantly decreased over the last decade with the use of better, lower risk gadolinium contrast agents and restriction of use with renal dysfunction.[20] An additional significant concern related to the use of gadolinium contrast agents is that several studies have indicated that use of these agents may result in gadolinium deposition in tissues, such as the brain, typically after several MR imaging studies with contrast.[21–23] No studies have been able to show any clinically significant outcome from this gadolinium deposition; however, long-term studies are needed to assess whether there are clinical effects of this deposition.

These advantages and disadvantages of iodinated and gadolinium-based contrast agents are important considerations that may factor into the decision to use CTA or MR imaging for the assessment of CLMs. Whatever imaging modality is selected, it is of outmost importance that a good-quality, angiographic study be obtained to adequately depict the presence of systemic feeding vessels.

CONGENITAL LUNG MALFORMATION IMAGING ALGORITHM

A summary of the postnatal imaging algorithm for the evaluation of CLMs is described in **Fig. 1**. Postnatal suspicion for a CLM may either arise secondary to a concern on prenatal imaging or from clinical symptoms, such as respiratory distress, tachypnea, cough, wheeze, or recurrent infections, either in an infant or child. Prenatal imaging alone is not sufficient for the evaluation and characterization of a CLM postnatally because of the limitations of prenatal imaging and the possible

evolution (and even regression) of CLMs during pregnancy and birth.[24–26] CLMs may re-gress and/or display different imaging characteristics on postnatal imaging after the physiologic changes of parturition. For example, postnatal inflation of the lungs significantly changes the imaging appearance of CLO. The optimal postnatal imaging algorithm for a CLM depends on careful consideration of three main aspects that interplay into the final patient management and clinical decision making: (1) institutional surgical standards, (2) imaging study types, and (3) symptom assessment.

Institutional Surgical Standards

Institutional surgical standards affect the postnatal imaging algorithm of pediatric patients with CLMs. Currently, most pediatric hospitals in the United States advocate cross-sectional imaging evaluation in symptomatic and asymptomatic infants and children with a suspected CLM based on prenatal imaging findings and/or postnatal symptoms. This preference for imaging symptomatic and asymptomatic children in the United States is because of a prevailing belief that asymptomatic CLMs can cause future symptoms, such as recurrent infections, and have a small reported risk of malignancy,[27] leading many American institutions to recommend surgical intervention, even in the case of currently asymptomatic CLMs. At other institutions, particularly in Europe, alternative imaging and management strategies exist for CLMs, with some recommending watchful waiting and only performing cross-sectional imaging in those children with a suspected CLM that develops symptoms.[6] At these institutions, surgical intervention is

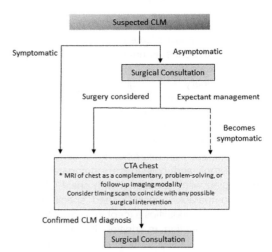

Fig. 1. Commonly used algorithm for postnatal work-up of congenital lung malformations.

only performed if the patient becomes symptomatic. Of note, asymptomatic CLMs are thought to become symptomatic in at least 30% of cases.[6] Consequently, at these institutions, cross-sectional imaging is not performed in asymptomatic infants and children who are suspected of having a CLM because it would not change management. Therefore, careful consideration of each institution's clinical standards toward CLM management is important for determining the postnatal imaging algorithm of pediatric patients with CLMs.

Types of Imaging Study

The second consideration in the imaging evaluation of a CLM is the type of imaging study. The most noninvasive and inexpensive screening modalities, radiography and ultrasound, are limited for the postnatal characterization of CLMs. Chest radiographs are often used as an initial imaging study; however, they lack sensitivity, specificity, and spatial resolution for the detection and characterization of CLMs.[28,29] Similarly, although ultrasound is used to characterize some CLMs and can demonstrate feeding vessels, it is challenging because air within the inflated lungs limits sonographic penetration and assessment.

In contrast, cross-sectional imaging modalities, specifically chest CTA and chest MR imaging, have high clinical utility in the postnatal assessment of CLMs. Both of these imaging modalities provide detailed anatomic information with substantial technical improvements in pediatric CT and MR imaging techniques over the past two decades. Chest CTA still remains the preferred imaging modality for evaluating CLMs, mainly because of its ability to completely evaluate lung parenchyma and identify associated subtle vascular abnormalities.[8,11,30] However, exposure to potentially harmful ionizing radiation and the need for sedation remains an important concern in infants and children. Fortunately, recent improvements in CT technologies have led to substantial reductions in radiation dose and faster scanning speeds, decreasing the need for sedation.[31–33]

Chest MR imaging remains an important, radiation-free imaging alternative to chest CTA. Similar to ultrasound, air within the lungs can cause substantial artifact and signal void on MR imaging, slightly decreasing its sensitivity for the detection of small CLMs within the aerated lungs. In addition, respiratory motion can also cause substantial motion artifact on chest MR imaging, further limiting evaluation. However, newer faster MR imaging sequences, such as steady-state acquisition and single-shot fast spin echo, can decrease motion artifact and also provide improved soft tissue characterization of CLMs.[13,34] If intravenous (IV) contrast is administered, chest MR imaging can also characterize the vasculature within CLMs. Furthermore, because parenchymal CLMs have been reported to have reduced enhancement compared with normal lung parenchyma, contrast sequestration at peak perfusion is useful for delineating CLMs.[13]

Symptom Assessment

Clinical symptoms also play an important role in determining the imaging approach for pediatric patients with a CLM. If severe respiratory distress is present perinatally, emergent postnatal cross-sectional imaging is typically performed to expedite diagnosis and aid in surgical planning. For pediatric patients with milder symptoms, such as cough, wheezing, or recurrent respiratory infections, with clinical concern for an underlying CLM, screening chest radiography may be performed initially, followed by cross-sectional imaging as close as possible to an appropriate age for surgical intervention. For example, in infants with mild symptoms, surgical intervention is typically preferred around 6 to 12 months after the development of active humoral immunity but before recurrent respiratory infections that could result in scarring or complicate surgical resection.[35]

PRACTICAL IMAGING APPROACH TO PEDIATRIC CONGENITAL LUNG MALFORMATIONS

The technical details of the currently available imaging modalities for evaluating CLMs in infants and children are beyond the scope of this article. The following section summarizes the utility of various imaging modalities for the detection of various CLMs, including characteristic postnatal imaging features.

Radiography

Radiography is often used as an initial screening imaging modality for detection of a CLM after birth. On chest radiographs, persistent opacities or lucencies, and recurrent infections in the same location (especially the left lower lobe for sequestration), raise suspicion for an underlying CLM. However, radiographs are insensitive for the detection of CLMs. Specifically, the lack of a visible abnormality on chest radiograph does not exclude a CLM. If there is strong clinical concern for a CLM, further evaluation with cross-sectional imaging is warranted for complete assessment.

Ultrasound

Ultrasound has limited utility for the postnatal detection of CLMs secondary to reduced penetration of sound waves through aerated lung (although it has been used in the past before improvements in other modalities). On ultrasound, a CLM may appear as a well-circumscribed focal lung abnormality with cystic, solid or mixed components, with or without associated abnormal vessels (best assessed with Doppler ultrasound imaging). Of note, a recent case report described the use of contrast-enhanced ultrasound to guide biopsy of a CPAM in an adult.[36] Use of contrast-enhanced ultrasound for this purpose in infants and children has yet to be fully evaluated.

Computed Tomography Angiography

With the highest spatial resolution and sensitivity for the postnatal detection of CLMs, chest CTA is the current gold standard for postnatal evaluation of CLMs. To maximize detection of abnormal vasculature often associated with CLMs, chest CTA technique is recommended, with the anatomic coverage extending from the lower neck to the mid-abdomen to fully capture the extent of any abnormal vasculature, which may arise or extend below the diaphragm. The need for sedation depends on patient age and ability to cooperate with breathing instructions; however, many chest CTA studies are able to be successfully completed within the first year of life without sedation. Our recent study, which directly compared the diagnostic quality of chest CTA without and with general anesthesia in appropriately screened infants and young children for the evaluation of congenital thoracic disorders using multidetector CT with turbo flash spiral mode and free-breathing technique, showed that only a small minority (3%) of chest CTA studies performed without general anesthesia had motion artifact severe enough to limit evaluation.[15] The results of this study support the use of chest CTA without general anesthesia (using turbo flash spiral mode and free-breathing technique) for detecting and evaluating CLMs.

In the authors' experience, in asymptomatic children, it is desirable not to image infants during the early neonatal period because delayed resorption of the expected fetal pulmonary fluid is challenging to distinguish from fluid-filled CPAM cysts. Furthermore, in cases of CLO, the expected hyperinflated lung distal to the abnormal bronchus may remain fluid-filled, not yet manifesting the characteristic hyperinflation.

Chest CTA post-processing techniques, such as multiplanar reformats and three-dimensional reconstructions of the airway and vasculature, are critical for the accurate characterization of CLMs. Lee and colleagues[37] showed that although axial multidetector CT images allow accurate diagnosis of CLM type, location, mass effect, and anomalous arteries of CLMs, supplemental multiplanar reformats and three-dimensional reconstructions of the vasculature add significant diagnostic value for the evaluations of CLMs with increased detection of anomalous vessels, a potentially important finding for surgical planning. Therefore, post-processing multiplanar (two-dimensional) reformats and three-dimensional reconstructions are routinely performed for evaluation of CLMs in the pediatric population.

MR Imaging

MR imaging is an attractive, alternative cross-sectional imaging modality, especially in light of newer faster sequences that allow improved detection of CLMs within the aerated lungs, such as steady-state acquisition and single-shot fast spin echo. MR imaging can often be performed without sedation during at least the first 6 months of life and in older children who can follow breathing instruction. For infants and young children between these two age groups, sedation may be necessary because of the length of a typical chest MR imaging study. Similar to CTA, chest MR imaging field of view typically extends from lower neck through mid-abdomen, with acquisitions performed in three planes, usually with IV contrast. Kellenberger and colleagues[13] recently found that chest MR imaging with contrast, including peak perfusion enhancement, was useful for deciphering the extent of CLMs. In addition, for CLMs with abnormal vasculature, MR imaging of the chest can be obtained while undergoing simultaneous cardiac MR imaging to assess for flow and shunting.

It has been shown that MR imaging has good sensitivity for accurately detecting soft tissue and fluid components within larger CLMs and is useful for surgical planning.[13,38] Typical MR imaging features of CLMs are described next and differ depending on the CLM type. However, Kellenberger and colleagues[13] described a useful imaging feature that all parenchymal CLMs demonstrated reduced enhancement at peak pulmonary perfusion after IV contrast administration.

SPECTRUM OF PEDIATRIC CONGENITAL LUNG MALFORMATIONS

Although this review focuses on imaging recommendations and guidelines for evaluation of CLMs, which does not substantially change depending on the suspected type of CLM (because standard

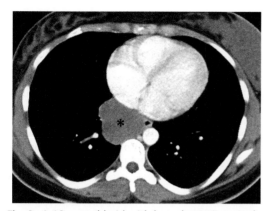

Fig. 2. A 16-year-old girl with bronchogenic cyst who presented with chest pain. Axial contrast-enhanced CT image shows a well-circumscribed and nonenhancing mediastinal cystic structure (*asterisk*) located posterior to heart. Hounsfield unit measurement was 9 consistent with water attenuation within the mass. Surgical pathology confirmed a bronchogenic cyst.

protocols should allow for diagnostic assessment of all CLM types), the following section briefly describes the salient imaging features of commonly encountered CLMs in children. In brief, for all of these CLMs, there are several imaging features that should be evaluated in all of these lesions for diagnosis and for surgical planning. These include the vascular supply and drainage of the CLM, the size of CLM, presence of aeration in the CLM (which typically occurs after 6–8 weeks of life), the presence of associated airway or bronchocele, and abnormal fissural anatomy (which plays an important role in surgical planning).[39]

Congenital Foregut Duplication Cyst

Congenital foregut duplication cysts comprise three main different types of malformations including bronchogenic, esophageal, and neurenteric duplication cysts (**Fig. 2**). During the first 4 weeks of gestation, the tracheal buds form from the ventral aspect of the primitive foregut.[40,41] Foregut duplication cysts are thought to derive from abnormal budding, either in this initial step or possibly later within subsequent development of the branches of the airway. In keeping with the hypothesis of abnormal budding, esophageal duplications cysts typically occur near or within the esophagus, and bronchogenic duplication cysts occur somewhere within or near the airway.[42] The esophagus is the second most common location for enteric duplication cysts after the ileum.[43] Foregut duplication cysts, specifically neurenteric cysts, may be associated with Klippel-Feil syndrome and hemivertebrae.[44,45] Affected pediatric

patients may present with dysphagia from mass effect on the esophagus and/or respiratory symptoms because of mass effect on adjacent airways.[46–50]

Large foregut duplication cysts may be visible on chest radiograph as a rounded mediastinal or lung opacity, although many are radiographically occult. On chest CTA, foregut duplication cysts appear as well-defined, low-attenuation, unilocular cystic mass, without internal enhancement or vascularity. Foregut duplication cysts are typically thin-walled with smooth or gently lobulated margins.[51] On MR imaging, foregut duplication cysts are well-circumscribed cystic structures that demonstrate low to intermediate T1 and high T2 signal, with only thin peripheral wall enhancement.[13] Foregut duplication cysts may become infected postnatally. In the setting of superinfection of a foregut duplication cyst, small internal foci of gas and/or the presence of surrounding inflammation, such as mediastinal fat stranding or thick peripheral rim-enhancement, is seen on contrast-enhanced CT or MR imaging.

Surgical resection is recommended for symptomatic foregut duplication cysts. Asymptomatic lesions are also often resected because of concern for possible future infection; however, management depends on institutional standards and parental preference.

Congenital Pulmonary Airway Malformation

CPAMs are the most common congenital lung anomaly, accounting for 30% to 40% of all CLMs (**Fig. 3**).[8,52] Reported to occur in up to 1 out of 7200 live births, CPAMs are cystic, solid, or mixed lesions that are postulated to result from early occlusion of the airway during development or abnormal bronchoalveolar development with hamartomatous proliferation of terminal respiratory units.[53–55] Children with CPAMs may present with respiratory symptoms, such as shortness of breath or recurrent pulmonary infections, depending on the size and location of the CPAM.

CPAMs have been divided into five subtypes using the updated Stocker classification system.[56] Type 0 CPAM is characterized as a large air-filled cystic structure, presumed to originate from the trachea or mainstem bronchi, but is considered incompatible with life.[57] Therefore, type 0 CPAM is usually seen on prenatal imaging studies. Type 1 CPAM typically presents with larger cysts (2–10 cm), whereas type 2 CPAM is composed of smaller cysts (<2 cm). Type 3 CPAM is composed of microcysts (<5 mm) with a solid appearance on imaging because microcysts are often too small to resolve on imaging studies. Type 4 is a rare

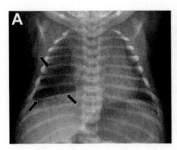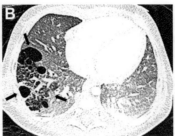

Fig. 3. A 3-month-old boy with congenital pulmonary airway malformation (CPAM) who presented with a prenatal diagnosis of a focal lung lesion. Surgical pathology confirmed the diagnosis of type 2 CPAM. (A) Frontal chest radiograph shows a multicystic lesion (*arrows*) in the right lower lobe. (B) Axial lung window CT image demonstrates a multicystic lesion with varying size of internal cystic components (*arrows*) in the right lower lobe.

subtype, characterized by large cysts thought to originate from the acinar structures of the lung.[57,58] Solid components, representing hamartomatous tissue, are found in any of the CPAM types, although are most commonly seen in type 3 CPAMs. Type 2 is the most common CPAM and has the strongest association with other congenital malformations, including renal agenesis, cardiovascular effects, diaphragmatic hernia, and esophageal atresia.[57] Of note, type 1 and type 4 CPAMs are considered radiographically indistinguishable from type I pleuropulmonary blas-toma.[59,60]

CPAMs may appear as a hyperlucent, air-filled mass on chest radiograph. Because the pores of Kohn allow air passage, these lesions can increase in size over time with subsequent air trapping. On CT, CPAMs appear as a well-defined cystic lung mass, containing multiple air-filled cysts, with cyst size depending on the subtype. On postnatal MR imaging, the fluid within the cystic spaces typically is replaced by air and appears as regions of susceptibility artifact.

CPAMs may frequently occur as part of a hybrid lesion, containing components of CPAM and a second CLM, most commonly bronchopulmonary sequestration. Hybrid CLMs are surprisingly common, accounting for approximately 20% to 30% of all CLMs.[8,11] On imaging, hybrid CPAM-sequestration lesions often demonstrate the dysplastic pulmonary tissue of the sequestration. In addition, a feeding systemic artery, a characteristic finding of a bronchopulmonary sequestration, is often present in hybrid CPAM-sequestration CLMs.[13] On MR imaging, these solid components can demonstrate enhancement but show reduced enhancement compared with normal lung parenchyma at peak pulmonary enhancement.[13]

Management of CPAMs depends largely on its size and associated mass effect. Symptomatic CPAMs are usually surgically resected. Additionally asymptomatic type 1 CPAM are often resected because of risk of superinfection and a small possible risk of malignancy[61,62] Treatment of asymptomatic CPAMs varies slightly with surgical institutional standards. One approach that some institutions follow is to check for a germline DICER1 mutation in any child with an asymptomatic cystic pulmonary malformation, because a germline DICER1 mutation indicates that cystic lesions are more likely to represent pleuropulmonary blastoma.[60] With this management algorithm, if the DICER1 mutation is not present, the patient is asymptomatic, and the cystic lesion was present on prenatal imaging, then monitoring rather than immediate resection is more likely to be considered. If symptomatic, not detected on prenatal imaging, or multilobar in location, these features are more likely to indicate pleuropulmonary blastoma for which resection is recommended.

Congenital Lobar Overinflation

CLO, previously known as congenital lobar emphysema, is a congenital pulmonary malformation that leads to hyperinflation of a segment or lobe that contains otherwise histologically normal lung parenchyma (**Fig. 4**). Reported to have a prevalence of 1 in 20 to 30,000 live births,[63] CLO has a predilection to affect males (3:1).[64] Although the exact cause is unknown, there are several different hypotheses, including internal or external compression of a lobar airway and incomplete bronchial cartilage ring formation, leading to collapse of the airway and air trapping during expiration.[64] However, 50% of cases are deemed idiopathic with the bronchus appearing normal on histopathology at the time of resection.[64] CLO has been associated with congenital heart disease (up to 24% of cases).[65] Affected pediatric patients typically present with shortness of breath or recurrent infections.

On imaging, CLO is characterized by pronounced hyperinflation of a lobe or segment. The left upper lobe is the most common location affected by CLO (43%), followed by the right middle (32%), and right upper lobes (21%).[64] Of note,

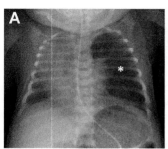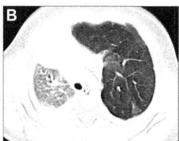

Fig. 4. A 3-day-old girl with congenital lobar overinflation (CLO) who presented with progressively worsening respiratory distress. Surgical pathology confirmed the diagnosis of left upper lobe CLO. (*A*) Frontal chest radiograph shows a hyperlucent left upper lobe (*asterisk*) with mild mediastinal shift toward contralateral side. Also seen are a left subclavian central venous line and a nasogastric tube. (*B*) Axial lung window CT image demonstrates hyperinflated left upper lobe with underlying attenuation of vessels and bronchi.

the lower lobes are rarely affected (less than 5% of CLO cases). Postnatally, CLO may be visible on chest radiograph as a region of hyperlucent, hyperinflated lung, often with mass effect on adjacent lobes and structures, including mediastinal shift and compressive atelectasis. The lobar nature of this lesion is more easily identified by CT, which can demonstrate hyperexpansion of a segment or lobe, with associated air-trapping, in otherwise normal-appearing lung parenchyma. Of note, there are no associated solid or cystic components. Mass effect, including mediastinal shift and compressive atelectasis in adjacent lung, is frequently present.

Symptomatic CLO is typically resected.

Bronchial Atresia

Bronchial atresia (BA) is a CLM that results from focal obliteration of a proximal segment of a bronchus and subsequent hyperinflation of the lung distal to this obliterated bronchus (**Fig. 5**). Although any lung segment can be affected, the left upper lobe apicoposterior segment is most frequently

affected.[66] At least two theories regarding the pathophysiology of BA exist: a disruption in the cells that develop into a segmental bronchus during development; and possible vascular injury to an already-formed bronchus during development.[66] Both would result in an obliterated bronchus (bronchocele or mucocele) and distal hyperinflation with or without mucoid proliferation. Up to two-thirds of children with BA are asymptomatic.[66] Symptomatic pediatric patients may present with shortness of breath or recurrent pulmonary infections.

BA may be visible on chest radiograph as a focal region of hyperlucent, hyperexpanded lung with an associated linear density (mucocele). Better characterized on CT, BA appears as a central branching tubular opacity, often extending out from the hilum, in keeping with mucocele, surrounded by distal hyperinflated segmental or lobar lung parenchyma. MR imaging typically shows a similar T2 hyperintense tubular lesion, extending from the hilum toward the peripheral lung, with hyperinflation of the distal lung. No internal vascularity or enhancing solid components are typically seen.

Treatment of BA includes lobectomy if symptomatic. If small and asymptomatic, expectant management may be appropriate, depending on institutional standards and patient preference.

Pulmonary Sequestration

Bronchopulmonary sequestration is a congenital malformation defined as a segment or lobe of a dysplastic lung with no connection to the tracheobronchial system that receives its blood supply from a feeding systemic artery, typically arising from the thoracic or abdominal aorta, instead of the pulmonary artery (**Figs. 6** and **7**).

Bronchopulmonary sequestrations are traditionally classified into two subtypes: intralobar and extralobar. Intralobar sequestrations are not encased by visceral pleura and typically drain via the pulmonary veins. Most intralobar sequestrations are found in the posterior basal segment of the left lobe,[67] although right-sided lesions have

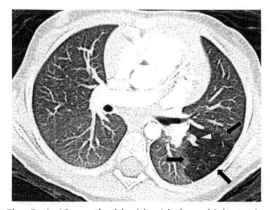

Fig. 5. A 16-month-old girl with bronchial atresia, seen on chest radiograph obtained for evaluation of pneumonia. Axial lung window CT image shows a nodular opacity (*arrowhead*) reflecting a bronchocele with surrounding hyperlucency (*arrows*) likely reflecting air trapping. Surgical pathology confirmed the diagnosis of bronchial atresia.

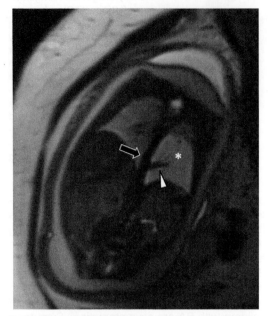

Fig. 6. A 37-week-gestational age male fetus with intralobar pulmonary sequestration. Coronal T2-weighted HASTE MR image obtained during fetal MR imaging shows an abnormal artery (*arrowhead*) arising from descending aorta (*arrow*) supplying blood flow to a large left lung mass (*asterisk*). Surgical pathology confirmed the diagnosis of left lower lobe pulmonary sequestration.

been described in association with scimitar syndrome.[68] In contrast, extralobar sequestrations have a separate visceral pleura and systemic venous drainage, typically into the inferior vena cava, azygous, or hemiazygos vein.[68,69] Extralobar sequestrations are typically found between the pleura and the adjacent diaphragm on the left, although

subdiaphragmatic sequestrations have been described.[70,71] Intralobar sequestration are more common, accounting for approximately 75% of sequestrations.[68] The prevailing theory is that in pulmonary sequestration, a supernumerary lung bud forms during development that derives its blood supply from the systemic system. If the bud forms before the development of the pleura, this results in an intralobar sequestration and an extralobar sequestration after pleural development.[68,72] Bronchopulmonary sequestration, especially extralobar sequestration, may be associated with multiple additional abnormalities, including scimitar syndrome, congenital heart disease, and congenital diaphragmatic hernia.[72]

The clinical presentation of bronchopulmonary sequestration depends on the type, with extralobar sequestration often presenting in infancy with respiratory distress and high output heart failure, and intralobar sequestration more commonly presenting in older children with recurrent respiratory infections, although these descriptions are more historical because sequestrations are nowadays often detected prenatally.

On chest radiographs, sequestration may present as a consolidative opacity. Chest CTA most clearly delineates the solid-appearing mass of dysplastic pulmonary tissue, with no definitive communication to the tracheobronchial tree, and the course of the abnormal systemic feeding artery. Chest CTA also assesses the venous drainage of the sequestration. MR imaging of the chest typically shows an enhancing, typically T2 bright mass with a systemic feeding vessel. Pulmonary sequestration may be seen as part of a hybrid lesion, most commonly in combination

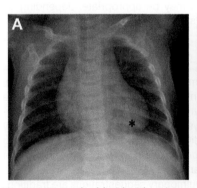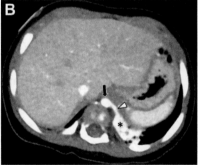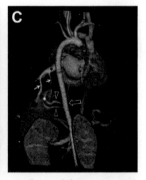

Fig. 7. A 5-month-old girl with pulmonary sequestration who presented with recurrent lower lobe pneumonia. Surgical pathology confirmed the diagnosis of intralobar pulmonary sequestration. (*A*) Frontal chest radiograph shows a subtle opacity (*asterisk*) in the left lower lobe. (*B*) Axial enhanced CT image demonstrates an enhancing pulmonary sequestration (*asterisk*) with systemic arterial supply (*arrowhead*) from descending aorta (*arrow*). (*C*) Three-dimensional volume-rendered CT image of the vascular structures shows a pulmonary sequestration (*white asterisk*) with two systemic feeding arteries (*arrowheads*) arising from the descending aorta (*thick arrow*) and two anomalous veins (*thin arrows*), draining into the left lower lobe pulmonary vein (*black asterisk*).

with CPAM. Consequently, assessment for findings of additional CLMs, such as cystic spaces, is important.

Treatment of bronchopulmonary sequestrations is usually surgical. Extralobar sequestration is often removed because of concern for left to right shunting. Intralobar sequestrations are also often resected because of concern for recurrent infection, which can complicate surgery.[73] Percutaneous closure of the systemic feeding artery, which has been reported to cause regression of the bronchopulmonary sequestration without significant complications, is continuing to be evaluated as a nonsurgical alternative.[74,75] Small asymptomatic bronchopulmonary sequestrations are not infrequently observed in adults and observation may be considered depending on institutional standards.

SUMMARY

CLMs in the pediatric population are increasingly detected early in life on fetal ultrasound and often further defined by fetal MR imaging. In children with suspected CLMs based on prenatal imaging or symptoms, CTA of the chest provides the best anatomic characterization of CLMs, including parenchymal findings and any associated vascular abnormalities. MR imaging is considered as a complementary or problem-solving imaging modality, although MR imaging has slightly reduced sensitivity and specificity compared with chest CTA for CLMs, and may be more useful for follow-up of known lesions. Optimal imaging characterization of CLMs is critical for timely and accurate diagnosis of CLMs and preoperative planning. Clear understanding of the imaging algorithm for CLMs and the characteristic imaging features of various CLMs is important for radiologists and clinicians treating children with suspected CLMs to expedite diagnosis and improve pediatric patient care.

CLINICS CARE POINTS

- The decision to perform cross-sectional imaging postnatally for a CLM is currently based on institutional surgical standards, types of imaging study, and symptom assessment.
- Chest CTA is the most appropriate imaging modality for assessing prenatally diagnosed or clinically suspected CLMs in infants and children.

- Chest MR imaging/MR angiography may be considered as a complementary, problem-solving, or follow-up imaging modality for evaluation of CLMs in the appropriate clinical circumstance.

DISCLOSURE

The authors have nothing to disclose.

REFERENCES

1. Biyyam DR, Chapman T, Ferguson MR, et al. Congenital lung abnormalities: embryologic features, prenatal diagnosis, and postnatal radiologic-pathologic correlation. Radiographics 2010;30(6):1721–38.
2. Laberge JM, Flageole H, Pugash D, et al. Outcome of the prenatally diagnosed congenital cystic adenomatoid lung malformation: a Canadian experience. Fetal Diagn Ther 2001;16(3):178–86.
3. Duncombe GJ, Dickinson JE, Kikiros CS. Prenatal diagnosis and management of congenital cystic adenomatoid malformation of the lung. Am J Obstet Gynecol 2002;187(4):950–4.
4. Stocker LJ, Wellesley DG, Stanton MP, et al. The increasing incidence of foetal echogenic congenital lung malformations: an observational study. Prenatal Diagn 2015;35(2):148–53.
5. Hammond PJ, Devdas JM, Ray B, et al. The outcome of expectant management of congenital cystic adenomatoid malformations (CCAM) of the lung. Eur J Pediatr Surg 2010;20(3):145–9.
6. Criss CN, Musili N, Matusko N, et al. Asymptomatic congenital lung malformations: is nonoperative management a viable alternative? J Pediatr Surg 2018;53(6):1092–7.
7. Thompson AJ, Sidebotham EL, Chetcuti PAJ, et al. Prenatally diagnosed congenital lung malformations: a long-term outcome study. Pediatr Pulmonol 2018;53(10):1442–6.
8. Mon RA, Johnson KN, Ladino-Torres M, et al. Diagnostic accuracy of imaging studies in congenital lung malformations. Arch Dis Child - Fetal Neonatal Ed 2019;104(4):F372–7.
9. Beydon N, Larroquet M, Coulomb A, et al. Comparison between US and MRI in the prenatal assessment of lung malformations. Pediatr Radiol 2013;43(6):685–96.
10. Zeidan S, Gorincour G, Potier A, et al. Congenital lung malformation: evaluation of prenatal and postnatal radiological findings. Respirology 2009;14(7):1005–11.
11. Alamo L, Reinberg O, Vial Y, et al. Comparison of foetal US and MRI in the characterisation of congenital lung anomalies. Eur J Radiol 2013;82(12):e860–6.

12. Zirpoli S, Munari AM, Primolevo A, et al. Agreement between magnetic resonance imaging and computed tomography in the postnatal evaluation of congenital lung malformations: a pilot study. Eur Radiol 2019;29(9):4544–54.

13. Kellenberger CJ, Amaxopoulou C, Moehrlen U, et al. Structural and perfusion magnetic resonance imaging of congenital lung malformations. Pediatr Radiol 2020;50(8):1083–94.

14. Newman B. Magnetic resonance imaging for congenital lung malformations. Pediatr Radiol 2021;1–11. https://doi.org/10.1007/s00247-021-05018-7.

15. Tivnan P, Winant AJ, Jonston P, et al. Thoracic CTA in infants and young children: image quality of dual-source CT (DSCT) with high-pitch spiral scan mode (turbo flash spiral mode) with or without general anesthesia with free-breathing. Pediatr Pulmonology 2021;56(8):2660–7.

16. Mellon RD, Simone AF, Rappaport BA. Use of anesthetic agents in neonates and young children. Anesth Analg 2007;104(3):509–20.

17. Research C for DE and. FDA Drug Safety Communication. FDA review results in new warnings about using general anesthetics and sedation drugs in young children and pregnant women. FDA. 2019. Available at: https://www.fda.gov/drugs/drug-safety-and-availability/fda-drug-safety-communication-fda-review-results-new-warnings-about-using-general-anesthetics-and. Accessed May 22, 2021.

18. Gilligan LA, Davenport MS, Trout AT, et al. Risk of acute kidney injury following contrast-enhanced CT in hospitalized pediatric patients: a propensity score analysis. Radiology 2020;294(3):548–56.

19. McGaha PK, Johnson J, Garwe T, et al. Computed tomography with intravenous contrast is not associated with development of acute kidney injury in severely injured pediatric patients. Am Surgeon 2019;85(1):1–5.

20. Ponrartana S, Moore MM, Chan SS, et al. Safety issues related to intravenous contrast agent use in magnetic resonance imaging. Pediatr Radiol 2021;51(5):736–47.

21. McDonald RJ, McDonald JS, Kallmes DF, et al. Gadolinium deposition in human brain tissues after contrast-enhanced MR imaging in adult patients without intracranial abnormalities. Radiology 2017;285(2):546–54.

22. Radbruch A, Richter H, Fingerhut S, et al. Gadolinium deposition in the brain in a large animal model: comparison of linear and macrocyclic gadolinium-based contrast agents. Invest Radiol 2019;54(9):531–6.

23. Zivadinov R, Bergsland N, Hagemeier J, et al. Cumulative gadodiamide administration leads to brain gadolinium deposition in early MS. Neurology 2019;93(6):e611–23.

24. Hadchouel A, Benachi A, Revillon Y, et al. Factors associated with partial and complete regression of fetal lung lesions. Ultrasound Obstet Gynecol 2011;38(1):88–93.

25. Bush A. Prenatal presentation and postnatal management of congenital thoracic malformations. Early Hum Dev 2009;85(11):679–84.

26. Illanes S, Hunter A, Evans M, et al. Prenatal diagnosis of echogenic lung: evolution and outcome. Ultrasound Obstet Gynecol 2005;26(2):145–9.

27. Casagrande A, Pederiva F. Association between congenital lung malformations and lung tumors in children and adults: a systematic review. J Thorac Oncol 2016;11(11):1837–45.

28. Calvert JK, Lakhoo K. Antenatally suspected congenital cystic adenomatoid malformation of the lung: postnatal investigation and timing of surgery. J Pediatr Surg 2007;42(2):411–4.

29. Parikh DH, Rasiah SV. Congenital lung lesions: postnatal management and outcome. Semin Pediatr Surg 2015;24(4):160–7.

30. Style CC, Cass DL, Verla MA, et al. Early vs late resection of asymptomatic congenital lung malformations. J Pediatr Surg 2019;54(1):70–4.

31. Agostini A, Mari A, Lanza C, et al. Trends in radiation dose and image quality for pediatric patients with a multidetector CT and a third-generation dual-source dual-energy CT. Radiol Med 2019;124(8):745–52.

32. Rompel O, Glöckler M, Janka R, et al. Third-generation dual-source 70-kVp chest CT angiography with advanced iterative reconstruction in young children: image quality and radiation dose reduction. Pediatr Radiol 2016;46(4):462–72.

33. Martine R-J, Santangelo T, Colas L, et al. Radiation dose levels in pediatric chest CT: experience in 499 children evaluated with dual-source single-energy CT. Pediatr Radiol 2017;47(2):161–8.

34. Gorkem SB, Coskun A, Yikilmaz A, et al. Evaluation of pediatric thoracic disorders: comparison of unenhanced fast-imaging-sequence 1.5-T MRI and contrast-enhanced MDCT. AJR Am J Roentgenol 2013;200(6):1352–7.

35. Saleh ME, Beshir H, Awad G, et al. Surgical outcomes for pediatric congenital lung malformation: 13 years' experience. Indian J Thorac Cardiovasc Surg 2020;36(6):1–11.

36. Xu W, Wen Q, Zha L, et al. Application of ultrasound in a congenital cystic adenomatoid malformation in an adult. Medicine (Baltimore) 2020;99(49):e23505.

37. Lee EY, Tracy DA, Mahmood SA, et al. Preoperative MDCT evaluation of congenital lung anomalies in children: comparison of axial, multiplanar, and 3D images. AJR Am J Roentgenol 2011;196(5):1040–6.

38. Martinez SC, Eghtesady P, Bhalla S, et al. Scimitar syndrome: multimodal imaging before and after repair. Tex Heart Inst J 2015;42(6):593–5.

39. Navallas M, Chiu P, Amirabadi A, et al. Preoperative delineation of pulmonary fissural anatomy at multi-

detector computed tomography in children with congenital pulmonary malformations and impact on surgical complications and postoperative course. Pediatr Radiol 2020;50(5):636–45.

40. Katz JM, Malik A, Basit H. Embryology, esophagus. In: StatPearls. StatPearls Publishing; 2021. Available at: http://www.ncbi.nlm.nih.gov/books/NBK542304/. Accessed April 11, 2021.

41. Staller K, Kuo B. Development, anatomy, and physiology of the esophagus. In: Shaker R, Belafsky P, Postma G, et al, editors. Principles of Deglutition. New York: Springer; 2013. doi:10.1007/978-1-4614-3794-9_19.

42. Liu R, Adler DG. Duplication cysts: diagnosis, management, and the role of endoscopic ultrasound. Endosc Ultrasound 2014;3(3):152–60.

43. Nebot CS, Salvador RL, Palacios EC, et al. Enteric duplication cysts in children: varied presentations, varied imaging findings. Insights Imaging 2018; 9(6):1097–106.

44. Pavone V, Praticò AD, Caltabiano R, et al. Cervical neurenteric cyst and Klippel-Feil syndrome: an abrupt onset of myelopathic signs in a young patient. J Pediatr Surg Case Rep 2017;24:12–6.

45. Oliveira RS de, Cinalli G, Roujeau T, et al. Neurenteric cysts in children: 16 consecutive cases and review of the literature. J Neurosurg Pediatr 2005; 103(6):512–23.

46. Sonthalia N, Jain SS, Surude RG, et al. Congenital esophageal duplication cyst: a rare cause of dysphagia in an adult. Gastroenterology Res 2016; 9(4–5):79–82.

47. Gupta B, Meher R, Raj A, et al. Duplication cyst of oesophagus: a case report. J Paediatr Child Health 2010;46(3):134–5.

48. Kaistha A, Levine J. An unusual cause of pediatric dysphagia: bronchogenic cyst. Glob Pediatr Health 2017;4. 2333794X16686492.

49. Nayan S, Nguyen LHP, Nguyen V-H, et al. Cervical esophageal duplication cyst: case report and review of the literature. J Pediatr Surg 2010;45(9):e1–5.

50. Moulton MStJ, Moir C, Matsumoto J, et al. Esophageal duplication cyst: a rare cause of biphasic stridor and feeding difficulty. Int J Pediatr Otorhinolaryngol 2005;69(8):1129–33.

51. McAdams HP, Kirejczyk WM, Rosado-de- Christenson ML, et al. Bronchogenic cyst: imaging features with clinical and histopathologic correlation. Radiology 2000;217(2):441–6.

52. Shanmugam G, MacArthur K, Pollock JC. Congenital lung malformations: antenatal and postnatal evaluation and management. Eur J Cardiothorac Surg 2005;27(1):45–52.

53. Lau CT, Kan A, Shek N, et al. Is congenital pulmonary airway malformation really a rare disease? Result of a prospective registry with universal antenatal screening program. Pediatr Surg Int 2017;33(1):105–8.

54. Ursini WP, Ponce CC. Congenital pulmonary airway malformation. Autops Case Rep 2018;8(2):e2018022.

55. Leblanc C, Baron M, Desselas E, et al. Congenital pulmonary airway malformations: state-of-the-art review for pediatrician's use. Eur J Pediatr 2017; 176(12):1559–71.

56. STOCKER JT. Congenital pulmonary airway malformation: a new name and expanded classification of congenital cystic adenomatoid malformation of the lung. Histopathology 2002;41(suppl2):424–31.

57. Mehta PA, Sharma G. Congenital pulmonary airway malformation. In: StatPearls. StatPearls Publishing; 2021. Available at: http://www.ncbi.nlm.nih.gov/books/NBK551664/. Accessed April 11, 2021.

58. Fowler DJ, Gould SJ. The pathology of congenital lung lesions. Semin Pediatr Surg 2015;24(4):176–82.

59. Haider F, Al Saad K, Al-Hashimi F, et al. It's rare so be aware: pleuropulmonary blastoma mimicking congenital pulmonary airway malformation. Thorac Cardiovasc Surg Rep 2017;6(1):e10–4.

60. Feinberg A, Hall NJ, Williams GM, et al. Can congenital pulmonary airway malformation be distinguished from type I pleuropulmonary blastoma based on clinical and radiological features? J Pediatr Surg 2016;51(1):33–7.

61. Koh J, Jung E, Jang SJ, et al. Case of mucinous adenocarcinoma of the lung associated with congenital pulmonary airway malformation in a neonate. Korean J Pediatr 2018;61(1):30–4.

62. Ioachimescu OC, Mehta AC. From cystic pulmonary airway malformation, to bronchioloalveolar carcinoma and adenocarcinoma of the lung. Eur Respir J 2005; 26(6):1181–7.

63. Thakral CL, Maji DC, Sajwani MJ. Congenital lobar emphysema: experience with 21 cases. Pediatr Surg Int 2001;17(2–3):88–91.

64. Mukhtar S, Trovela DAV. Congenital lobar emphysema. In: StatPearls. StatPearls Publishing; 2021. Available at: http://www.ncbi.nlm.nih.gov/books/NBK560602/. Accessed April 11, 2021.

65. Abdel-Bary M, Abdel-Naser M, Okasha A, et al. Clinical and surgical aspects of congenital lobar over-inflation: a single center retrospective study. J Cardiothorac Surg 2020;15(1):102.

66. Hutchison MJ, Winkler L. Bronchial atresia. In: StatPearls. StatPearls Publishing; 2021. Available at: http://www.ncbi.nlm.nih.gov/books/NBK537142/. Accessed April 11, 2021.

67. Wei Y, Li F. Pulmonary sequestration: a retrospective analysis of 2625 cases in China. Eur J Cardiothorac Surg 2011;40(1):e39–42.

68. Chakraborty RK, Modi P, Sharma S. Pulmonary sequestration. In: StatPearls. StatPearls Publishing;

2021. Available at: http://www.ncbi.nlm.nih.gov/books/NBK532314/. Accessed April 12, 2021.

69. Skrabski R, Royo Y, Di Crosta I, et al. Extralobar pulmonary sequestration with an unusual venous drainage to the portal vein: preoperative diagnosis and excision by video-assisted thoracoscopy. J Pediatr Surg 2012;47(10):e63–5.

70. Lager DJ, Kuper KA, Haake GK. Subdiaphragmatic extralobar pulmonary sequestration. Arch Pathol Lab Med 1991;115(5):536–8.

71. Obeidat N, Sallout B, ALAAli W. Isolated subdiaphragmatic extralobar pulmonary sequestration: masquerading as suprarenal mass with spontaneous resolution. Clin Exp Obstet Gynecol 2016;43(3):457–9.

72. Al-Salem AH. Bronchopulmonary sequestration. In: Atlas of Pediatric Surgery. Cham, Switzerland: Springer; 2020. doi:10.1007/978-3-030-29211-9_33.

73. Garrett-Cox R, MacKinlay G, Munro F, et al. Early experience of pediatric thoracoscopic lobectomy in the UK. J Laparoendosc Adv Surg Tech A 2008; 18(3):457–9.

74. Borgia F, Santamaria F, Mollica C, et al. Clinical benefits, echocardiographic and MRI assessment after pulmonary sequestration treatment. Int J Cardiol 2017;240:165–71.

75. Ríos-Méndez RE, Andrade-Herrera JN, Aráuz-Martínez ME. Short-term outcome of percutaneous treatment of pulmonary sequestration in a pediatric hospital in the Andes: a case series. Arch Bronconeumol 2017;53(3):163–4.

76. Merli L, Nanni L, Curatola A, et al. Congenital lung malformations: a novel application for lung ultrasound? J Ultrasound 2021;24(3):349–53.

77. Gallardo AM, Álvarez de la Rosa RM, De Luis EJF, et al. [Antenatal ultrasound diagnosis and neonatal results of the congenital cystic adenomatoid malformation of the lung]. Rev Chil Pediatr 2018;89(2): 224–30.

78. Epelman M, Kreiger PA, Servaes S, et al. Current imaging of prenatally diagnosed congenital lung lesions. Semin Ultrasound CT MR 2010;31(2):141–57.

79. Style CC, Mehollin-Ray AR, Verla MA, et al. Accuracy of prenatal and postnatal imaging for management of congenital lung malformations. J Pediatr Surg 2020;55(5):844–7.

Pediatric Pulmonary Nodules
Imaging Guidelines and Recommendations

Teresa I. Liang, MD, FRCPC[a],*, Edward Y. Lee, MD, MPH[b]

KEYWORDS

- Pediatric • Pulmonary • Nodules • Malignancy • Thoracic • Radiography
- Computed tomography (CT) • Magnetic resonance imaging (MR imaging)

KEY POINTS

- The status of an underlying malignancy is key in determining the appropriate algorithm to use in the pediatric population with an incidental pulmonary nodule.
- In the absence of an underlying malignancy, children with unexpected solid pulmonary nodules smaller than 5 mm should not require dedicated follow-up imaging, unless there is an underlying clinical concern.
- In children with extrathoracic malignancy, there remains conflicting literature and a variety of primary malignancies with different propensities for intrathoracic metastasis.
- Pulmonary nodules remain a diagnostic challenge in children with known extrathoracic malignancy, given the variable appearances and lack of standardized characteristics to determine benignity versus malignancy.
- Computed tomography is currently the best imaging modality to identify, evaluate, and perform follow-up of pediatric pulmonary nodules that cannot be visualized on chest radiography.

INTRODUCTION

Pulmonary nodules, when they are small, may be difficult to be identified on chest radiography. However, pulmonary nodules are not infrequently incidentally detected on computed tomography (CT) imaging in the pediatric population.[1] The increased availability and improved CT techniques in recent years, such as the use of multidetector CT, resulting in thinner slice sections and decreased motion artifacts,[2–4] have enabled the detection of smaller lung lesions,[2,5,6] resulting in more pulmonary nodules being identified incidentally. Although the Fleischner guidelines for directing follow-up imaging based on nodule size and a patient's risk for malignancy exists, this set of criteria is only applicable to the adult population older than 35 years old.[7,8] It currently recommends that the management of young patients should be made on a case-by-case basis and discourages the use of serial CT scans for follow-up.[8]

Unfortunately, no comparable universally accepted criteria for evaluating children with pulmonary nodules currently exists. A main reason for why no established criteria exists is the relative paucity of literature available and the conflicting data for the determination of a benign versus malignant appearance.[2,9,10] Additionally, owing to concerns regarding radiation exposure, a large proportion of the studies have been performed in children with extrapulmonary malignancies.[2,10–13] Only more recently have

Disclosures: The authors have nothing to disclose.
[a] Department of Radiology & Diagnostic Imaging, Stollery Children's Hospital and University of Alberta, 8440 112 Street NW, Edmonton, AB T6G 2B7, Canada; [b] Department of Radiology, Boston Children's Hospital, Harvard Medical School, 330 Longwood Avenue, Boston, MA 02115, USA
* Corresponding author.
E-mail address: til@ualberta.ca

Radiol Clin N Am 60 (2022) 55–67
https://doi.org/10.1016/j.rcl.2021.08.004
0033-8389/22/© 2021 Elsevier Inc. All rights reserved.

there been studies assessing the characteristics of pulmonary nodules incidentally detected in healthy children.[1,14-16]

Without established recommendations tailored for pediatric population, radiologists and clinicians may be inclined to inappropriately extrapolate data from the Fleischner guidelines when they encounter pediatric patients with pulmonary nodules on imaging studies. A previous survey of the Society of Thoracic Radiology members demonstrated that radiologists tend to be overly aggressive in follow-up imaging, most commonly recommending follow-up examinations in 3 to 6 months for small nodules (3–5 mm) in young patients with no history of malignancy.[9,17] Additionally, a 2014 survey of pediatric pulmonologists in the United States demonstrated a tendency for a more aggressive approach in managing children with incidentally detected pulmonary nodules.[9,18] For example, when presented with a small (<4 mm), noncalcified nodule, 21% recommended a 3- to 6-month follow-up and 27% recommended a 12-month follow-up.[9,18] Given that the probability of an incidental pulmonary nodule being malignant in an otherwise healthy child is extremely low, this finding suggests that many radiologists and clinicians may be inappropriately recommending follow-up CT studies, resulting in unnecessary radiation exposure and anesthesia.[19,20] As previously established, the lifetime radiation risks attributable to CT examinations are considerably higher in children[21,22] and, thus, it is imperative to avoid unnecessary CT follow-up scans for unproven clinical indications.

In 2015, the Society of Pediatric Radiology (SPR) Thoracic Imaging Committee had presented a recommended algorithm to aid clinical management of incidentally detected lung nodules in children.[23,24] As new literature has since become available, especially with the updated research including healthy children,[1,14-16] the purpose of this article is to provide an updated literature analysis and evidence-based imaging recommendations, as well as discuss a practical approach to the imaging of pediatric pulmonary nodules.

EVIDENCE-BASED IMAGING ALGORITHM
Pulmonary Nodules in Healthy Children

Within the scarcely available literature on pediatric pulmonary nodules, incidental pulmonary nodules are not infrequently encountered. Alves and colleagues[16] recently reviewed preoperative chest CT scans for pectus carinatum or pectus excavatum treatment and identified that 75% of the patients had at least 1 pulmonary nodule. Renne and colleagues[15] retrospectively reviewed 259 trauma chest CT scans in pediatric patients and demonstrated 86 patients (33%) with incidental pulmonary nodules. Similarly, Samim and colleagues reviewed chest CT scans in children with high-energy trauma and demonstrated a total of 27 (37.5%) patients with incidental pulmonary nodules in the 72 included patients.[1] Interestingly, Breen and colleagues[14] retrospectively reviewed abdominal CT scans performed at a single institution over a span of 7 years, and only detected pulmonary nodules in 1.2% of the 5234 patients.

Assefa and Atlas[18] previously reviewed 36 patients with incidentally identified pulmonary nodules on a variety of chest and abdominal CT scans and chest radiographs to review the natural history of incidentally identified pulmonary nodules in children with nonmalignant disease. A total of 46 nodules were identified, and 37 nodules (27 patients) were larger than 4 mm.[18] Within this subset of patients, 22 of the patients had follow-up chest imaging 3 to 12 months later, and 14 (54%) of the nodules remained unchanged, 5 (19%) had decreased in size, and 7 (27%) had resolved on a follow-up CT scan, with no obvious growth or enlargement over the study period identified to suggest malignancy.[18] Thus, the authors concluded the low risk of malignancy in these subcentimetric nodules and raised the concern for potential harm of repeated follow-up CT scans outweighing any potential clinical benefit.[18] Breen and colleagues[14] confirmed this finding, with no malignant pulmonary nodules identified in their pediatric patients with incidental pulmonary nodules without a history of known malignancy.

Recommendations in Healthy Children with Pulmonary Nodules

Recently, Barber and colleagues[25] have questioned the usefulness of a diagnostic workup for an incidental solitary pulmonary nodule in patients without oncologic diagnosis or symptoms, because no definitive diagnosis was identified in 94% of cases. In light of this finding, in addition to the combination of a frequent occurrence and low associated malignancy risk in otherwise healthy children, it is imperative that follow-up imaging for incidental pulmonary nodules in this population be recommended cautiously to minimize the potential harm from repeated imaging, such as radiation exposure with risk of malignancy and caregiver anxiety.

The 2015 SPR Thoracic Imaging guidelines suggested that, if an unexpected asymptomatic solid pulmonary nodule was identified with a negative clinical history, and with the presence of classic features of benignity such as a popcorn calcification, fat, or features to suggest an intrapulmonary lymph node (peripheral, triangular, elongated, smoothly marginated, or a pleural tag),[26] uniformly calcified or stability over time, no further imaging was required.[24] Since then, more recent literature examining dedicated populations of children without malignancies have suggested the usefulness of size to suggest benignity.[14–16,18] Breen and colleagues[14] identified that the malignant pulmonary nodules in their study were significantly larger than the benign pulmonary nodules, and a size of 7 mm or larger was recommended as an optimal cut-off to suggest high risk. Similarly, Alves and colleagues[16] noted that 95% of the pulmonary nodules within their study were less than 6 mm and concluded that under these limits, incidental nodules are very unlikely to be pathologic. Finally, Renne and colleagues[15] only identified incidental pulmonary nodules smaller than 5 mm, and thus concluded that 5 mm pulmonary nodules can be detected frequently in children without malignant disease. Therefore, upon review of the recent literature, a conservative recommendation would be that children with unexpected solid pulmonary nodules smaller than 5 mm in the absence of a malignancy, should not require dedicated follow-up CT scans unless there is an underlying clinical concern requiring further follow-up.

Pulmonary Nodules in Children with a Primary Extrathoracic Malignancy

In addition to the common presence of incidental pulmonary nodules in an otherwise healthy child, pulmonary nodules are also not uncommonly identified in the pediatric population with extrathoracic malignancies, including but not limited to Wilms tumors, osteosarcomas, soft tissue sarcomas, and embryonal tumors.[27] Previously, Grampp and colleagues[11] identified pulmonary nodules in 34% of patients with extrathoracic malignant tumors. Similarly, Silva and colleagues[2] reviewed 488 patients with a new diagnosis of a non–central nervous system solid tumor or lymphoma and identified 111 patients (23%) with pulmonary nodules on the presentation CT scan. Rissing and colleagues[28] prospectively reviewed 331 patients with sarcoma treated over a 5-year range, and identified 34 children, of whom 6 (18%) were identified to have indeterminate nodules on the initial CT scan. Recently, Vaarwerk and colleagues[29] reviewed the clinical significance of pediatric patients with rhabdomyosarcoma with indeterminate nodules over an 8-year clinical span, and of the 316 patients included with chest CT imaging, 67 patients (21.2%) were identified with least a single pulmonary nodule. Thus, like the incidental pulmonary nodules identified in healthy children, the conundrum of what to do with the pulmonary nodule in patients with a primary extrathoracic malignancy is not infrequently encountered and becomes a challenging situation.

In contrast with the healthy child, this situation is complicated by a whole spectrum of primary malignancies with a variety of intrathoracic metastasis risk and a diverse range of pulmonary metastasis appearance. Although a greater proportion of the literature has been evaluated in children with malignancies, the ultimate challenge remains in the ability to determine a benign incidental pulmonary nodule versus metastatic disease, which can evidently alter the patient's management, but unfortunately, which radiologists have done poorly.[10] Although increased size on serial imaging has been widely accepted to suggest metastatic disease,[13] given the concern for radiation risks, serial follow-up CT imaging should be avoided if possible.

The challenge remains in trying to direct management at initial diagnosis. Silva and colleagues[2] reviewed 111 infants and children with extrapulmonary malignancies who had lung nodules, and found that the distribution, attenuation, shape, margin, and presence or absence of calcifications were not useful to reliably differentiate benignity from malignancy. This finding is like the initial studies performed by Robertson and colleagues[13] in 1988, who concluded that pulmonary nodules smaller than 5 mm in diameter were no more likely to be benign than larger nodules. Similarly, McCarville and colleagues[10] reviewed 41 young patients with 81 pulmonary nodules and demonstrated that size was not associated with malignancy. Grampp and colleagues[11] have also cautioned the usefulness of size to determine malignancy; they demonstrated that 70% of solitary pulmonary nodules smaller than 5 mm in children at initial presentation with solid extrathoracic tumors may be benign.

In contrast, Rissing and colleagues[28] reviewed 331 patients with sarcoma, including a subset of 34 pediatric patients, and concluded that pulmonary nodules greater or equal to 5 mm were at increased risk for metastatic disease in comparison with the patients without pulmonary nodules or with pulmonary nodules smaller than 5 mm. Brader and colleagues[12] reviewed 30 pediatric patients with osteosarcoma who underwent a chest CT scan and had a total of 117 pulmonary nodules resected over a 5-year span. They demonstrated that, although most characteristics were not useful, nodule size of 5 mm or larger and the presence of calcifications were associated with a statistically significant increased probability of malignancy.[12]

Recommendations in Children with Primary Extrathoracic Malignancy and Pulmonary Nodules

Although the imaging characteristics are important for ultimate diagnosis and management, it does raise the ultimate question, namely, "Does having the diagnosis really change outcome?" This clinically important concept was very recently questioned by Vaarwerk and colleagues[29] of the Pediatric Soft Tissue Sarcoma Study Group who reviewed 316 patients with rhabdomyosarcoma, of whom 67 had indeterminate pulmonary nodules. Indeterminate pulmonary nodules were defined by the European Pediatric Soft Tissue Sarcoma Study Group rhabdomyosarcoma 2005 protocol as no more than 4 pulmonary nodules smaller than 5 mm size or 1 pulmonary nodule between 5 and 10 mm.[29] The authors concluded that the indeterminate pulmonary nodules at diagnosis did not affect outcomes in patients with localized rhabdomyosarcoma, and thus recommended against the need to biopsy or upstage these patients.[29] However, there has been conflicting data; in addition to demonstrating the increased risk of metastatic disease in patients with sarcoma with pulmonary nodules 5 mm or larger, Rissing and colleagues[28] demonstrated that this group was also associated with a worse 3-year disease-free survival, suggesting that the ultimate diagnosis of these pulmonary nodules do matter. However, this dataset did include a large proportion of adult patients; therefore, this data should be applied cautiously. Similarly, Zhou and colleagues[30] recently evaluated 88 patients with indeterminate pulmonary nodules in patients with high-grade localized osteosarcoma and demonstrated in their 34 pediatric patients a poorer event-free survival.

The 2015 SPR Thoracic Imaging guidelines previously suggested a conceptual framework to aid in management of pulmonary nodule on a CT scan in a child.[24] Ultimately, this algorithm emphasized the importance of individualized care for pediatric patients with a history of malignancy.[24] Even upon review of updated literature, given the conflicting results, a similar recommendation of a case-by-case individualized care is suggested. In challenging situations, a multidisciplinary discussion regarding the clinical team's concern, tolerance of caregivers, interpreting radiologist's comfort, surgical feasibility, and the possibility of altering the clinical outcome is recommended.

PRACTICAL IMAGING APPROACH TO PEDIATRIC PULMONARY NODULES

Because the recommendations of how to approach a child with an incidental pulmonary nodule has been previously discussed, this section discusses the benefits and challenges of the available imaging modalities and reviews the recommended definitions and descriptors and spectrum of imaging manifestations to allow the radiologist and clinician to become more familiar to practically approach the imaging of pediatric pulmonary nodules.

IMAGING MODALITIES

Three main imaging modalities currently used to evaluate pulmonary nodules in pediatric patients include chest radiography, CT scan, and MR imaging, which are discussed in this section.

Chest Radiography

Chest radiographs remain the first-line and most performed imaging examination in pediatric patients with suspected thoracic disorders, because it remains readily available, easy to acquire, relatively lower in radiation compared with a CT scan, and low in cost.[31] Although the recent pediatric pulmonary nodule literature typically discuss the findings and usefulness of a CT scan, it is important to recognize that radiographs are still continuously being used for assessment of other suspected thoracic abnormalities, such as pneumonia or long-term cancer surveillance,[32] and can also incidentally detect pulmonary nodules. In a recent study published in 2021 by Barber and colleagues,[25] it was noted that, of the 88 children with pulmonary nodules, 38% of them were identified initially with chest radiographs. Therefore, it is imperative that radiologists continue to scrutinize chest radiographs carefully to ensure that pulmonary nodules are not missed.

Computed Tomography Scans

A CT scan remains the most used imaging modality for the assessment of pulmonary nodules in both pediatric and adult populations. With the advent of high-resolution multidetector CT allowing faster acquisition times and thinner collimation and resulting in a greater spatial resolution, and additional postprocessed visualization techniques such as multiplanar reconstructions, maximum intensity projections (MIPs), and computer-aided detection, this has markedly improved the radiologist's ability to detect pulmonary nodules.[3–6,15,23,33–35] Encouragingly, CT technology continues to advance; recently Cho and colleagues[36] successfully differentiated metastatic from benign nodules in patients with osteosarcoma using 3-dimensional computerized texture analysis.

However, even with technological advances, there remain the inherent challenges of pulmonary nodule detection, especially in children, such as a smaller thoracic diameter, as well as respiratory and motion artifacts from faster respiratory and heart rates. This challenge is compounded by the desire to aggressively minimize radiation dose, resulting in increased background noise and worsened image quality,[37,38] although recent promising literature has demonstrated similar nodular detection accuracy with a simulated 60% dose reduction.[39] An additional challenge is that younger children, typically those less than 3 years old, may not be able to follow the breath-hold instructions, and thus require anesthetic to improve compliancy.[40] In recognition of the 2016 Food and Drug Administration warning about the risk of general anesthesia in children younger than 3 years,[41] whenever possible, anesthesia should be avoided; instead, in conjunction with the rapid acquisition times, gentle respiration should be encouraged.[40]

Although MIPs have demonstrably improved pulmonary nodule detection, there remains conflicting literature regarding which plane and thickness is optimal. In 2013, Kilburn-Toppin and colleagues[35] demonstrated the use of 10-mm axial MIPs in addition to axial source images to improve sensitivity and decrease reading time. However, Ozkan and colleagues[33] subsequently demonstrated that, although 5-mm axial MIP images had the fastest reading times, the highest advantage was with 5-mm coronal 5 MIP images. Verhagen and colleagues[42] recently confirmed that, although the detection of pulmonary nodules was improved with MIPs, inter-reader agreement remained only fair, and pulmonary nodule characterization remained best with 1-mm slice thickness CT images.

At our local institution, we typically perform chest CT studies via volumetric data acquisition protocol on a multidetector CT scanner (Siemens Somatom Definition Flash) at end-inspiration, with a reference peak kilovoltage range of 80 to 100 kVp, automatic tube current exposure control, collimation 128 × 0.6 mm, pitch of 3 (FLASH), and rotation time of 0.28 s. Multiplanar images are constructed with soft tissue and lung algorithms at 1 mm and 3 mm thickness, as well as axial and coronal 5-mm MIPs. If studies are performed with IV contrast, low-osmolar nonionic contrast material (iopamidol, Isoevue 370, Bracco) is administered on a weight-based dose (1.5–2.0 mL/kg) using a power injection method.

MR Imaging

Although CT scanning remains the gold standard for pulmonary nodule imaging, advances in chest MR imaging techniques have improved lung visualization, and remain an attractive, ionizing radiation-free alternative. The absence of ionizing radiation remains a desirable goal for pediatric patients with malignancies, because surveillance for metastases or recurrence is required routinely, and the cumulative dose may become damaging over time.[43–45] Additionally, these pediatric patients may possess an underlying increased potential for developing new malignancies related to risk or treatment-related factors.[43]

The current literature suggests that MR imaging can reliably detect pulmonary nodules 5 mm or larger with optimal conditions[43,46–48]; however, pulmonary nodules smaller than 3 mm remain a challenge with poor sensitivity.[43,49] An added challenge with MR imaging remains the calcified pulmonary nodules, such as with osteosarcoma metastasis with a resultant susceptibly-related loss of signal intensity and thus appearing occult on MR imaging.[43] Although the majority of the strategies have been adopted for 1.5 T scanners, with the increased availability of 3 T MR imaging, there has been discussion regarding the benefits of a higher magnetic field strength. However, although using a higher magnetic field strength would theoretically yield improved lesion detection and spatial resolution, this technique is thought to degrade image quality and decrease overall effectiveness owing to the increased susceptibility artifacts on MR imaging.[47] Other MR imaging techniques have also been investigated; for example, diffusion-weighted imaging and dynamic contrast-enhanced MR imaging have demonstrated some usefulness in the detection and characterization of pulmonary nodules in the adult population.[49–52]

SPECTRUM OF PEDIATRIC PULMONARY NODULES
Definition of a Pulmonary Nodule

Before the characterization of a pulmonary nodule on CT imaging, a radiologist must be familiar with the widely accepted definitions, as previously detailed by the Flesichner Society.[53] A pulmonary nodule is defined as a rounded opacity, well or poorly defined, measuring up to 3 cm in diameter, and can be ground glass, solid, or contain both solid and ground glass components.[53] Ground glass components are defined as hazy with an increased opacity and preservation of the bronchial and vascular margins, whereas a solid component is defined as soft tissue attenuation.[53]

Pulmonary Nodules in Healthy Children

As discussed elsewhere in this article, incidental pulmonary nodules in healthy children are not infrequently seen and can be a diagnostic challenge.

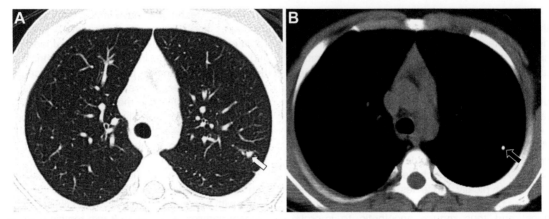

Fig. 1. A 11-year-old girl with a pulmonary granuloma. (*A*) Axial lung window CT image shows a tiny pulmonary nodule (*arrow*) in the left upper lobe. (*B*) Axial soft tissue window CT image confirms that the pulmonary nodule seen in *A* is calcified (*arrow*).

Pulmonary nodules in healthy children have been reported to have a large variety of characteristics, distributions, and sizes. Commonly reported shapes included round, triangular, and ovoid, and commonly reported margins include smooth, poorly defined, and irregular. The number of pulmonary nodules has also been reported to vary from a solitary nodule up to 4 nodules per patient.[15] Although there is no consensus on the most common location, the peripheral location and lower lobes have been reported as the most frequent locations.[1,14–16] Incidental pulmonary nodules are commonly identified in the perifissural location in addition to within the lung parenchyma.[15] The presence of calcification has also demonstrated to be variable ranging from 2% to 19% of the pulmonary nodules identified.[14,15]

In addition to the smaller size described elsewhere in this article to suggest a benign appearance, additional classic features of a benign appearance include uniform calcification, suggesting a granuloma (**Fig. 1**), the presence of fat and popcorn calcification, suggesting a hamartoma (**Fig. 2**), and long-term stability.[24] The presence of a nodule in a peripheral or perifissural location, with an oval or polygonal shape, and demonstrating a connection to pleura via linear extension (pleural tag) would be highly suggestive of an intrapulmonary lymph node (**Fig. 3**).

Pulmonary Nodules in Children with an Extrathoracic Malignancy

Pulmonary nodules remain a diagnostic challenge in children with extrathoracic malignancy, because there are a variety of appearances and no globally accepted characteristics to suggest benignity versus malignancy. Similarly, these pulmonary nodules can present as single or multiple and, like incidental nodules in healthy children, metastatic nodules tend to also be peripheral with a

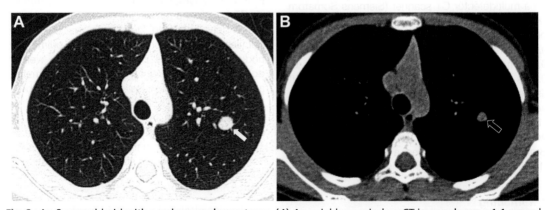

Fig. 2. An 8-year-old girl with a pulmonary hamartoma. (*A*) An axial lung window CT image shows a 1.1-cm pulmonary nodule (*arrow*) in the left upper lobe. (*B*) An axial soft tissue window CT image demonstrates punctate fat density (*arrow*), in keeping with a pulmonary hamartoma, which was stable on follow-up imaging evaluation.

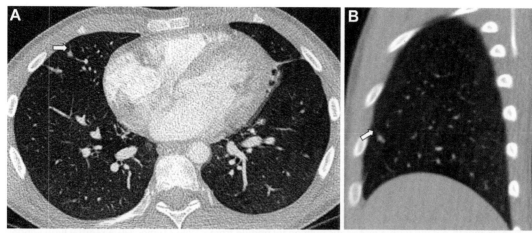

Fig. 3. A 13-year-old otherwise healthy boy who presented with chest pain and was found to have an incidental intrapulmonary lymph node. (*A*) An axial lung window CT image shows a triangular-shaped pulmonary nodule with a pleural tag (*arrow*) in the right middle lobe. (*B*) A coronal bone window CT image confirms an incidental triangular nodule with a pleural tag (*arrow*) in the right middle lobe.

lower lobe predilection owing to hematogenous spread (**Fig. 4**).[27] The presence of sharply defined margins in children has been reported to be suggestive of malignancy[10] (**Fig. 5**). This finding contrasts with the adult population, where spiculated or irregular margins are more suggestive of malignancy and is probably because pulmonary nodules are more likely metastases in children, but more likely to be primary lung cancer in adults.[10] An increased size of the pulmonary nodule has also been suggestive of malignancy (**Fig. 6**),[13] although an infectious nodule could also demonstrate short-term interval growth. The presence of calcification has been associated with an increased likelihood of malignancy in patients with osteosarcomas.[12] Atypical pulmonary metastases appearances include cavitary pulmonary

nodules (**Fig. 7**) most commonly in children with sarcomas, ground glass halos most commonly seen in children with highly vascular tumors, pulmonary nodules associated with adjacent pleural thickening (**Fig. 8**), miliary nodules associated with papillary thyroid carcinoma (**Fig. 9**), and lymphangitic carcinomatosis (**Fig. 10**).[27]

However, it is prudent to remember that a large proportion of the nodules identified within these children are benign, including fibrosis, drug reaction, chronic inflammation, scarring, and intrapulmonary lymph nodes.[2,10,24,54] Cho and colleagues[36] recently concluded that benign intrapulmonary lymph nodes in children with extrapulmonary solid malignancies most commonly are subcentimeter in size, with

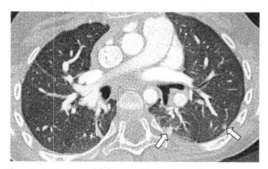

Fig. 4. A 4-year-old boy with metastatic pulmonary nodules from hepatoblastoma (not shown). An axial lung window CT image shows pulmonary nodules (*arrows*) in the left lower lobe. Surgical pathologic evaluation confirmed metastatic disease.

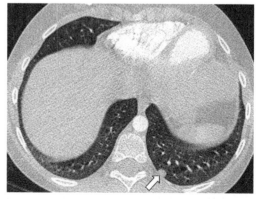

Fig. 5. A 7-year-old boy with a metastatic pulmonary nodule from a Wilms tumor. An axial lung window CT image shows a metastatic pulmonary nodule (*arrow*) with sharply defined margins in the left lower lobe.

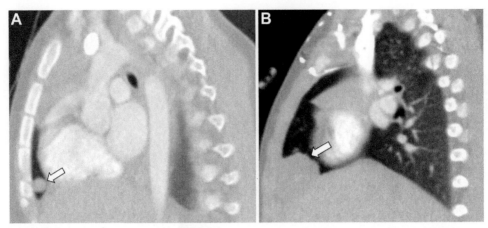

Fig. 6. A 25-month-old girl with a metastatic pulmonary nodule from a Wilms tumor. (*A*) A sagittal lung window CT image obtained as an initial staging evaluation shows a pulmonary nodule (*arrow*) in the right cardiophrenic angle. (*B*) A sagittal lung window CT image obtained as a follow-up evaluation demonstrates an interval increase in the size of the pulmonary nodule (*arrow*) in the right cardiophrenic angle, in keeping with metastatic disease.

smooth margins, noncalcified, solid, and a triangular shape.

Primary Pulmonary Neoplasms

Primary pediatric thoracic tumors are rare and with a narrow range of pathologies in children.[55] However, the majority of the primary pulmonary neoplasms present as a large pulmonary mass, cystic or endobronchial lesion rather than the pulmonary nodule appearance discussed elsewhere in this article. Nonetheless, it is important to review briefly the more common primary pulmonary malignancies, so that the radiologist can better recognize and distinguish the entities.

Pleuropulmonary blastoma (PPB) is most common primary lung malignancy of infancy and childhood, but remains a rare entity, and typically

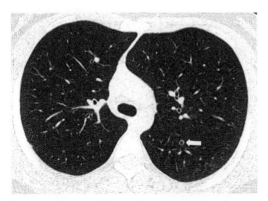

Fig. 7. A 15-year-old boy with a metastatic pulmonary nodule from an Ewing sarcoma. An axial lung window CT image shows a cavitary pulmonary nodule (*arrow*) in the left upper lobe in keeping with metastatic disease.

occurs in children younger than 6 years of age.[55] PPB contains blastomatous and sarcomatous elements and is thought to be associated with germline variants in the DICER1 gene.[55] There are 3 main subtypes defined in the literature: purely cystic (type 1), mixed cystic and solid (type 2; **Fig. 11**), and purely solid (type 3). The solid type PPBs are typically a large mass at the time of presentation, and thus would not be of diagnostic consideration in the setting of an incidental small pulmonary nodule in the pediatric population.[23] The cystic type 1 PPB can be small, but should not be misdiagnosed as a solid pulmonary nodule given the cystic nature.[23]

Inflammatory myofibroblastic tumor is the most common primary lung mass in children, representing approximately 16% to 38% of primary lung tumors.[55–57] Affected children often present with cough, fever, chest pain or hemoptysis.[55] These tumors are composed of spindle-cell proliferation and inflammatory components.[55] Imaging presentation can be highly variable, including a large pulmonary mass (**Fig. 12**) or an endobronchial lesion (**Fig. 13**). Calcification is common, estimated in 15% of cases (see **Fig. 12**). Again, if present as a solid pulmonary mass, typically these lesions are large at presentation and, thus, would not be of diagnostic consideration in the setting of an incidental small pulmonary nodule in the pediatric population.

Neoplasms of the large airway most commonly manifest as carcinoid tumors in the pediatric population.[55,56] Affected pediatric patients are almost always symptomatic at the time of diagnosis secondary to postobstructive atelectasis or pneumonitis.[23] Carcinoid tumors typically manifest as an

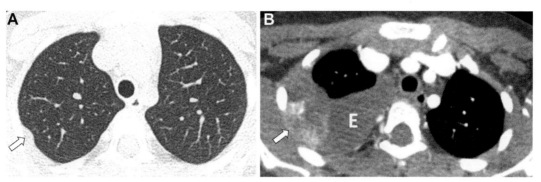

Fig. 8. A 7-year-old boy with a metastatic pulmonary nodule associated with pleural thickening from a primary osteosarcoma of the left distal femur status post chemotherapy and surgical resection. (*A*) An axial lung window CT image obtained as an initial evaluation shows new subtle pleural thickening (*arrow*) in the posterolateral right upper pleura. (*B*) An axial soft tissue window CT image obtained as a 3-month follow-up evaluation demonstrates a new, large, pleural-based calcified mass (*arrow*) and metastatic pleural effusion (E) in keeping with worsening metastatic disease.

endobronchial lesion in the central lung (**Fig. 14**), often with calcifications and avid enhancement.[55] There has been 1 reported case of a teenaged boy with Cushing's syndrome and a peripheral 2-cm pulmonary nodule in the middle lobe, pathologically diagnosed as an atypical bronchopulmonary carcinoid.[58] Therefore, although the differential for thoracic endoluminal tumors include salivary gland tumors such as mucoepidermoid tumors or possibly metastatic disease from gastrointestinal carcinoid lesions, in the setting of an incidental (asymptomatic) small pulmonary nodule, a carcinoid neoplasm would be highly unlikely.

Recurrent respiratory papillomatosis is a rare condition secondary to growth of benign squamous papillomas in the aerodigestive tract, caused by the human papillomavirus, usually subtypes 6 and 11.[55] Affected pediatric patients with recurrent respiratory papillomatosis may present with hoarseness or voice change, stridor, cough, recurrent respiratory infections, and dyspnea.[55] Pulmonary parenchymal disease is thought to be due to the aerial spread of the papilloma fragments related to surgical procedures, and typically present as scattered round nodules and cysts in the lung parenchyma (**Fig. 15**).[55] If solid, these nodules could potentially mimic the incidental solid pulmonary nodule, but there typically is a known exposure history and the presence of small nodules in the trachea and airways (see **Fig. 15**). Although low, there is a risk that these lesions may undergo malignant transformation to squamous cell carcinomas.[55,59] The

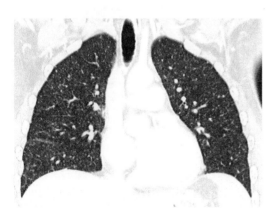

Fig. 9. A 16-year-old boy with metastatic numerous miliary pulmonary nodules from a primary thyroid malignancy. A coronal lung window CT image shows multiple tiny pulmonary nodules in both lungs.

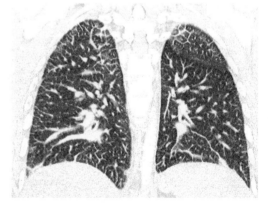

Fig. 10. A 13-year-old boy with lymphangitic carcinomatosis from a metastatic adenocarcinoma of an unknown primary. Coronal lung window CT image shows diffuse and extensive interlobular thickening in both lungs in keeping with lymphangitic carcinomatosis.

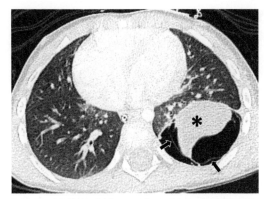

Fig. 11. A 4-year-old boy with a type 2 pleuropulmonary blastoma (PPB). Axial lung window CT image shows a large mass with both cystic and solid (*asterisk*) components as well as internal septations (*arrows*). Surgical pathology confirmed a type 2 PPB.

findings of a heterogeneous mass with central necrosis in a previously identified cyst, invasion of adjacent structures, or the presence of pleural effusion and lymphadenopathy is suggestive of malignant transformation.[57,60,61]

CONCLUSION

Since the SPR Thoracic Imaging Committee recommendations published in 2015, there have been multiple new studies evaluating the pediatric incidental pulmonary nodule. Based on the updated literature, in otherwise healthy children with unexpected solid pulmonary nodules smaller than 5 mm, no dedicated CT follow-up is recommended unless there is an underlying clinical concern. In contrast, in children with known extrathoracic malignancies, there remains conflicting literature and a variety of primary malignancies with different propensity for intrathoracic metastasis. Thus, like the 2015 SPR recommendations,

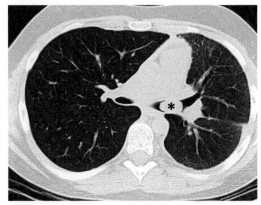

Fig. 13. An 11-year-old boy with an inflammatory myofibroblastic tumor who presented with shortness of breath and left-sided chest pain. An axial lung window CT image shows an ovoid, soft tissue mass (*asterisk*) in the left mainstem bronchus and postobstructive atelectasis/volume loss. Surgical resection and subsequent pathologic evaluation confirmed an inflammatory myofibroblastic tumor.

an ongoing careful case-by-case individualized care is suggested in these children.

Although MR imaging is an emerging modality and attractive owing to the lack of ionizing radiation, a CT scan remains the gold standard for the diagnosis, characterization, and follow-up of the pediatric pulmonary nodule. Recognition of the spectrum of pulmonary nodules in the pediatric population, as well as the benign nodule characteristics or typical characteristics of intrapulmonary lymph nodes, can be helpful in decreasing

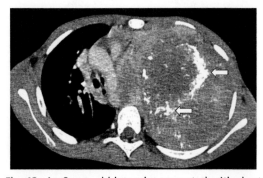

Fig. 12. An 8-year-old boy who presented with chest pain with a large partially calcified mass (*arrows*) in the left hemithorax with mass effect on the mediastinum, with surgical pathology in keeping with an inflammatory myofibroblastic tumor.

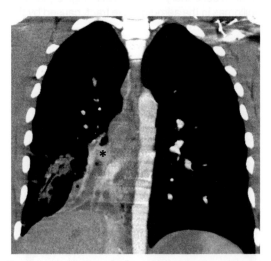

Fig. 14. An 11-year-old boy with a carcinoid tumor who presented with recurrent pneumonia. A coronal soft tissue window CT image demonstrates an enhancing soft tissue mass (*asterisk*) in the right lower lobe bronchus with dilated and fluid and mucousfilled bronchi distally.

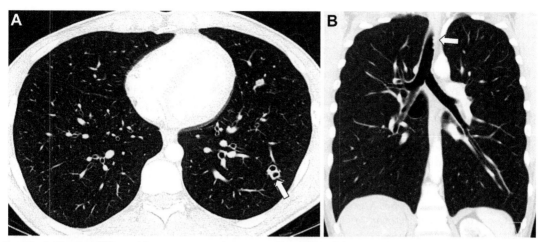

Fig. 15. A 17-year-old boy with recurrent respiratory papillomatosis. (*A*) An axial lung window CT image shows a small cavitary pulmonary nodule (*arrow*) in the left lower lobe. Multiple small pulmonary nodules are also noted in both lungs (not shown). (*B*) A coronal lung window CT image demonstrates multiple endotracheal nodules (*arrow*).

unnecessary follow-up imaging. Finally, being aware that primary pediatric lung malignancies typically present as large cystic or solid masses or endobronchial lesions rather than pulmonary nodules, can help to recognize that malignant lung nodules in children are more likely to be caused by metastatic disease rather than primary tumor, thus, allowing the radiologist to provide a more accurate and succinct differential diagnosis.

CLINICS CARE POINTS

- In the absence of an underlying malignancy, children with unexpected solid pulmonary nodules smaller than 5 mm should not require dedicated follow-up imaging unless there is an underlying clinical concern requiring further follow-up.

- In children with a known underlying malignancy, continued careful case-by-case individualized care is recommended.

- Although pulmonary nodules can have a large variety of appearances in children with extrathoracic malignancy, it is imperative to remember that a large proportion of the pulmonary nodules identified are benign and to avoid unnecessary follow-up imaging.

- Primary pulmonary malignancies typically present as large cystic or solid masses or endobronchial lesions rather than pulmonary nodules and thus should not typically be included in the differential diagnosis of an incidental pulmonary nodule.

- CT scan remains the current gold standard imaging modality for the identification, evaluation, and following-up pediatric pulmonary nodules.

REFERENCES

1. Samim A, Littooij AS, van den Heuvel-Eibrink MM, et al. Frequency and characteristics of pulmonary nodules in children at computed tomography. Pediatr Radiol 2017;47(13):1751–8.
2. Silva CT, Amaral JG, Moineddin R, et al. CT Characteristics of lung nodules present at diagnosis of extra pulmonary malignancy in children. AJR Am J Roentgenol 2010;194(3):772–8.
3. Ha HI, Goo HW, Seo JB, et al. Effects of high-resolution CT of the lung using partial versus full reconstruction on motion artifacts and image noise. AJR Am J Roentgenol 2006;187(3):618–22.
4. Girvin F, Ko J. Pulmonary nodules: detection, assessment, and CAD. AJR Am J Roentgenol 2008;191(4):1057–69.
5. Fischbach F, Knollmann F, Griesshaber V, et al. Detection of pulmonary nodules by multislice computed tomography: improved detection rate with reduced slice thickness. Eur Radiol 2003; 13(10):2378–83.
6. Kim JS, Kim JH, Cho G, et al. Automated detection of pulmonary nodules on CT images: effect of section thickness and reconstruction intervals – initial results. Radiology 2005;236(1):295–9.
7. MacMahon H, Austin JH, Gamsu G, et al. Guidelines for management of small pulmonary nodules

detected on CT scans: a statement from the Fleischner Society. Radiology 2005;237(2):395–400.

8. MacMahon H, Naidich DP, Goo JM, et al. Guidelines for management of incidental pulmonary nodules detected on CT images: from the Fleischner Society 2017. Radiology 2017;284(1):228–43.

9. Assefa D, Atlas AB. Natural history of incidental pulmonary nodules in children. Pediatr Pulmonol 2015; 50(5):456–9.

10. McCarville MB, Lederman HM, Santana VM, et al. Distinguishing benign from malignant pulmonary nodules with helical chest CT in children with malignant solid tumors. Radiology 2006;239:514–20.

11. Grampp S, Bankier AA, Zoubek A, et al. Spiral CT of the lung in children with malignant extra-thoracic tumors: distribution of benign vs malignant pulmonary nodules. Eur Radiol 2000;10:1318–22.

12. Brader P, Abramson SJ, Price AP, et al. Do characteristics of pulmonary nodules on computed tomography in children with known osteosarcoma help distinguish whether nodules are malignant or benign? J Pediatr Surg 2011;46(4):729–35.

13. Robertson PL, Boldt DW, De Campo JF. Paediatr Paediatric pulmonary nodules: a comparison of computed tomography, thoracotomy findings and histology. Clin Radiol 1988;39(6):607–10.

14. Breen M, Zurakowski D, Lee EY. Clinical significance of pulmonary nodules detected on abdominal CT in pediatric patients. Pediatr Radiol 2015;45: 1753–60.

15. Renne J, Linderkamp C, Wacker F, et al. Prevalence and configuration of pulmonary nodules on multi-row CT in children without malignant diseases. Eur Radiol 2015;25:2651–6.

16. Alves GRT, Marchiori E, Irion KL, et al. Mediastinal lymph nodes and pulmonary nodules in children: MDCT findings in a cohort of health subjects. AJR Am J Roentgenol 2015;204(1):35–7.

17. Munden RF, Hess KR. "Ditzels" on Chest CT. AJR Am J Roentgenol 2001;176(6):1363–9.

18. Assefa D, Atlas AB. Management of pulmonary nodules in pediatric patients. A survey of practicing pediatric pulmonologist in the USA. Am J Respir Crit Care Mrd 2014;189:A1801.

19. Feely MA, Hartman TE. Inappropriate application of nodule management guidelines in radiologist reports before and after revision of exclusion criteria. AJR Am J Roentgenol 2011;196(5):1115–9.

20. Swensen SJ, Duncan JR, Gibson R, et al. An appeal for safe and appropriate imaging of children. J Patient Saf 2014;10(3):121–4.

21. Slovis TL. Children computed tomography radiation dose, and the as low as reasonably achievable (ALARA) concept. Pediatrics 2003;112(4):971–2.

22. Brenner DJ, Elliston CD, Hall EJ, et al. Estimated risks of radiation-induced fatal cancer from pediatric CT. AJR Am J Roentgenol 2001;176(2):289–96.

23. Westra SJ, Brody AS, Mahani MG, et al. The incidental pulmonary nodule in a child. Part 1: recommendations from SPR Thoracic Imaging Committee regarding characterization, significance and follow up. Pediatr Radiol 2015;45(5):628–33.

24. Westra SJ, Thacker PG, Podberesky DJ, et al. The incidental pulmonary nodule in a child. Part 2: commentary and suggestions for clinical management, risk communication and prevention. Pediatr Radiol 2015;45(5):634–9.

25. Barber A, Passarelli P, Dworsky ZD, et al. Clinical implications of pulmonary nodules detected in children. Pediatr Pulm 2021;56:203–10.

26. Cho JY, Winant AJ, John JH, et al. CT features of benign intrapulmonary lymph nodes in pediatric patients with known extrapulmonary solid malignancy. AJR Am J Roentgenol 2021;216:1–6.

27. Gagnon MH, Wallace AB, Yedururi S, et al. Atypical pulmonary metastases in children: a pictorial review of imaging patterns. Pediatr Radiol 2021;51: 131–9.

28. Rissing S, Rougraff BT, Davis K. Indeterminate pulmonary nodules in patients with sarcoma affect survival. Clin Orthop Relat Res 2007;459:118–21.

29. Vaarwerk B, Bisogno G, McHugh K, et al. Indeterminate pulmonary nodules at diagnosis rhabdomyosarcoma: are they clinically significant? A report from the European Paediatric Soft Tissue Sarcoma Study Group. J Clin Oncol 2019;37:723–30.

30. Zhou C, Wang Y, Qian G, et al. Clinical significant of indeterminate pulmonary nodules on the clinical survival of 364 patients with nonmetastatic, high-grade, localized osteosarcoma: a 12-year retrospective cohort study. J Surg Oncol 2021;123(2):587–95.

31. Hart A, Lee EY. Pediatric chest disorders: practical imaging approach to diagnosis. In: Hodler J, Kubik-Huch RA, von Schulthess GK, editors. Diseases of the chest, breast, heart and vessels 2019-2022: diagnostic and interventional imaging [Internet]. Cham, CH: Springer; 2019. Chapter 10.

32. Servaes SE, Hoffer FA, Smith EA, et al. Imaging of Wilms tumor: an update. Pediatr Radiol 2019;49: 1441–52.

33. Ozkan MB, Tscheuner S, Ozkan E. Diagnostic accuracy of MIP slice modalities for small pulmonary nodules in paediatric oncology patients revisited: what is additional from the paediatric radiologist approach? Egypt J Radiol Nucl Med 2016;47: 1629–37.

34. Helm E, Silva CT, Roberts HC, et al. Computer-aided detection for the identification of pulmonary nodules in pediatric oncology patients: initial experience. Pediatr Radiol 2009;39:685–93.

35. Kilburn-Toppin F, Arthurs OJ, Tasker AD, et al. Detection of pulmonary nodules at paediatric CT: maximum intensity projections and axial source

images are complimentary. Pediatr Radiol 2013;43:820–6.

36. Cho YJ, Kim WS, Choi YH, et al. Computerized texture analysis of pulmonary nodules in pediatric patients with osteosarcoma: differentiation of pulmonary metastases from non-metastatic nodules. PLoS One 2019;14(2):e0211969.

37. Punwani S, Zhang J, Davies W, et al. Paediatric CT: the effects of increasing image noise on pulmonary nodule detection. Pediatr Radiol 2008;38:192–201.

38. Li X, Samei E, Barnhart HX, et al. Lung nodule detection in pediatric chest CT: quantitative relationship between image quality and radiologist performance. Med Phys 2011;38:2609–18.

39. Chapman T, Swanson JO, Phillips GS. Pediatric chest CT radiation dose reduction: protocol refinement based on noise injection for pulmonary nodule detection accuracy. Clin Imaging 2013;37:334–41.

40. Young C, Xie C, Owens CM. Paediatric multidetector row chest CT: what you really need to know. Insights Imaging 2012;3:229–46.

41. Derderian CA, Szmuk P, Derderian CK. Behind the Black Box: the evidence for the U.S. Food and Drug Administration warning about the risk of general anesthesia in children younger than 3 years. Plast Reconstr Surg 2017;140(4):782–92.

42. Verhagen MV, Smets AMJB, van Schuppen J, et al. The impact of reconstruction techniques on observer performance for the detection and characterization of small pulmonary nodules in chest CT of children under 13 years. Eur J Radiol 2018;100:142–6.

43. Baez JC, Ciet P, Mulkern R, et al. Pediatric chest MR imaging: lungs and airways. Magn Reson Imaging Clin N Am 2015;23:337–49.

44. De Jong PA, Mayo JR, Golmohammadi K, et al. Estimation of cancer mortality associated with repetitive computed tomography scanning. Am J Respir Crit Care Med 2006;173(2):199–203.

45. Chawla SC, Federman N, Zhang D, et al. Estimated cumulative radiation dose from PET/CT in children with malignancies: a 5-year retrospective review. Pediatr Radiol 2010;40(5):681–6.

46. Biederer J, Beer M, Hirsch W, et al. MRI of the lung (2/3). Why . when . how? Insights Imaging 2012;3(4):355–71.

47. Biederer J, Hintze C, Fabel M. MRI of pulmonary nodules: technique and diagnostic value. Cancer Imaging 2008;8:125–30.

48. Brazauskas KA, Ackman JB, Nelson B. Surveillance of actionable pulmonary nodules in children: the potential of thoracic MRI. Insights Chest Dis 2016;1:10.

49. Wu LM, Xu JR, Hua J, et al. Can diffusion weighted imaging be used as a reliable sequence in the detection of malignant pulmonary nodules and masses? Magn Reson Imaging 2013;31(2):235–46.

50. Regier M, Schwarz D, Henes FO, et al. Diffusion weighted MR-imaging for the detection of pulmonary nodules at 1.5 Tesla: intraindividual comparison with multidetector computed tomography. J Med Imaging Radiat Oncol 2011;55(3):266–74.

51. Schaefer JF, Vollmar J, Schick F, et al. Solitary pulmonary nodules: dynamic contrast-enhanced MR imaging – perfusion differences in malignant and benign lesions. Radiology 2004;232:544–53.

52. Kono R, Fujimoto K, Terasaki H, et al. Dynamic MRI of solitary pulmonary nodules: comparison of enhancement patterns of malignant and benign small peripheral lung lesions. AJR Am J Roentgenol 2007;188(1):26–36.

53. Hansell DM, Bankier AA, MacMahon H, et al. Fleischner Society: glossary of terms for thoracic imaging. Radiology 2008;246:697–722.

54. Rosenfield NS, Keller MS, Markowitz RI, et al. CT differentiation of benign and malignant lung nodules in children. J Pediatr Surg 1992;27:459–61.

55. Lichtenberger JP, Biko DM, Carter BW, et al. Primary lung tumors in children: radiologic-pathologic correlation from the Radiologic Pathology Archives. Radiographics 2018;38:2151–72.

56. Yu DC, Grabowski MJ, Kozakewich HP, et al. Primary lung tumors in children and adolescents: a 90-year experience. J Pediatr Surg 2010;45(6):1090–5.

57. Cohen MC, Kaschula RO. Primary pulmonary tumors in childhood: a review of 31 years' experience and the literature. Pediatr Pulmonol 1992;14(4):222–32.

58. De Matos LL, Trufelli DC, Das Neves-Pereira JC, et al. Cushing's syndrome secondary to bronchopulmonary carcinoid tumor: report of two cases and literature review. Lung Cancer 2006;53:381–6.

59. Gélinas JF, Manoukian J, Côté A. Lung involvement in juvenile onset recurrent respiratory papillomatosis: a systematic review of the literature. Int J Pediatr Otorhinolaryngol 2008;72(4):433–52.

60. Frauenfelder T, Marincek B, Wildermuth S. Pulmonary spread of recurrent respiratory papillomatosis with malignant transformation: CT-findings and airflow simulation. Eur J Radiol Extra 2005;56(1):11–6.

61. Knepper BR, Eklund MJ, Braithwaite KA. Malignant degeneration of pulmonary juvenile-onset recurrent respiratory papillomatosis. Pediatr Radiol 2015;45(7):1077–81.

Pediatric Pulmonary Embolism
Imaging Guidelines and Recommendations

Spencer G. Degerstedt, MD[a], Abbey J. Winant, MD[b],
Edward Y. Lee, MD, MPH[b],*

KEYWORDS

- Pulmonary embolism (PE) • Thrombosis • Radiography
- Computed tomography pulmonary angiography (CTPA) • Ventilation/perfusion (V/Q) scan
- Angiography • Pediatric

KEY POINTS

- Pulmonary embolism prevalence is much higher in children than thought; timely diagnosis is critical.
- There is a relative paucity of guidance on the imaging approach to diagnosing pulmonary embolism in children. Adult-based diagnostic algorithms are not applicable to the pediatric population.
- Pediatric-specific risk factor assessment is an important primary tool for guiding decision-making regarding imaging for pulmonary embolism, preferably with computed tomography pulmonary angiography.
- Most children diagnosed with pulmonary embolism have predisposing risk factors, including immobilization, a hypercoagulable state, an excess estrogen state, an indwelling central venous line, and prior pulmonary embolism and/or deep vein thrombosis.
- Radiologists need to work closely with referring clinicians to choose the most appropriate imaging modality and be familiar with recent imaging advancements to maximize the diagnostic yield, while minimizing radiation dose.

INTRODUCTION

The incidence of pulmonary embolism (PE) in the pediatric population and young adults is higher than previously thought.[1–4] If not diagnosed and treated promptly, PE poses a substantial risk of morbidity and mortality ($\leq$10%).[5,6] The clinical presentation of PE in children is highly variable and may even be clinically asymptomatic. Given their substantial cardiopulmonary reserve, children are unlikely to be symptomatic unless there is a greater than 50% obstruction of the pulmonary circulation or coexisting cardiopulmonary disease.[1,7] Therefore, high clinical suspicion, guided by pediatric-specific risk factor assessment, is

necessary for prompt diagnosis of pediatric PE. In addition, accurate imaging evaluation, which can directly or indirectly visualize PE, is essential for the initial detection and follow-up evaluation.

Multiple diagnostic algorithms and screening criteria for adults suspected of PE (i.e. Wells criteria,[8] Pulmonary Embolism Rule Out Criteria,[9] the Geneva score,[10] etc.) are currently available and widely used. However, there is a relative paucity of guidance for the diagnostic approach to PE in children. Therefore, the goal of this article is to present an up-to-date review of imaging techniques for pediatric PE, including the sensitivity and specificity of various modalities and characteristic radiologic findings, and to present an evidence-

[a] Department of Radiology, Beth Israel Deaconess Medical Center, Harvard Medical School, 330 Brookline Avenue, Boston, MA 02215, USA; [b] Department of Radiology, Boston Children's Hospital, Harvard Medical School, 300 Longwood Avenue, Boston, MA 02115, USA
* Corresponding author.
E-mail address: Edward.Lee@childrens.harvard.edu

Radiol Clin N Am 60 (2022) 69–82
https://doi.org/10.1016/j.rcl.2021.08.005

based algorithm to guide the imaging approach to detection of PE in children.

EVIDENCE-BASED IMAGING ALGORITHM

Five currently available imaging modalities for diagnosing PE in children are radiography, computed tomography pulmonary angiography (CTPA), nuclear medicine ventilation and perfusion (V/Q) scan, MR imaging, and conventional angiography. Given the paucity of scientifically proven data specifically for the pediatric population, the sensitivities and specificities of various imaging modalities for the detection of PE are still mainly based on information obtained in adult patients with PE. The sensitivity, specificity, advantages, and disadvantages of the currently available imaging modalities for diagnosing PE in children are summarized in Table 1.

PRACTICAL IMAGING APPROACH TO PEDIATRIC PULMONARY EMBOLISM

Survey Study Information on Current Imaging Modality for Evaluating Pulmonary Embolism

Lee and colleagues[11] published survey results collected in 2009 from 160 members of the Society of Pediatric Radiology spanning 118 institutions regarding the practices and policies for diagnosis of PE with emphasis on CTPA. Of the 118 respondents, 104 (88%) performed CTPA in children with clinical suspicion of PE and 93 (89%) of those 104 use CTPA as the first imaging choice. Ten respondents (10%) reported using a V/Q scan, and 1 (1%) reported conventional angiography as their usual study of choice in patients with suspected PE. Twenty-six respondents (25%) reported having a written policy or clinical pathway established for the diagnosis of PE. The majority of the respondents who reported using CTPA in children with suspected PE (64%) stated that obtaining a chest radiograph before the CTPA, whereas 7% did not obtain a chest radiograph before CTPA. The remaining 29% reported variably obtaining a chest radiograph before CTPA "depending on the clinical circumstances and/or ordering physician's preference."[11]

The demographics of the respondents and the frequency of CTPA performed in children, and the use of dose reduction techniques varied widely across institutions. Of the 118 respondents, 80 (68%) primarily worked in academic settings, 27 (23%) in a private practice setting, and 11 (9%) in combined academic and private settings. However, the frequency of CTPA examinations ordered between academic, private, or combined settings did not differ. The majority of respondents (58%) reported modifying CTPA protocols to decrease the radiation dose in children with the 3 most common measures, including mAs reduction, automatic exposure control, and a decreased kVp. However, a significantly higher percentage of radiation dose-reduction techniques were used within academic institutions compared with private institutions ($P = .03$).[11]

Current Imaging Techniques

Radiography

Chest radiographs are neither sensitive nor specific for the diagnosis of PE.[4,12] Because radiographs are widely available, relatively low cost, and have a relatively low radiation dose, chest radiography may be helpful for providing an alternative diagnosis for acute symptoms, such as pneumonia, pneumothorax, rib fracture, or pulmonary edema. For these reasons, chest radiographs are often the first step in the workup[11] of suspected pediatric PE; however, additional imaging studies are needed to definitively diagnose or exclude PE in the appropriate clinical scenario, especially when 2 or more established risk factors are present.[2]

Normal chest radiographs do not exclude the diagnosis of PE. For example, up to 12% of chest radiographs are normal in adult patients found to have a PE.[12] Several secondary radiographic signs of pediatric PE have been described, including the Westermark sign (oligemia), the prominent central pulmonary artery sign (Fleischner sign), pleural-based increased opacity (Hampton hump), and other noneponymous signs, such as vascular redistribution, pleural effusion, and an enlarged hilum. The sensitivity and specificity of these radiographic secondary signs of PE vary widely from 3% to 20% and 80% to 95%, respectively,[12] and most secondary signs, especially the latter, are considered nonspecific.

Computed tomography pulmonary angiography

After the PIOPED II study, multidetector CTPA emerged as the imaging modality of choice for the diagnosis of PE in adults and children owing to its fast scanning time, widespread availability, high spatial resolution, and high sensitivity and specificity.[7,13] PIOPED II is the largest study to date that compared CTPA with a composite reference standard, spanning 8 clinical centers; however, it is important to note that PIOPED II excluded patients younger than 18 years of age. Compared with conventional angiography, CTPA has also been demonstrated to be more sensitive in detection of subsegmental PE.[14] In addition, owing to the high anatomic detail provided by this cross-

Table 1
Summary of sensitivity, specificity, advantages, and disadvantages of currently available imaging modalities in the diagnosis of PE

Imaging Modality	Sensitivity	Specificity	Advantages	Disadvantages	References
Radiography	3%–20% (individual indirect signs of PE)	80%–95% (individual indirect signs of PE)	Low radiation dose, widely available, alternative diagnosis	Lack of sensitivity	PIOPED I (Worsley)[12]
CTPA	83%–100%	89%–97%	Noninvasive, relatively fast/available, sensitive and specific, alternative diagnosis	Relatively high radiation dose, iodinated contrast	PIOPED II (Hayashino),[53] Stein,[54] Patel,[55] Coche,[56] Qanadli,[57] Winer-Muram[58]
V/Q scan	78%[a]	98%[a]	Alternative to iodinated contrast tests, noninvasive	Difficult technique in children <5 y of age, may require more specific testing, relatively high radiation dose	PIOPED II (Sostman),[32] Patocka,[33] Zaidi[34]
MR imaging	84%[b]	~100%[b]	No radiation, noninvasive, alternative diagnosis	Sedation often required, high cost, lack of availability and scanner time	Kalb B,[35] Benson[13]
Angiography	32%[c]–99%	~100%	Role for thrombectomy/thrombolysis	Invasive, radiation dose varies, can miss subsegmental PE	Wittram (PIOPED II),[14] Stein[39]

Abbreviations: PIOPED, prospective investigation of PE diagnosis.
[a] Excludes intermediate and low risk, often leading to further testing. Gold standard in these cases either digital subtraction angiography or CTPA in combination with Wells criteria.
[b] In 22 adult patients when using combination of conventional bolus-triggered 3-D MR pulmonary angiography, respiratory-triggered cardiac-gated true fast imaging with steady-state precession, and contrast-enhanced low–flip-angle 3-D gradient-echo sequences.
[c] MDCT was shown to be more sensitive in diagnosis of subsegmental pulmonary emboli compared with conventional angiography.

sectional imaging modality, CTPA may also demonstrate alternative diagnoses that may clinically mimic the nonspecific symptoms of PE in children, such as pneumonia, atelectasis, malignancy, congenital heart disease, and, less co-mmonly, pericardial effusion, rib fractures, right atrial thrombus, and fat embolism.[15] Furthermore, faster scanning times of newer MDCT scanners has decreased the number of children requiring sedation for CTPA scans,[1] substantially decreasing the need for sedation and the cost of using anesthesia resources.

Computed tomography pulmonary angiography parameters CTPA parameters depend on institutional imaging guidelines. However, in general, collimation size decreases depending on the number of detectors of the scanner, such that an 0.75 mm collimation is typically used for 16 MDCT, an 0.625 mm collimation for 32 MDCT, and 0.60 mm for 64 MDCT. A high pitch range between 1.0 and 1.5 is recommended. Weight-based low-kilovoltage scanning simultaneously decreases the radiation dose and increases the detection of both central and peripheral pulmonary emboli.[16] In both children and adults, the use of sagittal and coronal multiplanar reformats as well as 3D reconstruction of the pulmonary vasculature have been found to result in significantly increased detection of PE and interobserver agreement.[16,17]

Contrast optimization Optimal contrast enhancement of the pulmonary arteries is critical for the detection of PE (**Fig. 1**). One large study found that 80% of CTPA studies in children are limited in the evaluation of subsegmental pulmonary arteries owing to suboptimal contrast opacification.[6] Before performing a CTPA, it is essential to carefully review the underlying cardiac anatomy and tailor the CT technique to optimize contrast enhancement of the pulmonary arteries (**Fig. 2**). Nonionic iodinated intravenous contrast at a dose of 2 to 4 mL/kg (volume to not exceed 125 mL), preferably administered via power injector at rates specific to intravenous catheter size (3.0 mL/s for 20G, 1.5–2.0 mL/s for 22G, 1.0 mL/s for catheters smaller than 22G or in the hand or foot).[1] Faster injection rates are preferred for optimal pulmonary arterial enhancement.[1]

Bolus tracking methods, in which a region of interest is placed over the pulmonary outflow tract to trigger the start of scanning when attenuation within the region of interest reaches more than 150 Hounsfield units, are preferred.[1,11] The use of a weight-based empiric scan delay method (starting scan approximately 12–25 seconds after the end of the intravenous contrast injection) has been found to be associated with higher rates of suboptimal pulmonary arterial enhancement, likely owing to wide variation in pediatric heart rates.[1] Shallow free breathing is recommended during CTPA scanning, because pulmonary arterial enhancement is affected by the respiratory cycle. Inspiratory scanning often results in increased dilution from increased venous return (owing to negative

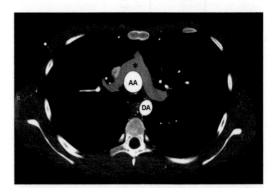

Fig. 2. Nondiagnostic CTPA study in a 14-year-old boy who presented with a prior surgical history of arterial switch operation owing to D-transposition of great arteries, chest pain, and shortness of breath. Axial enhanced CT image shows main pulmonary artery (*asterisk*), which is located anterior to the ascending aorta (AA) as the result of LeCompte maneuver. Suboptimal level (Hounsfield units = 86) of contrast enhancement within the main and proximal bilateral pulmonary arteries is seen, which underscores importance of understanding the underlying postcardiac surgery anatomy before performing CTPA study. DA, Descending aorta.

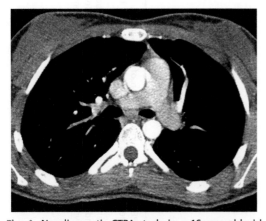

Fig. 1. Nondiagnostic CTPA study in a 16-year-old girl who presented with shortness of breath and an elevated D-dimer level. Axial enhanced CT image shows suboptimal level (Hounsfield units = 99) of contrast en-hancement within the main and proximal bilateral pulmonary arteries owing to intravenous catheter malfunction during the contrast ad-ministration.

intrathoracic pressure during inspiration) and decreased pulmonary blood flow in full inspiration.[1,18,19]

CTPA technique should be adapted for patients with congenital heart disease who have undergone the Fontan procedure, especially with bidirectional Glenn shunt, given the very sluggish flow within the Fontan pathway (**Fig. 3**). Simultaneous intravenous contrast injection from both the upper and lower extremities can help to decrease suboptimal enhancement and false positives related to a mixing artifact.[20] Furthermore, the use of a second delayed scan and bolus tracking may also help to optimize the enhancement of the pulmonary arteries in this setting.[20]

Ideally, imaging review of CTPA images for PE evaluation is performed with an organized search pattern, with a window width of 700 and level of 200. Additional postprocessing techniques, especially the use of sagittal and coronal 2-dimensional reformats and 3-dimensional (3D) vascular reconstructions, improve diagnostic accuracy.[17]

Postprocessing Techniques

Multiplanar Reformation Imaging Using the initial thin-slice axial data, multiplanar reformation imaging and maximal intensity projection imaging can be used to help increase the diagnostic yield of CTPA. In both children and adults, the use of sagittal and coronal multiplanar reformats and 3D reconstruction of the pulmonary vasculature has demonstrated a significant increase in detection and interobserver agreement for the detection of PE.[16,17] One inherent drawback to this method is the increased interpretation time of the study.

Maximum Intensity Projection Imaging Maximum intensity projection reconstruction improves angiographic imaging detection of vascular caliber, focal narrowing, and filling defects. This volume-rendering technique is broadly used and involves displaying the highest attenuation voxel within an algorithmically

selected ray. Slab editing increases the utility of MIP images by removing other high-attenuation voxels not of interest, such as calcifications, bones, surgical material, and so on.[21]

Dual Energy Computed Tomography Applcation Dual-energy CT is a novel imaging technique that combines functional and high-resolution anatomic information in a single scan by exploiting the unique attenuation properties (photoelectric absorption and Compton scattering) of tissues at different energies (80 kVp and 140 kVp).[1,22,23] Specifically, iodine perfusion maps are created in a postprocessing technique, which differentiates lung parenchyma perfusion from iodinated contrast (ideally, within pulmonary arteries). However, the timing of the scan should be optimized for the enhancement of the pulmonary arteries, which may not match the timing of maximal lung perfusion.[24] Dual energy CT lung perfusion abnormalities have been shown to correlate well with nuclear medicine scans (planar scintigraphy, single-photon emission CT [SPECT], and SPECT/CT), which remain the gold standard for lung perfusion imaging.[25,26] A dual-energy CT scan has been shown to increase the detection of peripheral PE, compared with conventional CTPA, in a canine model.[27]

There has yet to be a large role for combination of CT perfusion and ventilation imaging (using xenon) in the diagnosis of PE in children, but this modality has been used in other applications, such as congenital lung malformations, bronchiolitis obliterans, asthma, bronchopleural fistula, and chronic obstructive pulmonary disease.[26]

Artificial intelligence application There are multiple potential artificial intelligence (AI) applications being developed for the diagnosis of PE in children however, none are available broadly or used in standard clinical practice. Although there has been much discussion of the use of AI in radiology in the popular media, at present, there are very few AI applications

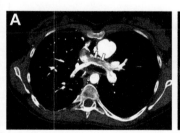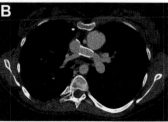

Fig. 3. Mixture of contrast and nonopacified blood mimicking PE in a 16-year-old girl who is status post Fontan procedure for hypoplastic left heart syndrome. (*A*) Axial enhanced CT image shows the mixture of contrast and nonopacified blood (*arrows*) within the left main pulmonary artery. Also noted is the metallic stent in the left main pulmonary artery. (*B*) Axial enhanced delayed second CT image obtained 60 seconds after the first scan demonstrates homogeneous contrast enhancement within the left main pulmonary artery, confirming the absence of PE. Again noted is the metallic stent in the left main pulmonary artery.

used in pediatric radiology in general.[28] One application of AI in pediatric radiology includes the Bone-Xpert software, which can provide rapid automatic assessment of bone age in hand radiographs according to Greulich and Pyle,[29] also with estimated standard deviation, which is used at some institutions.[30]

There are reported AI-powered algorithms that have been shown in adults to detect PE on CTPA. Weikert and colleagues[31] describe an AI-powered algorithm that correctly identified 215 of 232 examinations positive for PE (sensitivity, 92.7%; 95% confidence interval, 88.3%–95.5%) while correctly identifying 1178 of 1233 examinations negative for PE (specificity, 95.5%; 95% confidence interval, 94.2%–96.6%). The PE detection algorithm was based on 1-mm images in soft tissue reconstruction, a deep convolutional neural network of Resnet architecture, and trained and validated on 28,000 CTPAs from different institutions. The majority of false positives reported were related to contrast flow-related artifacts, pulmonary veins, and lymph nodes.[31] Unfortunately, the ages of these patients were not reported and likely were mostly adults. Currently, there is no significant role for AI applications in the diagnosis of PE in children.

Nuclear medicine study (ventilation and perfusion scan)

Before the adoption of CTPA, nuclear medicine V/Q scans were the primary noninvasive tests for diagnosis of PE in children and adults. However, the relatively low sensitivity and specificity of V/Q scans (planar scintigraphy, SPECT, and SPECT/CT) compared with CTPA, as well as the technically demanding proper inhalation of radiolabeled gas, limits its usefulness in pediatrics.[32] However, there are clinical scenarios in which other imaging modalities, such as CTPA or conventional angiography, may be contraindicated, such as in severe iodinated contrast allergy or acute kidney injury. Nuclear medicine scans remain the gold standard for the noninvasive imaging detection of lung perfusion abnormalities, despite the recent advent of dual-energy CT perfusion scans.[26]

V/Q scans are usually performed using radioisotope-labeled gas for the ventilation imaging, such as an aerosolized Tc-99m DTPA or xenon-133 gas via a nonrebreathing mask. This step is particularly challenging in young children and in other clinical scenarios in which patients cannot follow specific breathing instructions. The perfusion step involves intravenous injection of Tc-99m macroaggregated albumin particles (approximately 0.03 mCi/kg). Approximately 1 in 1000 particles lodges in the pulmonary capillaries (0.1%)

during the examination. Concurrent chest radiographs are crucial for correlation with po-ssible areas of mismatch in perfusion and ventilation. V/Q scans are then rated in probability of PE from very low, low, intermediate, or high risk.

In the PIOPED II study, the sensitivity and specificity of V/Q scans in diagnosis of PE (in adults) was 78% and 95%, respectively; however, this report excludes intermediate and low probability scans. The gold standard in these cases was either digital subtraction conventional angiography or CTPA in combination with Wells criteria. In general, V/Q scans, especially when indeterminate or low risk, usually lead to more testing and the majority of scans yield a low or intermediate probability of PE.[33,34] Consequently, V/Q scans are only clinically useful if they are normal or demonstrate high probability (85% chance) of PE.

MR Imaging

Noncontrast MR angiography (MRA) and contrast-enhanced MRA are additional noninvasive imaging techniques for diagnosing PE that avoid the use of iodinated contrast and ionizing radiation, and maintain a high sensitivity and specificity.[35] MRA may be a suitable alternative to CTPA in certain clinical settings. MRA is contraindicated in critically ill patients, despite advances in scan times and the potential to move patients out of the magnet for resuscitation.[13] There are also currently limited data to specifically support the use of MRA in children for the diagnosis of PE.

Similar to CTPA, the goal of contrast-enhanced MRA is to adequately opacify the pulmonary arteries to detect filling defects, such as pulmonary emboli.[13] There are various protocols for the MR imaging detection of PE (Table 2), most widely used is an approach by Benson and colleagues[13] using a gadolinium-based contrast agent, gabobenate dimeglumine (Multihance, Bracco Inc, NJ), at 0.1 mmol/kg, diluted with normal saline for

Table 2	
MR imaging protocol for PE (from Boston Children's Hospital)	
Plane	**Sequence**
Axial	TrueFISP
Axial	PROPELLER FSE PD
Coronal	MRA
Axial	VIBE FS

Abbreviations: FS, fat suppression; FSE, fast spine echo; PD, proton density; PROPELLER, periodically rotated overlapping parallel lines with enhanced reconstruction; TrueFISP, true fast imaging with steady state precession; VIBE, volumetric interpolated breath-hold examination.
Contrast – Gadvist (0.1 mL/kg).

total volume of 30 mL, injected at 1.5 mL/s to ensure uniform bolus throughout the pulmonary arteries during the k-space acquisition. After this, proper breath holding and 2-dimensional autocalibrated parallel imaging may be acquired with greater than 3.5× acceleration, shortening acquisition times and breath holds.[13] Similar to the CT bolus tracking technique, autotriggering can be used with rapid 2-dimensional gradient echo technique with a region of interest at the pulmonary outflow tract (using a signal threshold of approximately 20%).[36]

Similar to dual-energy CT imaging, pulmonary perfusion with dynamic contrast-enhanced MRA can be assessed using a rapid volumetric imaging sequence (i.e., 3D spoiled gradient echo time resolved MR imaging) either during a breath hold or shallow breathing.[13] In the case of severe contrast allergy or pregnancy, noncontrast techniques may be used, such as bright blood-balanced steady free precession to assess central and lobar arteries;[35,37] however, contrast-enhanced MRA is superior for evaluation of smaller pulmonary arteries (segmental and subsegmental).

Drawbacks of MRA techniques include longer scanning times, limited utility in pediatric patients unable to breath-hold, a relatively increased cost, and a relative lack of availability compared with CTPA.

Catheter-based conventional angiography

Catheter-based conventional angiography was formerly the gold standard for diagnosis of PE before PIOPED II, which resulted in CTPA being adopted as the gold standard.[7] CTPA has replaced conventional angiography in this regard because conventional angiography is invasive, expensive, and time consuming, with additional risks, including a high ionizing radiation dose, bleeding, infection, and heart block, with morbidity and mortality as high as 4.0% and 0.5%,[38,39] respectively. During conventional angiographic evaluation for PE, a pigtail catheter is advanced into the pulmonary arteries and approximately 10 to 50 mL of low-osmolar nonionic contrast is injected at rates of 10 to 25 mL/s,[7] usually with digital subtraction angiography to assess for filling defects. It is important to note that conventional angiography may be insensitive to the detection of subsegmental PE, with a sensitivity of only 32%,[14] compared with CTPA (which was used as the gold standard). Conventional angiography still plays a crucial role in the diagnosis and treatment of acute massive and submassive PE (hemodynamic instability) with therapeutic and catheter-directed modalities, such as ultrasound-assisted thrombolysis and mechanical embolectomy.[33,34,40,41]

Risk Factor Analysis for Pulmonary Embolism in Children and Young Adults

The incidence of PE in the pediatric population has traditionally been considered low, ranging from 0.73% to 4.20%.[42,43] However, multiple recent studies have found a substantially higher incidence of PE in the pediatric population (16% in patients aged 0–18 years of age)[2] (Table 3) and young adults (14% in patients aged 19–25 years of age)[3] (Table 4) at Boston Children's Hospital and in children and young adults (14% in patients aged 0–21 years) at the Children's Hospital of Philadelphia.[4] Although the general pediatric and young adult population varies widely from the population of patients at tertiary referral centers, clear risk factors and trends have been identified that help to guide the diagnostic approach to the detection of PE in children and young adults. The patients in these studies were very unlikely to have PE unless 1 or more risk factors were present. In addition, in multiple studies of pediatric PE, elevated D-dimer was not found to be statistically significant risk factor for pediatric PE; in fact, elevated D-dimer values did not consistently distinguish pediatric patients with PE from those without,[2,4,44,45] unlike in adults.

At the Children's Hospital of Philadelphia, there were 3 comorbidities that were statistically significantly associated with increased PE risk compared with a matched control group, including surgery or an orthopedic procedure, thrombophilia, and oral contraception use.[4] At Boston Children's Hospital, there were 5 significant independent risk factors for pediatric PE identified, including immobilization, a hypercoagulable state, an excess estrogen state, an indwelling central venous line,

Table 3		
Simplified algorithm of number of risk factors and probability of PE in children (aged 0–18 years)		
No. of Risk Factors[a]	**Probability of PE (%)**	**95% Confidence Interval (%)**
None	0.5	0.1–2.0
Any 1	8	5–15
Any 2	62	46–76
Any 3 or more	89	87–99

[a] Risk factors were immobilization, hypercoagulable state, excess estrogen state, indwelling CVL, and prior PE and/or deep vein thrombosis.

From Lee EY, Tse SKS, Zurakowski D, et al. Children suspected of having pulmonary embolism: multidetector CT pulmonary angiography – thromboembolic risk factors and implications for appropriate use. Radiology 2012; 262(1):249.

and prior PE and/or deep vein thrombosis.[2] The probability of detecting PE in this pediatric population without any of these risk factors was very low (0.5%), and sharply increased from 1 to 2 risk factors present (8% for any one risk factor, 62% for any 2, and 89% for any 3, see **Table 2**).[2] Similarly, in young adults (aged 19–25 years), there was a very low probability of PE without any of these risk factors (0.6%), but a dramatic increase between 1 and 2 risk factors, which varied, depending on the combination of risk factors (see **Table 4**).[3] For example, the combinations of immobilization and cardiac disease or immobilization and prior PE and/or deep vein thrombosis demonstrated an 80.1% or 80.2% risk, respectively, whereas the combination of cardiac disease and prior PE and/or deep vein thrombosis posed a risk of 54.9% and immobilization alone posed a 21.4% chance of PE compared with 7.4% chance with the other 2 risk factors.[3] These risk factors detailed elsewhere in this article had excellent discriminatory value in the diagnosis of PE.

SPECTRUM OF PEDIATRIC PULMONARY EMBOLISM IMAGING FINDINGS
Vascular Findings

Acute pulmonary embolism
Direct radiologic signs of acute PE are similar in children and adults.[1] Three well-described direct radiologic signs are (1) complete pulmonary arterial occlusion via vascular filling defect, in which the filling defect has a lower attenuation (Hounsfield units) than the surrounding contrast-opacified blood with or without lack of opacification in distal br-anches or asymmetric enlargement of the affected pulmonary artery and branches; (2) nonocclusive thrombus with central filling defect and peripheral opacification with contrast (the so-called doughnut sign when seen en face), with our without contrast opacification in distal vessels; and (3) an eccentric int-

raluminal filling defect with acute angle in relationship to the vessel wall (**Figs. 4–7**). PE should be confirmed with at least 2 consecutive slices and in multiple planes.[1] The majority of acute PE tend to be bilateral, segmental, and/or lobar, with a proclivity for the lower lobes, most commonly the right.[3,6] These findings are not as well-described on MRA, but generally hold true across modalities, manifesting on MRA as nonenhancing or low signal intensity filling defects within otherwise opacified pulmonary arteries.[1,13]

Chronic pulmonary embolism
Direct radiologic signs of chronic PE are variable, related to the variety of appearances of recanalization of the pulmonary artery, although some chronic PE do not recanalize.[1,46] Chronic PE may appear to be identical to acute PE, but persist for longer than 3 months. Chronic PE may appear as an eccentric intraluminal filling defect with obtuse angle (as opposed to an acute angle in acute PE), as an occluded vessel compared with adjacent or branching vessels, an intraluminal web, band, or arterial wall thickening or irregular lumen, and may occasionally calcify[1] (**Fig. 8**). These findings are also described similarly in MR imaging/MRA.[13] Poststenotic dilatation of the pulmonary arteries related to partial obstruction, systemic bronchial artery collateralization, and other findings of endothelialized fibrous tissue have been described and are also detected on MR imaging/MRA.[13,47]

Extravascular Findings

Although radiographic secondary signs of PE vary widely in sensitivity and specificity, they may increase the index of suspicion and pretest probability for PE. Radiographic secondary signs of PE include the Westermark sign (focal oligemia), the prominent central pulmonary artery sign (Fleischner sign), and the Hampton hump, a pleural-based

Table 4
Significant independent risk factors for PE in young adults aged 19–25 years

Risk Factor[a]	β Coefficient	Likelihood Ratio Test[b]	P	Odds Ratio (95% Confidence Interval)
Immobilization	3.89	28.6	<.001	49.1 (8.0–300)
Prior PE or DVT	2.69	10.7	.001	14.8 (2.9–92)
Cardiac disease	2.70	8.5	.004	14.9 (2.2–103)

Abbreviations: DVT, deep venous thrombosis.
 [a] Hypercoagulable state ($P = .68$) and central venous line placement ($P = .15$) were tested and not retained in the final multivariable model.
 [b] Based on χ^2 test with 1 degree of freedom.
 From Lee EY, Neuman MI, Lee NJ, et al. Pulmonary Embolism Detected by Pulmonary MDCT Angiography in Older Children and Young Adults: Risk Factor Assessment. *Am J Roentgenol.* 2012;198(6):1431-1437.

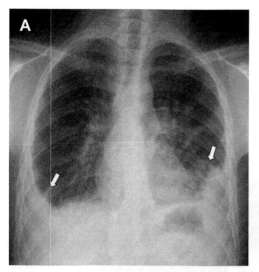
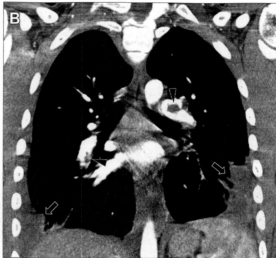
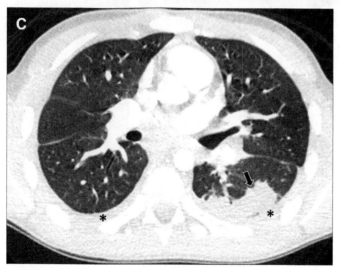

Fig. 4. Pulmonary infracts owing to PE in a 14-year-old boy who presented with shortness of breath and chest pain. (*A*) Frontal chest radiograph shows bilateral peripheral airspace opacities (*arrows*) representing pulmonary infarcts. (*B*) Coronal enhanced CT image demonstrates bilateral PE (*arrowheads*). Also noted are bilateral peripheral airspace opacities (*arrows*) representing pulmonary infarcts. (*C*) Axial lung window CT image shows pulmonary infarcts (*arrow*) and small bilateral pleural effusions (*asterisk*).

wedge-shaped opacity.[12] There are other non-eponynmous signs, such as vascular redistribution, pleural effusion and enlarged hilum, which are nonspecific.[12,22]

Cross-sectional imaging may also be helpful for the detection of extravascular findings of PE. According to Lee and colleagues,[48] the most common lung finding associated with acute PE in children is peripheral wedge-shaped areas of consolidation, likely reflecting pulmonary infarcts. Right heart strain is an important prognostic factor in acute PE, which can be manifest on imaging as straightening of the interventricular septum, right atrial enlargement, and right ventricular dilation with a ratio of the right to left ventricular width on a short axis or 4-chamber view of greater than 1.0.[22]

In chronic PE, indirect radiologic signs are fairly nonspecific, however mosaic attenuation of the affected lung (distal to the chronic PE) secondary to mosaic perfusion is the most common CT lung parenchymal finding.[1] In addition, pulmonary arterial hypertension may manifest as a complication of chronic PE, with right-sided heart enlargement and dilatation of the main pulmonary artery.

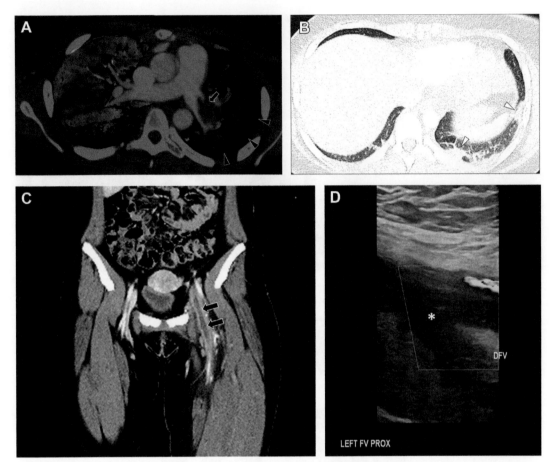

Fig. 5. Pulmonary embolism in a 17-year-old girl with an elevated estrogen level owing to oral contraceptive use who presented with shortness of breath and left groin and upper leg swelling and pain (*A*). Axial enhanced CT image using iodine map (i.e., perfusion CT image) shows a PE (*arrow*) in the left pulmonary artery with perfusion defects (*arrowheads*). (*B*) Axial lung window CT image demonstrates pulmonary infarcts (*arrowheads*) in the left lower lobe. (*C*) Coronal enhanced CT image shows thrombosis (*arrows*) in the left femoral vein. (*D*). Longitudinal Doppler ultrasound examination demonstrates a lack of blood flow (*asterisk*) in the left femoral vein, consistent with thrombosis.

Alternative Diagnoses

There are other acute or chronic entities that can present similarly to PE. When using the Wells criteria in the emergency setting in adults, identifying an alternative cause of symptoms is used to justify a lower clinical suspicion for PE.[8] The added benefit of many of the previously described imaging techniques is the ability to identify an alternative cause, particularly in CTPA, MRA, and radiography. For example, CTPA provides a thorough evaluation of the intrathoracic structures, including the chest wall and portions of the upper abdomen. For example, CTPA frequently identifies an alternative diagnosis when PE is excluded in 59% of children and in 25% of adults with suspected PE.[15,49] In these cases of suspected but excluded PE in children, pneumonia and atelectasis are the most

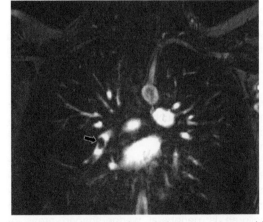

Fig. 6. Pulmonary embolism (PE) in an 18-year-old woman with thrombosis in the right upper extremity who presented with shortness of breath. Coronal MRA image shows a filling defect (*arrow*) in the right inferior pulmonary vein consistent with a PE.

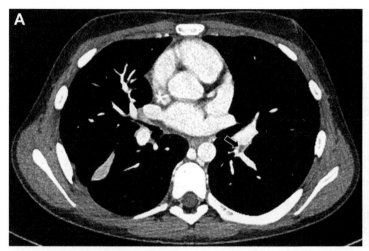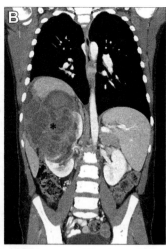

Fig. 7. Incidental pulmonary embolism (PE) in a 12-year-old boy with renal cell carcinoma who presented with chest pain, hematuria, and right flank pain. (*A*) Axial enhanced CT image shows a filling defect (*arrow*), representing the PE in the left pulmonary artery. (*B*) Coronal enhanced CT image demonstrates a large heterogeneous mass (*asterisk*) arising from the right kidney.

common alternative diagnoses made in 39% of cases, and also the 2 most common alternative diagnoses found in adults with suspected but excluded PE.[15,50,51] In addition, pleural effusion is a relatively common alternative diagnosis in up to 30% of cases of clinically suspected but excluded PE, although it is almost always seen in conjunction with pneumonia and/or atelectasis. Lee and colleagues[15] identified additional alternative diagnoses in children with suspected, but excluded PE, including malignancy, congenital heart disease,

fat embolism, pulmonary hypertension, right atrial thrombus, and rib fractures. Although not as well-characterized, MRA has been shown to have similar value in identifying actionable, alternative findings compared with CTPA.[52] Consequently, it is critical to search for alternative diagnoses outside of the pulmonary arteries when reviewing the imaging of patients with clinically suspected PE, especially when using cross-sectional imaging modalities, such as a CT scan and MR imaging.

SUMMARY

PE is more common than previously thought in children and young adults, associated with significant morbidity and mortality, and remains a clinically challenging diagnosis owing to nonspecific symptoms and variable clinical presentation of PE in children. There is a relative paucity of diagnostic algorithms for pediatric PE; however, the use of a pediatric-specific risk factor analysis can help to streamline the diagnostic approach and avoid unnecessary exposure to ionizing radiation in the vulnerable pediatric population. Although CTPA is the preferred imaging modality in diagnosing PE, MRA may be a suitable alternative cross-sectional modality in certain clinical circumstances. Both of these modalities may provide an alternative diagnosis if PE is clinically suspected, but excluded. Advancements in imaging, such as dual-energy CT scans, also provide functional information and increase diagnostic yield, without substantial increase in radiation exposure.

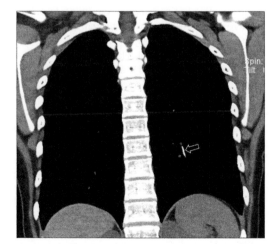

Fig. 8. Calcification in the pulmonary artery owing to chronic pulmonary embolism in a 16-year-old boy. Coronal CT image shows calcification (*arrow*) in the left inferior segmental pulmonary vein.

CLINICS CARE POINTS

- Previously established pediatric-specific independent risk factors should be used to guide the decision to image a pediatric or young adult patient when PE is suspected. The risk of PE substantially increases when one or more risk factors are present.

- CTPA is the preferred imaging modality for the diagnosis of PE in both children and adults. If available, a dual-energy CT scan may increase the detection of peripheral PE.

- An elevated D-dimer is not a statistically significant risk factor for PE in children, and has no predictive value in the pretest probability in the diagnosis of PE in children, unlike in adults.

- MRA may be a suitable alternative to CTPA when CT imaging is contraindicated (severe iodinated contrast allergy or acute kidney injury) that avoids ionizing radiation, but may involve sedation, longer scan times, and decreased availability.

- Although radiographs are neither sensitive nor specific in the diagnosis of PE, they are recommended as a part of the initial evaluation of PE, because they are low cost, low radiation, and may provide an alternative diagnosis.

- V/Q scans are generally not suitable for young children (<5 years of age) or children who cannot follow breathing instructions. V/Q scans are generally only clinically useful when they show a very low or high risk for PE.

- Therapeutic applications of conventional angiography should be explored with interventionalists on a case-by-case basis depending on hemodynamic status. However, conventional angiography is not routinely recommended for the primary diagnosis of PE, given the relatively high associated morbidity and mortality, and improved detection of subsegmental PE with CTPA.

DISCLOSURE

The authors have nothing to disclose.

REFERENCES

1. Thacker PG, Lee EY. Advances in multidetector CT diagnosis of pediatric pulmonary thromboembolism. Korean J Radiol 2016;17(2):198.

2. Lee EY, Tse SKS, Zurakowski D, et al. Children suspected of having pulmonary embolism. Pediatr Imaging 2012;262(1):10.

3. Lee EY, Neuman MI, Lee NJ, et al. Pulmonary embolism detected by pulmonary MDCT angiography in older children and young adults: risk factor assessment. Am J Roentgenol 2012;198(6):1431–7.

4. Victoria T, Mong A, Altes T, et al. Evaluation of pulmonary embolism in a pediatric population with high clinical suspicion. Pediatr Radiol 2009;39(1):35–41.

5. Hennelly KE, Baskin MN, Monuteaux MC, et al. Detection of pulmonary embolism in high-risk children. J Pediatr 2016;178:214–8.e3.

6. Kritsaneepaiboon S, Lee EY, Zurakowski D, et al. MDCT pulmonary angiography evaluation of pulmonary embolism in children. Am J Roentgenol 2009; 192(5):1246–52.

7. Thacker PG, Lee EY. Pulmonary embolism in children. Am J Roentgenol 2015;204(6):1278–88.

8. Wells PS, Anderson DR, Rodger M, et al. Excluding pulmonary embolism at the bedside without diagnostic imaging: management of patients with suspected pulmonary embolism presenting to the emergency department by using a simple clinical model and d-dimer. Ann Intern Med 2001;135(2): 98–107.

9. Kline JA, Wells PS. Methodology for a rapid protocol to rule out pulmonary embolism in the emergency department. Ann Emerg Med 2003;42(2):266–75.

10. Prediction of pulmonary embolism in the emergency department: the Revised Geneva Score | Annals of Internal Medicine. Available at: https://www-acpjournals-org.ezp-prod1.hul.harvard.edu/doi/10.7326/0003-4819-144-3-200602070-00004. Accessed June 23, 2021.

11. Lee EY, Zurakowski D, Boiselle PM. Pulmonary embolism in pediatric patients survey of CT pulmonary angiography practices and policies. Acad Radiol 2010;17(12):1543–9.

12. Worsley DF, Alavi A, Aronchick JM, et al. Chest radiographic findings in patients with acute pulmonary embolism: observations from the PIOPED Study. Radiology 1993;189(1):133–6.

13. Benson DG, Schiebler ML, Nagle SK, et al. Magnetic resonance imaging for the evaluation of pulmonary embolism. Top Magn Reson Imaging 2017;26(4): 145–51.

14. Wittram C, Waltman AC, Shepard J-AO, et al. Discordance between CT and Angiography in the PIOPED II Study. Radiology 2007;244(3):883–9.

15. Lee EY, Kritsaneepaiboon S, Zurakowski D, et al. Beyond the pulmonary arteries: alternative diagnoses in children with MDCT pulmonary angiography negative for pulmonary embolism. Am J Roentgenol 2009;193(3):888–94.

16. Schueller-Weidekamm C, Schaefer-Prokop CM, Weber M, et al. CT angiography of pulmonary arteries to detect pulmonary embolism: improvement of vascular enhancement with low kilovoltage settings. Radiology 2006;241(3):899–907.

17. Lee EY, Zucker EJ, Tsai J, et al. Pulmonary MDCT angiography: value of multiplanar reformatted images in detecting pulmonary embolism in children. Am J Roentgenol 2011;197(6):1460–5.

18. Renne J, Falck C, Ringe KI, et al. CT angiography for pulmonary embolism detection: the effect of breathing on pulmonary artery enhancement using a 64-row detector system. Acta Radiol 2014;55(8):932–7.

19. Bauer RW, Schell B, Beeres M, et al. High-pitch dual-source computed tomography pulmonary angiography in freely breathing patients. J Thorac Imaging 2012;27(6):376–81.

20. Prabhu SP, Mahmood S, Sena L, et al. MDCT evaluation of pulmonary embolism in children and young adults following a lateral tunnel Fontan procedure: optimizing contrast-enhancement techniques. Pediatr Radiol 2009;39(9):938–44.

21. Fishman EK, Ney DR, Heath DG, et al. Volume rendering versus maximum intensity projection in CT angiography: what works best, when, and why. Radiographics 2006;26(3):905–22.

22. Tang CX, Schoepf UJ, Chowdhury SM, et al. Multidetector computed tomography pulmonary angiography in childhood acute pulmonary embolism. Pediatr Radiol 2015;45(10):1431–9.

23. Zhang LJ, Zhou CS, Schoepf UJ, et al. Dual-energy CT lung ventilation/perfusion imaging for diagnosing pulmonary embolism. Eur Radiol 2013;23(10):2666–75.

24. Goo HW. Dual-energy lung perfusion and ventilation CT in children. Pediatr Radiol 2013;43(3):298–307.

25. Thieme SF, Becker CR, Hacker M, et al. Dual energy CT for the assessment of lung perfusion–correlation to scintigraphy. Eur J Radiol 2008;68(3):369–74.

26. Thieme SF, Graute V, Nikolaou K, et al. Dual Energy CT lung perfusion imaging–correlation with SPECT/CT. Eur J Radiol 2012;81(2):360–5.

27. Tang CX, Zhang LJ, Han ZH, et al. Dual-energy CT based vascular iodine analysis improves sensitivity for peripheral pulmonary artery thrombus detection: an experimental study in canines. Eur J Radiol 2013;82(12):2270–8.

28. Davendralingam N, Sebire NJ, Arthurs OJ, et al. Artificial intelligence in paediatric radiology: future opportunities. Br J Radiol 2021;94(1117):20200975.

29. Greulich WW, Pyle SI. Radiographic atlas of skeletal development of the hand and wrist. Stanford (CA): Stanford University Press; 1959.

30. Thodberg HH, Kreiborg S, Juul A, et al. The Bone-Xpert method for automated determination of skeletal maturity. IEEE Trans Med Imaging 2009;28(1):52–66.

31. Weikert T, Winkel DJ, Bremerich J, et al. Automated detection of pulmonary embolism in CT pulmonary angiograms using an AI-powered algorithm. Eur Radiol 2020;30(12):6545–53.

32. Sostman HD, Miniati M, Gottschalk A, et al. Sensitivity and specificity of perfusion scintigraphy combined with chest radiography for acute pulmonary embolism in PIOPED II. J Nucl Med 2008;49(11):1741–8.

33. Patocka C, Nemeth J. Pulmonary embolism in pediatrics. J Emerg Med 2012;42(1):105–16.

34. Zaidi AU, Hutchins KK, Rajpurkar M. Pulmonary embolism in children. Front Pediatr 2017;5:170.

35. Kalb B, Sharma P, Tigges S, et al. MR imaging of pulmonary embolism: diagnostic accuracy of contrast-enhanced 3D MR pulmonary angiography, contrast-enhanced low-flip angle 3D GRE, and non-enhanced free-induction FISP sequences. Radiology 2012;263(1):271–8.

36. Riederer SJ, Bernstein MA, Breen JF, et al. Three-dimensional contrast-enhanced MR angiography with real-time fluoroscopic triggering: design specifications and technical reliability in 330 patient studies. Radiology 2000;215(2):584–93.

37. Herédia V, Altun E, Ramalho M, et al. MRI of pregnant patients for suspected pulmonary embolism: steady-state free precession vs postgadolinium 3D-GRE. Acta Med Port 2012;25(6):359–67.

38. Mills SR, Jackson DC, Older RA, et al. The incidence, etiologies, and avoidance of complications of pulmonary angiography in a large series. Radiology 1980;136(2):295–9.

39. Stein PD, Athanasoulis C, Alavi A, et al. Complications and validity of pulmonary angiography in acute pulmonary embolism. Circulation 1992;85(2):462–8.

40. Navanandan N, Stein J, Mistry RD. Pulmonary embolism in children. Pediatr Emerg Care 2019;35(2):143–51.

41. Bavare AC, Naik SX, Lin PH, et al. Catheter-directed thrombolysis for severe pulmonary embolism in pediatric patients. Ann Vasc Surg 2014;28(7):1794.e1–7.

42. Byard RW, Cutz E. Sudden and unexpected death in infancy and childhood due to pulmonary thromboembolism. An autopsy study. Arch Pathol Lab Med 1990;114(2):142–4.

43. Buck JR, Connors RH, Coon WW, et al. Pulmonary embolism in children. J Pediatr Surg 1981;16(3):385–91.

44. Rajpurkar M, Warrier I, Chitlur M, et al. Pulmonary embolism-experience at a single children's hospital. Thromb Res 2007;119(6):699–703.

45. Biss TT, Brandão LR, Kahr WHA, et al. Clinical probability score and D-dimer estimation lack utility in the diagnosis of childhood pulmonary embolism. J Thromb Haemost 2009;7(10):1633–8.

46. Castañer E, Gallardo X, Ballesteros E, et al. CT diagnosis of chronic pulmonary thromboembolism. Radiographics 2009;29(1):31–50.

47. Doğan H, de Roos A, Geleijins J, et al. The role of computed tomography in the diagnosis of acute and chronic pulmonary embolism. Diagn Interv Radiol Ank Turk 2015;21(4):307–16.

48. Lee EY, Zurakowski D, Diperna S, et al. Parenchymal and pleural abnormalities in children with and without pulmonary embolism at MDCT pulmonary angiography. Pediatr Radiol 2010;40(2):173–81.

49. Strijen MJLV, Bloem JL, Monyé WD, et al. Helical computed tomography and alternative diagnosis in patients with excluded pulmonary embolism. J Thromb Haemost 2005;3(11):2449–56.

50. Shah AA, Davis SD, Gamsu G, et al. Parenchymal and pleural findings in patients with and patients without acute pulmonary embolism detected at Spiral CT. Radiology 1999;211(1):147–53.

51. Tsai K-L, Gupta E, Haramati LB. Pulmonary atelectasis: a frequent alternative diagnosis in patients undergoing CT-PA for suspected pulmonary embolism. Emerg Radiol 2004;10(5):282–6.

52. Schiebler ML, Ahuja J, Repplinger MD, et al. Incidence of actionable findings on contrast enhanced magnetic resonance angiography ordered for pulmonary embolism evaluation. Eur J Radiol 2016; 85(8):1383–9.

53. Hayashino Y, Goto M, Noguchi Y, et al. Ventilation-perfusion scanning and helical CT in suspected pulmonary embolism: meta-analysis of diagnostic performance. Radiology 2005;234(3):740–8.

54. Stein PD, Fowler SE, Goodman LR, et al. Multidetector computed tomography for acute pulmonary embolism. N Engl J Med 2006;354(22):2317–27.

55. Patel S, Kazerooni EA, Cascade PN. Pulmonary embolism: optimization of small pulmonary artery visualization at multi-detector row CT. Radiology 2003; 227(2):455–60.

56. Coche E, Verschuren F, Keyeux A, et al. Diagnosis of acute pulmonary embolism in outpatients: comparison of thin-collimation multi-detector row spiral CT and planar ventilation-perfusion scintigraphy. Radiology 2003;229(3):757–65.

57. Qanadli SD, Hajjam ME, Mesurolle B, et al. Pulmonary embolism detection: prospective evaluation of dual-section helical CT versus selective pulmonary arteriography in 157 patients. Radiology 2000; 217(2):447–55.

58. Winer-Muram HT, Rydberg J, Johnson MS, et al. Suspected acute pulmonary embolism: evaluation with multi-detector row CT versus digital subtraction pulmonary arteriography. Radiology 2004;233(3):806–15.

Childhood Interstitial Lung Disease
Imaging Guidelines and Recommendations

Thomas Semple, MDres, FRCR, MBBS, BSc[a], Abbey J. Winant, MD[b],
Edward Y. Lee, MD, MPH[b],*

KEYWORDS

- Childhood interstitial lung disease (ChILD) • Imaging study • Computed tomography
- Classification system • Infant • Children

KEY POINTS

- Childhood interstitial lung disease (ChILD) is an umbrella term referring to a diverse group of diffuse lung diseases occurring in childhood.
- ChILD differs in appearance from adult ILD with common, important confounding features that must be recognized, which include respiratory motion mimicking ground glass opacification and reversible "bronchiectasis" in the context of acute or recent viral infection.
- Computed tomography (CT) remains the current gold standard imaging modality for the confirmation and characterization of suspected ChILD after chest radiography because of its high sensitivity and increased likelihood of providing a specific diagnosis.
- Optimal CT technique is crucial to ChILD imaging with diagnostic-quality CT images often possible in free-breathing nonsedated infants.
- A clear understanding of the characteristic imaging findings of certain ChILD entities is imperative for timely diagnosis and optimal patient management.

INTRODUCTION

Childhood interstitial lung disease (ChILD) is an umbrella term encompassing a diverse group of diffuse lung diseases affecting infants and children. Although the timely and accurate diagnosis of ChILD is often challenging, it is optimally achieved through the multidisciplinary integration of imaging findings with clinical data, genetics, and possibly lung biopsy. This article reviews the definition and classification of ChILD; the role of imaging, pathology, and genetics in ChILD diagnosis; treatment options; and future goals. In addition, a practical approach to ChILD imaging based on the latest available research and the characteristic imaging appearance of ChILD entities are presented.

CHILDHOOD INTERSTITIAL LUNG DISEASE DEFINITION AND CLASSIFICATION

The term *interstitial lung disease* (ILD) refers to a large, heterogeneous group of diffuse parenchymal lung diseases. In adult practice, these conditions are generally well characterized. Adult ILDs are broadly divided into 3 groups: (1) the major idiopathic interstitial pneumonias such as idiopathic pulmonary fibrosis (IPF), nonspecific interstitial pneumonia (NSIP), organizing pneumonia, etc; (2) the rare idiopathic interstitial pneumonias such as

a Department of Radiology, The Royal Brompton Hospital, London and Centre for Paediatrics and Child Health, Imperial College London, Sydney Street, London SW3 6NP, UK; b Department of Radiology, Boston Children's Hospital, Harvard Medical School, Boston, MA 02115, USA
* Corresponding author.
E-mail address: Edward.Lee@childrens.harvard.edu

Radiol Clin N Am 60 (2022) 83–111
https://doi.org/10.1016/j.rcl.2021.08.009
0033-8389/22/© 2021 Elsevier Inc. All rights reserved.

lymphocytic interstitial pneumonia (LIP) and pleuroparenchymal fibroelastosis (PPFE); and (3) the unclassifiable idiopathic interstitial pneumonias.[1]

In adult ILD, the diagnostic emphasis is on distinguishing fibrotic from inflammatory entities, in particular distinguishing the specific diagnosis of IPF—defined by the histologic pattern known as *usual interstitial pneumonia* (UIP)—from other ILD diagnoses.[1–3] The underlying need for this distinction is based on well-established evidence of differences in prognosis and, more recently, differences in treatment of each condition.

A comparative study published in 2000 is an important example of the evidence required to advance adult ILD care to its current state. Nicholson and colleagues[4] reviewed the histopathology specimens from 78 patients diagnosed with cryptogenic fibrosing alveolitis (CFA) in the late 1970s to the 1980s. CFA is a now an outdated term more recently subdivided into separate specific entities, and as such Nicholson and colleagues[4] reclassified these patients into UIP, NSIP, and desquamative interstitial pneumonia/respiratory bronchiolitis-associated interstitial lung disease (DIP/RBILD, the smoking-related ILDs) diagnoses. More than 85% of the patients they examined had clinical follow-up to death or to 10 years postbiopsy, with significantly higher mortality demonstrated in UIP than NSIP ($P<.01$), no deaths in the DIP/RBILD group, and more frequent treatment response in DIP/RBILD than in either NSIP or UIP ($P<.01$ and $<.001$, respectively).[4] This distinction in diagnosis and the accompanying knowledge of prognosis and expected treatment response is of critical value to those involved in adult ILD care.

Unfortunately, the knowledge and evidence base available to those working with ILD in the pediatric population is a very different story. Childhood ILD (neatly abbreviated as ChILD) is an umbrella term encompassing more than 200 rare diffuse lung diseases that affect children.[5] Although variably reported, the incidence of ChILD is less than 1 per 100,000 population, 60 to 80 times less frequent than adult ILD.[6,7] Although a few specific ILD diagnoses are common to both adults and children, the disease severity and clinical course are often different and there are many ILD diagnoses unique to the pediatric population.[8] As such, the classification of ChILD differs from adult ILD classification systems. In 2007, Deutsch and colleagues[8] devised a classification system distinguishing between ChILD entities based on patient age at presentation, dividing conditions into those that generally present in infancy and those that are not specific to infancy (**Box 1**).

This classification system was revisited and recommended for routine use by the 2013 American Thoracic Society (ATS) clinical practice guidelines.[9] Griese and colleagues[10] tested the classification system by assigning diagnoses to 100 randomly selected patients from the "Kids Lung Register," the registry of the European ChILD-EU initiative. Cases were initially classified based on a multidisciplinary team of subspecialty pediatric pulmonologists, radiologists, and pathologists. Reclassification of these same patients several years later by 2 pediatric pulmonologists demonstrated more than 80% agreement with initial diagnoses.[10] Just as in adult ILD practice, this multidisciplinary approach to ChILD diagnosis is critical to accurate and reproducible classification of individual ChILD diagnoses, requiring integration of all available information from clinical history, laboratory tests, imaging, bronchoalveolar lavage (BAL), and lung biopsy. This fact is highlighted by a study by Jacobs and colleagues[11] in which experienced subspecialty expert ChILD radiologists and pulmonologists categorized 84 ChILD

Box 1
The 2007 childhood interstitial lung disease classification from Deutsch and colleagues as part of the US Children's Interstitial and Diffuse Lung Disease Research Network

1. Disorders more prevalent in infancy
   a. Diffuse developmental disorders
   b. Lung growth abnormalities
   c. Specific conditions of undefined etiology
   d. Surfactant dysfunction mutations and related disorders

2. Disorders not specific to infancy
   a. Disorders of the normal host
   b. Disorders related to systemic disease processes
   c. Disorders of the immunocompromised host
   d. Disorders masquerading as interstitial lung disease

3. Unclassified

Data from Deutsch, G. H., Young, L. R., Deterding, R. R., Fan, L. L., Dell, S. D., Bean, J. A., Brody, A. S., Nogee, L. M., Trapnell, B. C., Langston, C., Albright, E. A., Askin, F. B., Baker, P., Chou, P. M., Cool, C. M., Coventry, S. C., Cutz, E., Davis, M. M., Dishop, M. K., Galambos, C., Patterson, K., Travis, W. D., Wert, S. E. & White, F. V. Diffuse lung disease in young children: Application of a novel classification scheme. *Am. J. Respir. Crit. Care Med.* 2007; **176**: 1120 – 1128

cases into broad groups and then more specific etiologies, based solely on imaging appearance with no further clinical information. Compared with the 80% agreement in the multidisciplinary study of Griese and colleagues,[10] this CT-alone approach yielded, at best, fair interobserver agreement in diagnosis, with Fleiss kappa values ranging from 0.16 to 0.44.[11] Consequently, a multidisciplinary approach to ChILD classification is critical for the accurate diagnosis and understanding of disease processes.

THE ROLE OF IMAGING, GENETICS, AND PATHOLOGY IN CHILDHOOD INTERSTITIAL LUNG DISEASE DIAGNOSIS

The 2013 ATS guidelines present 3 diagnostic algorithms, 2 for infants presenting with severe respiratory disease in the neonatal period (altered depending on the presence or absence of a family history of ILD) and 1 for children presenting after 1 month of age. All three algorithms for ChILD diagnosis feature imaging early in the diagnostic pathway, as soon as more common non-ChILD diagnoses (infection, cardiovascular disease, immunodeficiency, cystic fibrosis, and aspiration) have been excluded.

Genetic testing is a more recent addition to the multidisciplinary ChILD diagnostic process. Genetic testing is of increasing importance, particularly when ChILD presents in infancy and even more so when there is a strong family history. The aim of both imaging and genetic studies is to arrive at a specific diagnosis without invasive testing, with each algorithm ending with surgical lung biopsy if no specific diagnosis can otherwise be reached.

Even if imaging does not lead to a specific ChILD diagnosis, its role in multidisciplinary practice remains a key factor. Many diffuse lung diseases demonstrate nonhomogeneous lung involvement with geographic regions of sparing or differing disease patterns. Consequently, prebiopsy imaging is vital to guide the surgeon to an area of involved lung and in the subsequent interpretation of biopsy results.[12]

A 2004 study by a European Respiratory Society task force identified ChILD cases across Europe, examining among other things, the success of the diagnostic pathway. Of 185 patients, a specific diagnosis was reached in 177 (96%), with diagnosis reached without surgical biopsy in 78 (45%).[13] The success of noninvasive diagnosis in any cohort clearly depends on the prevalence of individual disease entities contained therein. In addition, one major, albeit understandable, limitation of ChILD research to date is the paucity of studies into the diagnosis and management of individual ChILD entities, with many studies investigating the prognosis and treatment responses of ChILD as a single entity.

TREATMENT OPTIONS AND FUTURE GOALS

Because such a broad variety of entities fall under the umbrella term ChILD, it is not helpful to consider treatment of ChILD as a single diagnosis. However, the rarity of individual diagnoses and the relatively recent application and availability of genetic studies severely limits the ability to reach the level of evidence-based practice seen in adult ILD care. Outside of a few specific ChILD disorders with specific treatments (mostly those with rheumatologic associations), the mainstay of ChILD treatment includes reduction in inflammation with corticosteroids, hydroxychloroquine, and azithromycin; supportive care with oxygen, noninvasive and invasive ventilation, extracorporeal membrane oxygenation (ECMO), and transplantation; and preventative measures, such as management of chronic aspiration and/or reflux, routine immunizations, and the avoidance of exposure to air pollutants.[7,14]

Future imaging goals include larger, multicenter, and international cohort studies of the imaging features of specific individual ChILD entities, complete with extensive clinical characterization (including detailed genetic analysis), to enable better understanding of the clinical significance of differing imaging phenotypes. Any cohort study across international borders is likely to include numerous different scanners and different scan protocols, and to attempt to standardize computed tomographic (CT) imaging for ChILD would likely result in a "race to the bottom" with suboptimal imaging quality on older scanners and far higher than necessary doses on newer scanners. Rather, a focus on site-specific tailoring of CT protocols, with input from medical physics experts and routine image quality and dose audit, is likely to result in appropriate diagnostic quality imaging being achieved. Furthermore, it can subsequently enable analysis and comparison across centers. ChILD-specific organizations, such as ChILD-EU and the US Children's Interstitial and Diffuse Lung Disease Research Network (ChILDRN), are likely to play a key role in enabling sufficient cross-border collaboration for the formation of sufficiently large patient cohorts.

A review of imaging technique and of the imaging features of specific ChILD disorders follows. Based on the aforementioned facts, our suggested algorithm for the investigation of suspected ChILD is presented in **Fig. 1**.

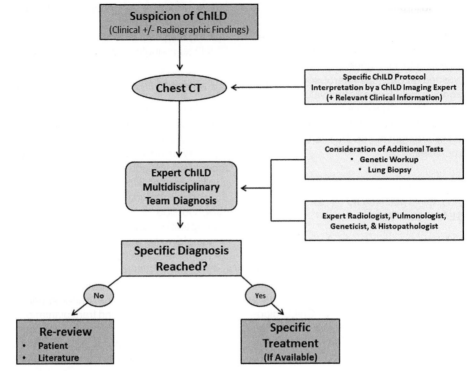

Fig. 1. Suggested diagnostic algorithm for evaluating ChILD.

PRACTICAL IMAGING APPROACH TO PEDIATRIC INTERSTITIAL LUNG DISEASE

Various imaging modalities are currently available with radiography and CT as the 2 most important and widely available imaging modalities for evaluating ChILD. A brief summary of their current roles along with relevant advantages and disadvantages are discussed in the following section.

Radiography

The chest radiograph is the most commonly performed respiratory imaging investigation worldwide, providing a single image overview of the entire thorax. In both children and adults, the sensitivity of chest radiography to ILD is lower than that of CT, with normal radiographic appearances of ChILD at initial presentation variably reported in 10% to 42% of children with later proven ILD.[15,16] However, it is often the radiographic appearance that leads to further more sensitive and specific cross-sectional imaging evaluation of ChILD.[15,16] In clinical practice, it is rare to encounter a request for CT for suspected ChILD without a prior chest radiograph for reference. Although less detailed than CT, a diagnostic-quality chest radiograph can provide an easily available, low dose form of follow-up imaging without the higher ionizing radiation exposure that would be required for frequent

follow-up via CT. Therefore, chest radiography should be reviewed before initial CT assessment and considered as the first-line follow-up imaging modality in the absence of substantial clinical decline of children with ILD.

There are several clinically relevant diagnoses that can be made on chest radiography in the setting of suspected ChILD. For example, when the diffuse granular appearance of typical surfactant deficiency of prematurity is seen in a term neonate, this may suggest underlying congenital surfactant dysfunction (eg, SPFB or adenosine triphosphate-binding cassette transporter A3 [ABCA3] mutations). In premature infants, chronic lung disease of prematurity, previously known as *bronchopulmonary dysplasia* (BPD), has an almost pathognomonic radiographic appearance characterized by alternating foci of hyperinflation and atelectasis, nearly as readily appreciable on chest radiography as on CT.[17] Another radiographic appearance worth mentioning is that of atelectasis and coarse peribronchial thickening with a bilateral lower lobe and right upper lobe distribution, an appearance often encountered in the setting of chronic aspiration. Aspiration alone can present as respiratory distress mimicking ChILD, but perhaps more clinically importantly, feeding issues are reported in as many as 73% of patients with a ChILD diagnosis with 35% requiring long-term gastrostomy feeding and 14% reporting oral aversion suggesting the possibility of chronic aspiration.[18] If undiagnosed and/or left untreated, chronic aspiration is a substantial additional risk to patients with ChILD.

Given the aforementioned facts, the roles of chest radiography in ChILD assessment include (1) initial suggestion of a ChILD diagnosis, (2) primary evaluation of disease distribution and appearance before CT imaging is available, (3) investigation of extrapulmonary features of specific ChILD entities, (4) detection of features of chronic aspiration (as a primary or exacerbating pathologic condition), and (5) as a follow-up evaluation imaging modality (ideally as part of a routine assessment akin to the annual evaluation in cystic fibrosis care). It is important to recognize that, given the reduced relative sensitivity and specificity, a normal chest radiograph should not be seen as excluding ChILD and CT should always be performed where there is ongoing clinical suspicion in the clinical setting of persistent or worsening symptoms.

Computed Tomography

As discussed previously, the superior anatomic detail provided by CT in combination with utilization of multiplanar reformats and 3D reconstructions leads to a far higher sensitivity for the diagnosis of ChILD compared with chest radiography. Furthermore, if lung biopsy is required, CT can guide the surgeon to an appropriate biopsy site, limiting the possibility of a nondiagnostic or nonrepresentative biopsy sample.[9,16]

While the ATS guidelines emphasize the important role of CT as the gold-standard imaging modality in ChILD diagnosis, there have been some advances, particularly in CT technique. The ATS guidelines recommend the use of "controlled ventilation high-resolution CT," with deep breaths delivered to a sedated child via a mask; this results in a short period of apnea during which imaging can be acquired with minimal respiratory motion.[19] Modern CT scanners are now far faster than their historic equivalents with top-end CT scanners capable of imaging the entire thorax of an adult in a fraction of a second.[20] In infants and small children, this means that it is now possible to acquire diagnostic-quality lung imaging during free breathing, without the need for sedation. It is well known that sedation and anesthesia result in the rapid accumulation of atelectasis in the dependent portion of the lungs, obscuring underlying pathologic conditions and mimicking the appearance of chronic aspiration (Fig. 2). Awake, free-breathing imaging can eliminate this risk and ensures that the resultant CT images demonstrate the lungs in their normal physiologic state.

If anesthesia is required, for example, in noncompliant patients, typically age 2-5 years old or those with developmental delay, or when utilizing a CT scanner that is not capable of sufficiently rapid imaging), the use of lung recruitment maneuvers before CT imaging is essential in reducing dependent atelectasis and maximizing the quality of the CT. At the Royal Brompton Hospital, if anaesthesia is required, a standard CT protocol for ChILD involves at least 4 slow lung inflations followed by a held inspiration at around 25 cm H_2O at the time of inspiratory CT imaging.

The ATS guidelines also mention the use of additional prone and decubitus positioning.[19,21,22] Decubitus imaging can be useful in producing expiratory imaging in noncompliant pediatric patients (the more dependent lung is relatively expiratory compared with the nondependant lung), and prone imaging is occasionally used to reduce dependent atelectasis at the lung bases from mimicking subtle subpleural ground glass opacification. The inclusion of expiratory imaging in ChILD CT protocols is a current topic of debate. In the context of constrictive/obliterative bronchiolitis (COB), for example, as a complication of prior adenovirus infection or as a manifestation of graft-versus-host disease (GVHD), expiratory CT imaging is useful in demonstrating subtle mosaic attenuation. However, if this appearance is demonstrated on the inspiratory CT images, additional expiratory CT imaging adds little more than extra radiation exposure and should be reserved for research settings where low attenuation is being quantified at a strictly controlled point in the respiratory cycle, ideally with the use of spirometer guidance.[23] In general, if COB is not the expected diagnosis, the routine inclusion of expiratory imaging in ChILD protocols may not be necessary. Prone positioning is almost never required in pediatric ILD imaging.

Along with improvements in the speed of CT acquisitions, there have been substantial reductions in the radiation dose required for diagnostic CT imaging. Modern CT scanners use advanced forms of 3D tube current modulation, kilovolt selection, and reconstruction algorithms that produce diagnostic-quality CT images from doses that would result in nondiagnostic, heavily noise-affected CT images using conventional CT image reconstruction methods. This improvement has led to the advent of low- and ultralow-dose CT protocols for lung imaging. Although these low dose CT techniques are useful for clinical settings in which low-resolution imaging is appropriate (eg, cystic fibrosis, infection, lung cancer screening in adults), it is the high-resolution capabilities of CT that make it central to the diagnosis of ChILD. As such, it is appropriate to have a slightly higher

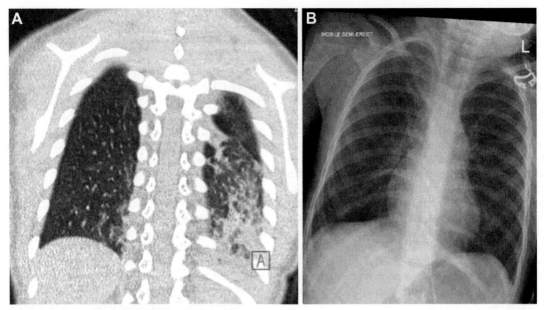

Fig. 2. Effect of sedation or general anesthesia on lung inflation in a 3-year-old male. (*A*) Coronal lung window CT image through the posterior, dependent portions of the lungs. Despite the anesthetic being "light" enough for spontaneous ventilation via a laryngeal mask airway, the degree of sedation is enough to decrease inspiratory effort and result in the substantial dependent atelectasis demonstrated. (*B*) Frontal chest radiograph obtained 1 day before CT demonstrates clear lungs, suggesting that the atelectasis seen on CT (*A*) is not pathologic. The use of recruitment maneuvers before CT acquisition can reduce the likelihood of sedation- or general anaesthesia-related atelectasis.

radiation dose, higher diagnostic yield, and higher confidence protocol specifically for use in the initial diagnosis of ChILD (ie, a single diagnostic-quality CT is preferred to an initial low-dose non-diagnostic CT that must be repeated because of too low radiation dose or overinterpretation of apparent diffuse ground glass opacification due to increased noise (**Fig. 3**). The Royal Brompton Hospital's pediatric pulmonary CT protocols are included in **Table 1**. CT scan parameters should be matched to individual CT scanners with the input of a local medical physics expert. The inclusion of these protocols in this article is merely intended to demonstrate a tailored approach to pulmonary CT protocols.

The goals of CT studies in children with suspected ChILD include confirmation of the presence of an ILD, demonstration of imaging findings of specific ChILD diagnoses, and guidance of potential future surgical biopsy. Specific diagnoses and their imaging appearances of ChILD are further discussed in the following sections; however, the imaging features of fibrotic disease bear mention here. In adult ILD, imaging features such as traction bronchiectasis, architectural distortion, volume loss (generally appreciated by displacement of the interlobar fissures), and the presence of honeycombing are generally accepted as being in keeping with the

presence of a fibrotic ILD.[24] Several key differences between adult ILD and ChILD disease processes and imaging features are important to keep in mind. The presence of acute infection at the time of imaging may result in the appearance of bronchial dilatation, thickening, ground glass opacification, and mosaic attenuation, closely mimicking the appearance of COB (**Fig. 4**). Therefore, it is crucial to avoid diagnostic imaging for the evaluation for ChILD during times of acute infection if the imaging is specifically intended to characterize an ILD.

Another crucial consideration is normal growth and development. Progression in the severity or extent of imaging features in adult ILD is taken as evidence of progression of the causative disease process.[24] However, in childhood, it is quite feasible that a single insult to the lung in infancy may be followed by substantial changes in the subsequent imaging appearance throughout childhood, not necessarily due to progression of disease, but possibly secondary to progression of lung growth around static disease. At present, very little longitudinal imaging data exist to characterize the expected imaging progression of ChILD, and consequently it is challenging to use structural imaging alone as the solitary means of assessing disease progression or treatment response in the setting of an interventional trial. Imaging

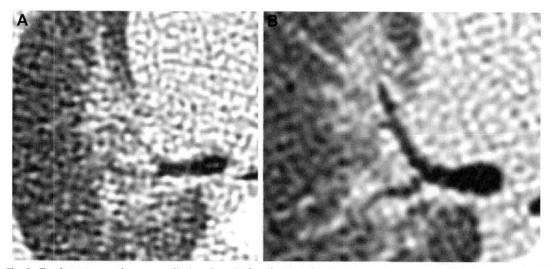

Fig. 3. Too low versus adequate radiation dose CT for ChILD evaluation in a male newborn. Axial CT images (A, B) on the same window width and level, using the same reconstruction Kernel, both acquired at 80kV on a Siemens Definition FLASH CT scanner (Siemens, Erlangen, Germany). The ILD protocol (*B*) used 20 mAs compared with16 mAs (*A*) on the initial acquisition, with a resultant DLP of 5 mGy.cm versus 4 mGy.cm (CTDIvol 0.34 vs 0.27). Although the change of mAs is small, the difference in image quality in a newborn is substantial. (*A*) Low-dose CT protocol (designed for evaluation of cystic fibrosis) mistakenly used in a 13-day-old boy with suspected ILD. Axial lung window CT image demonstrates too much image noise for confident assessment, particularly for distinguishing true ground glass opacification from respiratory motion artifact and image noise. (*B*) Repeat CT the next day using a specific ChILD protocol (higher tube current), less affected by noise and more convincingly demonstrating peribronchial ground glass opacification with mild associated bronchial distortion. The patient was later found to have a surfactant protein B mutation.

appearance must be interpreted in tandem with clinical markers of disease severity (**Fig. 5**).

A further relevant consideration when reporting CT findings in the setting of a ChILD is the importance of standardized language. The Fleischner Society glossary of terms, published in 2008, provides a set of internationally agreed upon terms and definitions that are essential to the classification of disease and the reproducibility of ILD imaging diagnosis. Varied use of terminology between adult and pediatric ILD imaging can become the source of considerable confusion. For example, the Fleischner Society definition of honeycombing includes "usually subpleural" "clustered cystic airspaces" and specifically mentions the need for caution in using the term because it is considered a specific imaging finding of UIP pattern fibrosis and its presence may impact patient care.[25] One common pitfall to avoid is the misinterpretation of cysts seen in surfactant protein dysfunction as honeycombing, particularly by those less familiar with adult ILD practice; this has the potential to be misleading because the UIP pattern fibrosis seen in adult fibrotic lung disease is almost never encountered in pediatric ILD.

A retrospective review of biopsies of children with ChILD secondary to surfactant protein C mutations demonstrated 2 patterns of disease on histology: (1) alveolar macrophage accumulation with inflammatory cells and cholesterol clefts, type II pneumatocyte hyperplasia, and alveolar septal thickening by mesenchymal cells and lymphocytes and (2) respiratory bronchiole and duct dilatation with muscular hyperplasia. None demonstrated interstitial fibrosis, but cysts were demonstrated on CT in 40% at presentation and paraseptal emphysema in 13% with new cyst formation or increased cyst extent demonstrated on follow-up CT in most patients.[26] Furthermore, although highly variable, the life expectancy and expected clinical course of children and adults with genetic disorders of surfactant function is generally different to the rapid decline seen in adults with progressive fibrosis as part of IPF. Therefore, the term *honeycombing* should be avoided in pediatric practice outside of those rare occasions in which multiple layers of subpleural cysts (adult pattern of UIP fibrosis) are demonstrated.

Ultrasonography

There is a growing trend, particularly among emergency and intensive care practitioners, of using ultrasonography as a primary modality for lung imaging, using the presence of differing artifacts (eg, ring-down or reverberation artifacts) at the pleural surface

Table 1
Royal Brompton Hospital thoracic CT protocol parameters in children and adults

Protocol	Parameters
Low dose	Free breathing 80 kV CareDose On: QrefmAs 80 Pitch 3
0–10 kg ILD	Free breathing 80 kV CareDose On: QrefmAs 150 Pitch 3
10–50 kg ILD	Breath hold if compliant, otherwise free breathing 100 kV CareDose On: QrefmAs 130 Pitch 3
Adult ILD	Breath hold at full inspiration 120 kV CareDose On: QrefmAs 110 Pitch 0.6

The pediatric acquisitions are high-pitch dual-source spiral scans to reduce respiratory motion artifact in free breathing children. Lower-pitch scanning in more compliant adults allows higher signal-to-noise ratio and an appearance more akin to traditional high-resolution CT, but is susceptible to respiratory motion artifact and, as such, requires reliable breath holding. Note that infants are scanned at low kV, but that the ILD protocol has a significantly higher tube current than the low-dose protocol, resulting in a better signal-to-noise ratio and more confident assessment of subtle parenchymal disease and differentiation of ground glass opacification from respiratory motion artifact.

as a surrogate for the presence or absence of underlying lung disease.[27] Although the technique may have some merits in low-resource settings, its inability to distinguish ILD from any other pathologic entity expanding the interstitium (eg, pulmonary edema or subsegmental atelectasis) renders it completely inadequate for the assessment of suspected ChILD (Fig. 6).

There is, however, a clear role for ultrasonography in the assessment of extrapulmonary disease, which may in some cases prove vital to forming a specific diagnosis. Examples include (1) thymic and thyroid lesions that may be present in infantile Langerhans cell histiocytosis (LCH), (2) duodenal dilatation often seen in alveolar capillary dysplasia, (3) enlarged peripheral lymph nodes and hepatosplenomegaly characteristic of immunodeficiencies and hematologic malignancy, and (4) calcified liver lesions seen in Gaucher disease.[28–30] In any patient presenting with ChILD with no specific diagnosis reached via CT, ultrasound examination of any relevant extrapulmonary viscera should be considered.

MR Imaging

Although pulmonary imaging by MR imaging has historically been limited by poor signal, high levels of susceptibility artifact at air-tissue interfaces, and the need for general anesthesia, there has been substantial advancement in the field of pulmonary MR imaging in recent years.[31–37] Follow-up of structural lung abnormality by MR imaging is becoming more commonplace in the setting of specific lung diseases with gross structural pathology, particularly the bronchiectasis, marked bronchial wall thickening, and mucous plugging encountered in cystic fibrosis.[31] The subtler structural abnormalities encountered in the setting of ChILD (eg, ground glass opacification and thin-walled pulmonary cysts) is far more difficult to appreciate with a conventional MR imaging scanner, but the recent advent of a low-field-strength (0.55 T) clinical MR unit with modern coil technology and sequences offers potential for the demonstration of structural ILD features in the near future.[38] However, at present, the far higher spatial resolution of CT and the ability to perform ultrafast free breathing imaging even in newborns mean that MR imaging is unlikely to replace CT as the gold-standard imaging modality for the detection of ChILD for the foreseeable future. Instead, rather than structural assessment, arguably the most appealing use of MR imaging in the setting of ChILD research is the application of ventilation and pulmonary perfusion MR imaging techniques.

Methods of imaging ventilation via MR include the use of hyperpolarized noble gases, fluorinated gases, or even oxygen as contrast agents. Oxygen is weakly paramagnetic in its dissolved state and changes in signal result from local partial pressure of oxygen. Fluorinated and hyperpolarized gasses have the advantage of providing signal without being dissolved in fluid within the lungs, therefore providing a pure ventilation signal (oxygen-enhanced MR imaging outputs are a composite of ventilation and perfusion). Both oxygen and fluorinated gasses can be used to produce maps of ventilation and relative times for gas wash in and washout, akin to those measured via multiple breath washout lung function testing, likely of more use in airways disease than in ILD imaging.[39–46]

An advantage of hyperpolarized noble gas imaging is the ability to quantify microscopic motion of a tracer gas within space. This imaging has been used to measure the size of individual airspaces with studies able to demonstrate catchup alveolarization far later in development than was previously thought possible in a cohort of teenagers with a history of premature birth.[47] Furthermore,

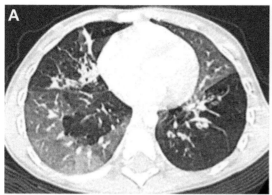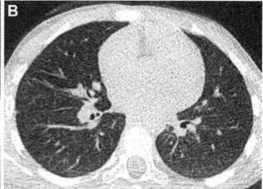

Fig. 4. CT imaging during active infection in a 2-year-old female referred for review of imaging. The provided clinical history was "adenovirus infection, suspected constrictive obliterative bronchiolitis." (*A*) Axial lung window CT image shows extensive low attenuation areas (air-trapping) with bronchial dilatation, wall thickening, and mucous plugging. Although the CT imaging appearance is in keeping with constrictive obliterative bronchiolitis, it became clear that the initial CT had been acquired at the time of the acute, severe adenovirus bronchiolitis. (*B*) Axial lung window follow-up CT image obtained several years later demonstrates complete interval resolution of the CT findings in (*A*). Constrictive obliterative bronchiolitis (COB) is an irreversible condition, and the prior CT appearance was clearly secondary to acute bronchiolitis, not COB; this highlights the importance of interpreting CT imaging findings within their clinical context as well as avoiding CT imaging for ChILD assessment during times of acute infection, risking the inappropriate labeling of a patient with ChILD.

the Larmor frequency of xenon shifts as it changes in state from gaseous to dissolved form, and again as it binds to hemoglobin. This shift has allowed in vivo, spatially localized measurements of the process of gaseous diffusion at the alveolar membrane in healthy and diseased lungs, including adults with IPF.[48–50] Although access to hyperpolarized gas MR imaging is currently limited to a handful of research centers worldwide, it is likely that the technique, alongside other methods of ventilation MR imaging, will have a substantial impact on the future of pulmonary imaging in both adult and pediatric patient populations.

Pulmonary perfusion can also be imaged in several different ways. Contrast media can be injected with static or dynamic MR acquisitions demonstrating pulmonary arterial and parenchymal enhancement, often forming part of routine assessment in adults with pulmonary hypertension. Arterial spin labeling has also been used as a noncontrast method of pulmonary vascular imaging in children. Fourier decomposition imaging is another noncontrast MR technique for assessing ventilation and pulmonary perfusion in children by using the amplitude of signal changes at respiratory and pulse frequencies to form maps of pulmonary ventilation and perfusion without any injected or inhaled contrast media, requiring only 15 seconds per free breathing acquisition.[51,52]

Last, MR lymphangiography is an increasingly well-established technique for assessing the pulmonary lymphatic system. Noncontrast techniques allow structural assessment of the central lymphatic system, and dynamic acquisitions following intranodal administration of contrast media are able to demonstrate the rate and direction of lymphatic flow (**Fig. 7**). In fact, MR imaging is now capable of identifying pulmonary lymphatic pathology, such as lymphangiectasia and lymphangiomatosis, in fetal life with further characterization possible when contrast media can be delivered as a newborn.[53–55]

Nuclear Medicine

A clear role has appeared for nuclear medicine in the monitoring of multisystem disease activity in adults with sarcoidosis.[56] However, although some suggest a role in disease staging in pediatric LCH, there is currently little clinical utility of nuclear medicine studies in childhood ILD practice.[57]

Interventional Radiology

Although transbronchial cryobiopsy has a possible role in adult ILD diagnosis, the size of the biopsy device precludes its use in ChILD diagnosis. Rarely, a specific ChILD may be diagnosable via image-guided biopsy of extrapulmonary tissues, for example, ultrasound-guided thyroid fine-needle aspiration in infantile LCH or peripheral lymph node biopsy in granulomatous lymphocytic ILD (GLILD).[28]

An additional role for interventional radiology in ChILD is pneumothorax drainage and management. Children with diffuse lung disease may suffer frequent pneumothoraces and may require

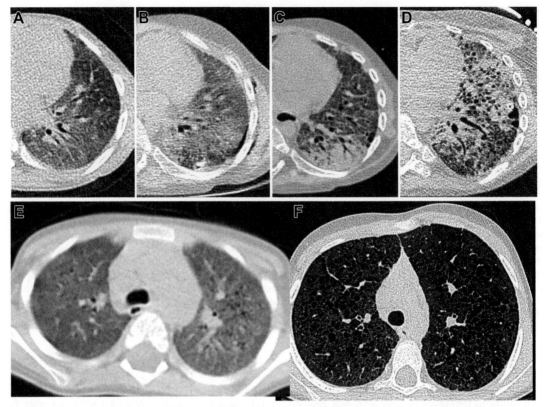

Fig. 5. Disease progression versus lung growth in a pediatric patient with STING-associated vasculitis with onset in infancy (SAVI) (*A–D*) compared with a pediatric patient with an ABCA3 mutation (*E, F*). (*A–D*) At 2 years of age (*A*), there is diffuse ground glass opacification. Over the subsequent years, imaged at ages 5 years (*B*), 6 years (*C*), and 7 years (*D*), there is increasingly dense ground glass opacification with progressive formation of emphysema-like cysts accompanied by recurrent pneumothoraces. There was clear clinical progression in symptoms over this period. (*E–F*) At 2 years of age (*E*), there is diffuse ground glass opacification with tiny, scattered cysts, and by 9 years of age (*F*), the ground glass opacification has largely resolved with the emergence of diffuse emphysema-like cysts throughout the entire lung. This change in appearance was associated with no clinical alteration in symptoms or oxygen requirement. This imaging progression from ground glass opacification to emphysema-like cyst formation is a relatively well-known phenomenon in children with disorders of surfactant protein function and may not represent true disease progression.

interventional radiology placement of thoracic drains into small pneumothoraces made clinically important as a result of their extensive parenchymal disease. For these pediatric patients, a specific, very-low-dose protocol should be used because diagnostic image quality is not required (**Fig. 8**).

SPECTRUM OF PEDIATRIC INTERSTITIAL LUNG DISEASE

As discussed previously, the ChILD classification system mainly categorizes ILDs that occur in the pediatric population into 2 categories: disorders with onset in infancy and disorders not specific to infancy. In the following section, these 2 main

categories of ChILD are systematically discussed alongside more recently described infant-onset ChILD entities not included within the most recent ATS classification.

Disorders with Onset in Infancy

The disorders with onset in infancy category is subdivided into (1) diffuse developmental disorders, (2) lung growth abnormalities, (3) specific disorders of undefined etiology, and (4) surfactant dysfunction disorders.

Diffuse developmental disorders

Diffuse developmental disorders are disorders of basic pulmonary development, characterized by the stage of developmental arrest. Typical clinical

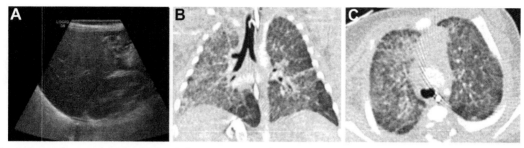

Fig. 6. Lung ultrasonography in ChILD diagnosis in an infant male with hypothyroidism and respiratory distress secondary to an Nkx2.1 (TTF1) mutation (so-called brain-thyroid-lung syndrome). (*A*) Longitudinal ultrasonographic image of the right lung base (using the liver as a sonographic window) shows sheet-like B-lines. This ultrasonographic appearance could represent any diffuse pathology of the interstitium (eg, pulmonary edema) and is entirely nonspecific. (*B, C*) Coronal (*B*) and axial (*C*) lung window CT images show the entire lung (as opposed to merely the immediately subpleural lung seen with ultrasonography) and demonstrate diffuse coarse interlobular septal thickening and ground glass opacification in keeping with ChILD.

presentation varies with type, but is generally severe respiratory distress at or shortly after birth. The 2 main diffuse pulmonary developmental disorders are acinar dysplasia and alveolar capillary dysplasia with malalignment of the pulmonary veins (ACD-MPV).

Early developmental arrest results in acinar dysplasia, the complete lack of alveolar development, with affected infants surviving only hours postnatally. ACD-MPV is a misnomer because the pulmonary veins are not malaligned. The

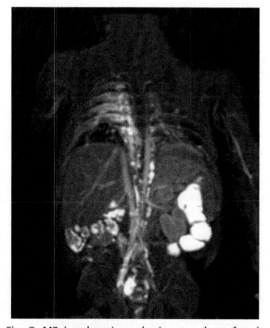

Fig. 7. MR lymphangiography in a newborn female with congenital right chylothorax. Coronal dynamic MR lymphangiography after intranodal contrast injection demonstrates abnormal lymphatic flow (increased MR imaging signal intensity) to the right pleura.

histopathologic appearance of transposition of the veins from their normal peripheral position in the interlobular septa to a centrilobular position is actually the result of dilated bronchial veins. There are well-known associations with FOXF1 mutations (up to 40% of reported ACD-MPV cases), and 80% are reported to have associated cardiac, renal, gastrointestinal, limb, or ocular malformations. The prognosis is generally bleak, with the affected patient often rapidly progressing to ECMO while the diagnosis is confirmed and one-way weaning.[58–60] There are, however, reports of ACD-MPV presenting at several months of age, and prolonged survival has been reported in those with patchy disease.[61] Despite the dramatic clinical presentation, CT imaging in ACD-MPV can be essentially normal, but a third of FOXF1 cases are reported to have concomitant pulmonary lymphangiectasia with resultant interlobular septal thickening and pleural effusions[62] (**Fig. 9**).

Lung growth abnormalities
The most common lung growth abnormality is chronic lung disease of prematurity. Exposure of underdeveloped lung to high-pressure mechanical ventilation and oxygen results in airway muscle hypertrophy, peribronchial fibrosis, COB, and hypertensive vasculopathy with the appearance of the so-called classic form of BPD. Modern neonatal intensive care with maternal steroid administration, avoidance of exposure to high concentrations of inspired oxygen, and low-pressure or oscillatory ventilation has resulted in a dramatic reduction in the incidence of classic BPD and an increased incidence of survival of extremely premature neonates with a "new" BPD with more subtle disease, but histology consistent with arrested lung development. Imaging generally demonstrates alternating bands of atelectasis and areas of lobular

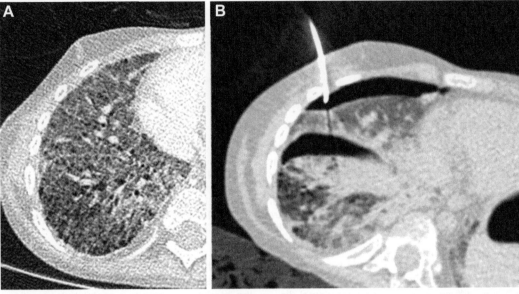

Fig. 8. Appropriate CT dose for diagnostic imaging versus appropriate dose for interventional procedure guidance in a 6-year-old female with ChILD due to underlying STING-associated vasculitis with onset in infancy. (*A*) Axial lung window CT image obtained for diagnostic purposes clearly demonstrates multiple cysts and diffuse ground glass opacification. (*B*) Axial lung window CT image obtained for guidance of chest tube placement for spontaneous pneumothorax. Note the loss of detail within the image. Diagnostic-quality CT imaging is not required in this situation, and, as such, decreasing CT dose settings (both kV and mAs) is appropriate.

hyperinflation with triangular subpleural opacities.[17,63–67] In fact, the appearance of the classic form of BPD with extensive disease should now raise suspicion for an additional genetic cause of surfactant dysfunction, particularly if the severity of disease is out of keeping with the gestational age and level of support required at birth.

Pulmonary hypoplasia can result from several insults, including insufficient thoracic space (eg, diaphragmatic hernia, short rib dysplasia, and large developmental congenital thoracic malformation) or by severe oligohydramnios (eg, secondary to bilateral renal agenesis, posterior urethral valves, or other severe urinary tract anomalies).[68]

Another important disorder of lung growth abnormality is the cystic dysplasia frequently encountered in those with trisomies (most commonly trisomy 21). Trisomy 21 is known to be associated with decreased alveolar number (58%–83% of normal).[69] As many as 36% of children with trisomy 21 have multiple 1- to 4-mm subpleural cysts, easily appreciable on CT imaging, variably extending around the periphery of the lung and along the interlobar fissures. These cysts communicate with distal airways and are thought to result from a lung growth abnormality. Although more common in those born prematurely, no clear association has been demonstrated with a need for chronic ventilation, the presence of congenital heart disease, or

the need for ECMO support.[70,71] Their importance is likely limited to accurate recognition and avoidance of being labeled as part of an alternative pathologic condition (**Fig. 10**).

Specific disorders of undefined etiology

Two important diagnoses of undefined etiology of the ChILD classification system are neuroendocrine cell hyperplasia of infancy (NEHI) and pulmonary interstitial glycogenosis (PIG).

Neuroendocrine cell hyperplasia of infancy NEHI typically presents in a term infant with a combination of tachypnea, retractions, inspiratory crackles, and/or hypoxemia, generally persisting until around 1 year of age before spontaneously resolving. When performed, lung biopsy demonstrates an increased number of bombesin stain-positive neuroendocrine cells around the distal airways, but normal-appearing lung on hematoxylin-and-eosin staining.[61] It is worth noting, however, that neuroendocrine cells are present around the airways in healthy lung and there is no agreed upper limit to the numbers of neuroendocrine cells con-sidered to be normal. It has been demonstrated that neuroendocrine cells decrease in number with increasing age. Therefore, it has been suggested that the increased number of neuroendocrine cells present around the airways in affected infants relates to

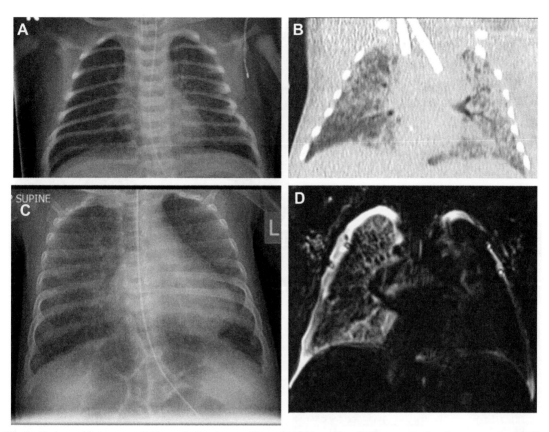

Fig. 9. Early and late presentation of alveolar capillary dysplasia with misalignment of pulmonary veins (ACD-MPV) in a term newborn male (*A, B*) who presented with severe respiratory distress and pulmonary hypertension on echocardiography at 24 hours of life and a 23-month-old term infant female (*C, D*) who presented with right chylothorax and pulmonary hypertension at 23 months of life. (*A*) Frontal chest radiograph shows diffuse coarse interstitial markings bilaterally. Also noted are endotracheal and nasogastric tubes. (*B*) Coronal lung window CT image demonstrates a diffuse interstitial lung disease characterized by ground glass opacification and interlobular septal thickening. Also note the cannulae for ECMO support. Lung biopsy confirmed ACD-MPV with a FOXF1 mutation later demonstrated on genetic analysis. (*C*) Frontal chest radiograph shows interstitial thickening and hyperinflation. (*D*) Coronal noncontrast MR lymphangiography demonstrates the "nutmeg" appearance of interlobular septal thickening throughout the right lung, in keeping with pulmonary lymphangiectasia/lymphangiomatosis. Retrograde pulmonary lymphatic perfusion was demonstrated on dynamic intranodal contrast MR lymphangiography (not shown). A large FOXF1-C1 deletion was demonstrated on genetic analysis in keeping with the late presentation of ACD-MPV.

dysmaturation of fetal airways (ie, delayed airways development).[61,72–74]

The CT appearance of NEHI is reportedly 100% specific, with ground glass opacification in a right middle lobe- and lingula-predominant distribution, and additional ground glass opacification coursing along the medial lung immediately adjacent to the mediastinum[75] (**Fig. 11**). There is a correlation between the extent of ground glass opacification and clinical phenotype, with significantly more ground glass opacification in NEHI patients requiring continuous oxygen than those with only nighttime oxygen support.[76] However, whereas the specificity of the CT appearance is high for NEHI, the sensitivity in the original study was only 78%.[75] A larger

study by Rauch and colleagues[77] examined the outcome of 80 infants with ground glass opacification on CT, dividing them into those with typical versus atypical NEHI appearances, with no differences in clinical outcome between the 2 groups. As a result of this characteristic presentation and CT appearance, open lung biopsy is now rarely performed in infants with a typical NEHI appearance on CT. However, although typical NEHI may present with atypical imaging appearances, there are instances in which the clinical picture is atypical. In these patients, CT appearance should be interpreted with care. NEHI with symptoms progressing beyond age 1 year is now frequently encountered, and there is at least one case report of 4 members

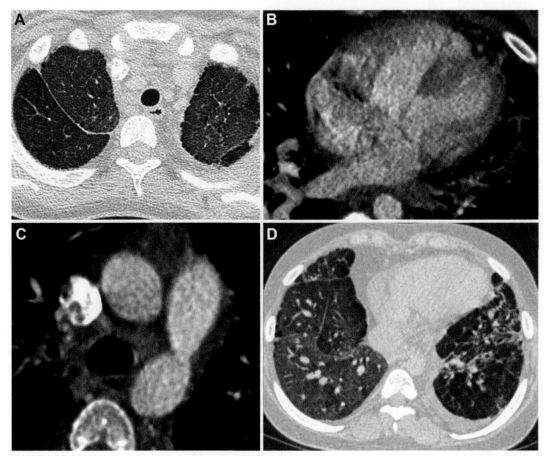

Fig. 10. Subpleural cysts in a 13-year-old boy with trisomy 21 referred for the evaluation of "undiagnosed interstitial lung disease with pulmonary hypertension." (*A*) Axial lung window CT image through the lung apices shows multiple subpleural and perilobular cysts within both lungs. (*B*) Axial enhanced soft tissue window CT image demonstrates atrioventricular septal defect and occlusion of the left pulmonary veins. (*C*) Axial enhanced soft tissue window CT image shows a large patent ductus arteriosus (PDA). (*D*) Axial lung window CT image through the lung bases demonstrates a lucent left lung base with thickened bronchi, interlobular septal thickening, and pleural effusion due to left pulmonary venous occlusion and left pulmonary arterial hypoplasia. Also note the relative enlargement of the right peripheral pulmonary arteries and right lower lobe ground glass opacification due to segmental pulmonary hypertension of the right lung. The left pulmonary artery hypoplasia, PDA, and pulmonary venous occlusion are likely to be of far more clinical importance than the cystic lung growth abnormality.

of a family with hereditary NEHI, found to have a mutation in Nkx2.1 (encoding TTF-1), with typical (if subtle) NEHI appearances on CT persisting to the age of 61 years and abnormal spirometry (significant obstruction and air trapping) demonstrated in a 32-year-old.[78]

Pulmonary interstitial glycogenosis Deposition of glycogen granules within the pulmonary interstitium of infants with tachypnea or respiratory distress has been termed PIG.[61] Like NEHI, there have been efforts to describe typical features, with Weinman and colleagues demonstrating that ground glass opacification, cysts, and interlobular septal thickening were the dominant CT findings (93%, 73%,

and 67%, respectively) in 15 infants with biopsy-proven PIG.[79] However, similar to the case of NEHI, it has been suggested that rather than a disease entity in its own right, PIG merely represents a marker of mesenchymal dysmaturity with diffuse or patchy PIG reported in biopsies from infants with lung growth abnormalities, twin-twin transfusion syndrome, Noonan syndrome, congenital thoracic malformations, congenital heart disease, and trisomy 21.[61,80–83]

Surfactant dysfunction disorders
A crucial role of type II pneumatocytes is the production of surfactant proteins. Surfactant proteins A and D contribute to innate host defence, whereas

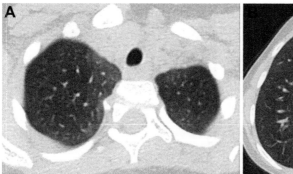
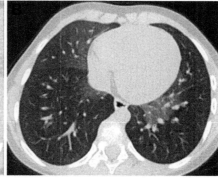

Fig. 11. Neuroendocrine cell hyperplasia of infancy (NEHI) in a 5-year-old boy. (*A*) Axial lung window CT image shows characteristic ground glass opacification in the apical paramediastinal regions. (*B*) Axial lung window CT image demonstrates characteristic medial right middle lobe and lingula ground glass opacification with further paramediastinal involvement.

surfactant proteins B and C (encoded by the SFTPB and SFTPC genes, respectively) are essential in regulating alveolar surface tension, preventing alveolar collapse on exhalation. Transcription of these proteins is regulated by TTF-1 (encoded by the Nkx2.1 gene) with surfactant manufactured in the endoplasmic reticulum and transported to the lamellar bodies for storage, via the ABCA3.[84,85] Mutations within any of the surfactant protein B or C, ABCA3, or Nkx2.1 genes may result in an ILD with varied age of onset, pathologic pattern, and resulting disease severity depending on the gene involved. Biopsy samples from differing parts of the lung may show different histopathologic patterns, and imaging patterns of disease may change over time[86] (**Fig. 12**). These mutations are reported to be the cause of up to 25% of severe refractory diffuse lung diseases presenting in infancy.[9]

SFTPB mutations generally present at or near birth with severe respiratory distress and are generally fatal in early infancy. The histopathologic pattern is often that of pulmonary alveolar proteinosis (PAP) with the imaging appearance of "crazy-paving"—ground glass opacification with superimposed interlobular septal thickening.

SFTPC mutations have a more varied age of onset and may even present in early adulthood. Indeed, SFTPC mutations are said to represent 17% of all ChILD entities presenting beyond infancy.[87–89] The pattern is often a chronic pneumonitis of infancy, DIP, or cellular NSIP. A case series by Mechri and colleagues[26] found ground glass opacification and pulmonary cysts to be the predominant CT findings (93% and 40%, respective) in 15 patients with ChILD secondary to confirmed SFTPC mutations.

ABCA3 mutations generally have a similar CT appearance to SFTPB mutations, with PAP commonly demonstrated, but with a less severe disease course. Doan and colleagues[86] examined

the follow-up imaging, and interestingly repeat histology (ie, repeat biopsy or tissue subsequently acquired at transplant or postmortem) demonstrated mixed histopathologic patterns, predominantly PAP, but with additional DIP and NSIP. Initial CT demonstrated ground glass opacification, but follow-up imaging showed a "reduction in intensity" of ground glass opacification, not corresponding to a change in symptom severity, with formation of interlobular septal thickening in all patients and cysts in 5 of 9 patients examined. The investigators also described a now well-recognized association with the development of a pectus excavatum deformity. The patients with repeat histology demonstrated progressive lobular remodeling, but less reactive interstitial widening and the later development of an endogenous lipoid pneumonia.[86]

As TTF-1 regulates surfactant production by type II pneumatocytes, Nkx2.1 mutations result in a reduction of formation of all forms of surfactant with variable resulting histopathologic patterns of disease.[90] However, as TTF-1 is also expressed in thyroid and neural tissue, affected pediatric patients generally present with congenital hypothyroidism and neurology (choreoathetosis and atonia) with lung disease relatively less common. The extrapulmonary symptoms provide crucial clues to the cause of their underlying disease, reducing the need for lung biopsy.[90–94]

Just as important as the production of functioning surfactant by type II pneumatocytes is the clearance of degraded surfactant proteins by alveolar macrophages. Mutations in the colony-stimulating factor receptor subunits 2A and B (encoded by CSF2RA and CSF2RB), particularly in Turner syndrome, result in inadequate alveolar macrophage function and a typically later presentation with PAP.[95] Further genetic causes of disordered surfactant protein catabolism include mutations in GATA-2, OAS1, SLC7A7, and MARS.[96–101]

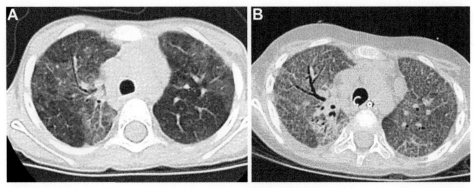

Fig. 12. Changing imaging pattern of disease in a 4-year-old boy with ChILD that has been proved to be secondary to an ABCA3 mutation. (A) Axial lung window CT image shows coarse ground glass opacification and mild bronchial distortion. (B) Axial lung window CT image obtained as a follow-up evaluation demonstrates a change in appearance with the development of an extensive classic "crazy-paving" appearance in keeping with pulmonary alveolar proteinosis with increased bronchial dilatation and distortion. In addition, the more consolidative opacity at the posterior right upper lobe is suspicious for sequela of aspiration, an important and potentially treatable exacerbating factor.

More Recently Described Infant-Onset Childhood Interstitial Lung Disease

As previously discussed, substantial advances in and wider access to genetic medicine has led to the discovery of several monogenetic causes of ChILD. The actin-binding protein filamin A (encoded by FLNA) is involved in cell signaling, maintenance of cell shape, and in cell motility.[102] Mutations have long been known to result in disordered neuronal migration (nodular periventricular gray matter heterotopia) and vascular and connective tissue integrity (aneurysmal patent ductus arteriosus and innominate artery aneurysms). However, more recently case series have been published with FLNA-associated respiratory disease with a characteristic multilobar overinflation with coarse interlobular septal thickening and patchy atelectasis, with variable clinical outcomes including long-term oxygen requirement and even death in infancy[103] (**Fig. 13**). Of note, the condition is X-linked and therefore generally only encountered in female patients (there is a single case report of FLNA lung disease in a male infant with mosaic expression of an FLNA mutation).[104]

There are several recently described infant-onset syndromes with ChILD in association with renal and skin disease. Although rare, these bear mentioning due to the severity and progressive nature of the lung disease and the potential for specific treatment in some cases. Mutations affecting the transmembrane receptor integrin A3 result in diffuse ILD manifesting as extensive architectural distortion, interlobular septal thickening, and ground glass opacification on CT in association with nephrotic syndrome and skin and nail lesions resembling epidermolysis bullosa[105] (**Fig. 14**). STING-associated vasculopathy of infancy (SAVI) is caused by a gain of function of the TMEM173 gene resulting in upregulation of the interferon pathway via the stimulator of interferon gene (STING).[106] SAVI results in infant onset of ChILD with progressive ground glass opacification and mediastinal lymphadenopathy, often in association with rash and/or necrotic skin lesions, recurrent fever, and renal disease.[107,108] Mutations in the coatomer subunit alpha (COPA) gene result in severe ChILD associated with rheumatoid factor, antinuclear and antineutrophil cytoplasm antibodies, arthritis, and renal disease.[109] COPA mutations have recently been found to act via STING-induced interferon signaling, explaining the similarities with SAVI, and are potentially treatable with immunosuppression and the Janus kinase (JAK) inhibitor ruxolitinib.[110,111]

Disorders Not Specific to Infancy

ChILD that occurs beyond infancy is categorized under the "disorders not specific to infancy" category within the ChILD classification system. This group is subdivided into: (1) disorders of the normal host, (2) disorders related to systemic disease, and (3) disorders of the immunocompromised host, which are discussed in the following section.

Disorders of the normal host
Among the various ChILD disorders that occur in normal children, 4 clinically important disorders

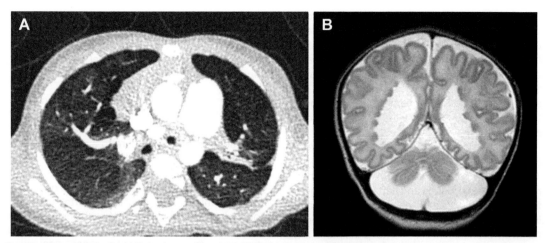

Fig. 13. Mutations in the X-linked gene filamin A (FLNA) in a 9-month-old female who presented with pulmonary hypertension. (*A*) Axial lung window CT image shows bilateral multilobar hyperinflation. (*B*) Coronal brain MR image demonstrates nodular periventricular gray matter heterotopia.

include obliterative bronchiolitis, hypersensitivity pneumonitis, inhalational lung disease, and exogenous lipoid pneumonia.

Constrictive/obliterative bronchiolitis Obliterative bronchiolitis is characterized histologically by irreversible fibrosis of the terminal respiratory bronchioles following insult to the lower respiratory tract. Two histologic forms are described: a proliferative form with airway obstruction by polypoid granulation tissue and a constrictive form with partial or complete airway obstruction via lumen narrowing resulting from peribronchial fibrosis with more response to corticosteroid in the proliferative form.[112,113]

Clinically, there are 3 main forms of constrictive obliterative bronchiolitis that occur in pediatric patients, which include (1) postinfectious bronchiolitis obliterans (PIBO), (2) post–lung transplant bronchiolitis obliterans (BO), and (3) post–hematopoietic stem cell transplant (HSCT) BO. The latter 2 are often referred to as bronchiolitis obliterans syndrome (BOS), although strictly speaking, this is the descriptor for obliterative bronchiolitis diagnosed with histopathologic correlation.[112]

The most common form in the pediatric population is PIBO, typically following adenovirus infection, although other organisms, such as *Mycoplasma pneumoniae*, can also be responsible. Genetic susceptibility and immune response are implicated, with PIBO encountered far more commonly in South American children and in the Southern hemisphere in general.[114]

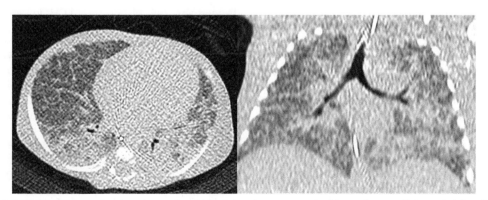

Fig. 14. Integrin A3 mutation in a 4-months-old female who presented with respiratory distress. Axial and coronal lung window CT images show extensive ground glass opacification, interlobular septal thickening, and dependent atelectasis and/or consolidation in keeping with ChILD. The diagnosis was made via genetic testing.

Post–lung transplant BO is a form of chronic lung allograft dysfunction and affects at least 50% of those surviving beyond 5 years posttransplant.[115] BO is reported in 2% to 6% of pediatric patients following HSCT[112] and has an association with viral infection around the time of HSCT. BO has been reported to be present in 100% of pediatric patients with HSCT with previous chronic GVHD.[116,117]

Consistent with the obstructive defect on spirometry, the predominant chest radiograph finding of BO is pulmonary overinflation with resultant hyperlucent-appearing lungs and flattening of the hemidiaphragms. In addition, there is frequently large airways involvement, with bronchial wall thickening and even bronchiectasis.[118] The principal CT finding of BO is mosaic attenuation with alternating hypolucent pulmonary lobules with markedly reduced caliber of the centrilobular pulmonary arterioles (Fig. 15). Indeed, the combination of this typical imaging finding in a pediatric patient with prior adenovirus infection and clinical suspicion of PIBO is said to be 67% sensitive and 100% specific for the diagnosis.[119] As such, in this setting of concordant clinical and imaging findings, it is now commonplace to make the diagnosis of PIBO without surgical biopsy confirmation. Although exaggerated by expiratory-phase CT imaging, mosaic attenuation and air trapping is generally appreciable on inspiratory imaging, and as described previously, additional expiratory or decubitus acquisitions may not be necessary in clinical practice.

Hypersensitivity pneumonitis More commonly encountered in adults, hypersensitivity pneumonitis (HP) may present in childhood (generally in mid to late teenage years) and shares the clinical and imaging features with adult HP. The most common causative exposure is to avian antigens, with less common reported causative exposures including mold spores, paints, glues, and insecticides.[120]

Imaging findings of hypersensitivity pneumonitis typically progress from ill-defined centrilobular nodularity and ground glass opacification (96% and 73% of a German study of 23 children) in the acute phase, to more well-defined centrilobular nodularity in the subacute phase, and ultimately progressing to coarse interlobular septal thickening, architectural distortion (fibrosis), and variable ground glass opacification in the chronic phase, often with areas of lobular hypoattenuation.[121–123]

If no causative exposure is identified, mutations in part of the telomere homeostasis pathway, such as telomere reverse transcriptase (TERT), telomerase RNA component (TERC), dyskerin 1, regulator of telomere elongation helicase 1 (RTEL1), and poly (A)-specific ribonuclease (PARN), should be considered, because these mutations have been found to predispose to hypersensitivity pneumonitis and are associated with a worse clinical outcome[124,125] (Fig. 16).

Inhalational lung disease Inhalational lung disease in children has been reported in the context of an outbreak of ChILD in Korea, later discovered to be secondary to exposure to air humidifier disinfectants. Imaging of inhalational lung injury typically shows a progression from initial ground glass and consolidation to centrilobular opacities, then becoming fainter over time. Mortality was reported to be as high as 58% with the extent of consolidation, centrilobular opacities, and ground glass opacification (more than 30%, 60%. and 70% of the lung, respectively) on CT found to predict mortality (hazard ratio 3.5, 0.2, and 3.5, respectively).[126,127]

Lipoid pneumonia Another example of a regional outbreak of ChILD is the series of florid exogenous lipoid pneumonia in children of Zimbabwean immigrants in South Africa, secondary to aspiration of oils administered as prophylaxis against constipation. Imaging findings of lipoid pneumonia are variable, but include extensive, masslike consolidation, potentially with internal areas of low attenuation on CT (Fig. 17). Diagnostic confirmation is possible via broncho-alveolar lavage (BAL), with gross demonstration of oils floating on the retrieved BAL fluid. Colonization of these oils has been reported, particularly with nontuberculous mycobacteria.[128,129]

Disorders related to systemic disease

LCH, vasculitides, collagen vascular disease, and storage disorders fall within the "disorders related to systemic disease" category and are discussed in the following sections.

Langerhans cell histiocytosis LCH in adults is generally encountered as a lung disease of young male smokers, whereas pediatric LCH is a multisystem disorder akin to a malignancy with involvement of bone, skin, liver, spleen, bone marrow, lung, and brain[130] (Fig. 18). Pulmonary involvement is reported in up to approximately 50% of cases, but pulmonary-predominant presentations are rare. Childhood onset of LCH in a large French registry ranged from 2 weeks to 16 years with around 50% of pediatric patients reported to have mutations in BRAF^{V600E}.[131] Pulmonary imaging findings of pediatric pulmonary LCH mimic those of adults affected with LCH, varying from small nodules to thick-walled cysts and parenchymal destruction. However, a substantial difference is

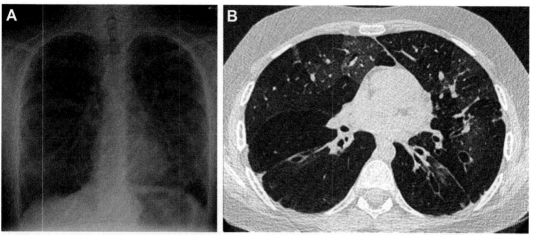

Fig. 15. Postinfective bronchiolitis obliterans (PIBO) in a 13-year-old boy who presented with shortness of breath. This child was diagnosed with PIBO at age 2 years following a severe adenovirus infection. (*A*) Frontal chest radiograph shows bilateral hyperinflation and bronchiectasis. (*B*) Axial lung window CT image confirms marked mosaic attenuation and bronchiectasis in both lungs.

that the lung bases are generally spared in adults, whereas the lung bases are almost always involved in childhood pulmonary LCH.[131–133] Treatment of severe disease is aggressive, often with a combination of vinblastine/prednisolone and mercaptopurine.[134]

Vasculitides Pediatric vasculitides are a remarkably diverse group of conditions, many of which demonstrate pulmonary involvement. Many pediatric vasculitides can present with pulmonary abnormalities, but the antineutrophil cytoplasmic antibody-associated vasculitides are most common (**Fig. 19**). In addition, alongside renal involvement, pulmonary disease is common in granulomatous polyangiitis (GPA). GPA is generally more severe in pediatric-onset disease than in adults and more commonly involves large airways (eg, subglottic, tracheal or bronchial stenosis) as well as the pulmonary parenchyma.[135,136] On imaging, nodules may

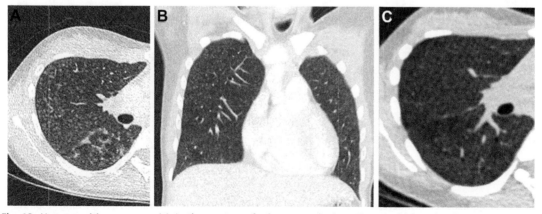

Fig. 16. Hypersensitive pneumonitis in the context of telomeropathy in a 13-year-old female who presented with respiratory symptoms. No convincing exposure was identified; however, the patient was discovered to have a deletion in the regulator of telomere elongation helicase 1 gene RTEL1. (*A, B*) Axial and coronal lung window CT images show coarse centrilobular ground glass nodules and interlobular septal thickening. (*C*) Axial lung window CT image obtained at age 15 years demonstrates interval regression with only subtle residual centrilobular ground glass nodules.

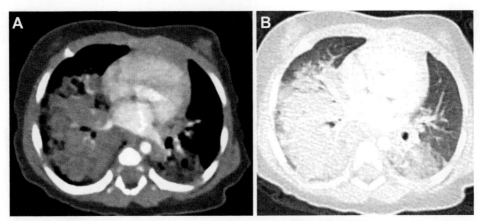

Fig. 17. Exogenous lipoid pneumonia in a 5-month-old female of Zimbabwean origin who recently migrated to the United Kingdom. (*A, B*) Axial enhanced soft tissue window CT image (*A*) and axial lung window CT image (*B*) show dense, masslike consolidation in the dependent portion of both lung bases, a frequent distribution of aspiration-related lung disease. Lung biopsy demonstrated lipoid pneumonia and confirmed the presence of *Mycobacterium abscessus*. Where possible, biopsy should be avoided owing to the risk of post operative pleural infection and osteomyelitis from non-tuberculous mycobacteria and other organisms within the aspirated oil.

be demonstrated, possibly cavitating, and potentially signs of pulmonary hemorrhage ranging from a halo of ground glass opacification around nodules to widespread consolidation in more extensive hemorrhage. When biopsies are performed, histology demonstrates necrotizing granulomatous inflammation.[137,138]

Eosinophilic granulomatous polyangiitis is a rare vasculitis that almost always features pulmonary involvement and progresses from an allergic phase (asthma ± sinusitis), through an eosinophilic phase, and finally to a vasculitic phase with cutaneous, neurologic, cardiac, and gastrointestinal manifestations. Pulmonary disease, polyneuropathy, and cardiomyopathy are 3 important causes of morbidity and mortality.[135,139–141]

Other causes of pulmonary hemorrhage include Goodpasture syndrome, systemic lupus eryth-

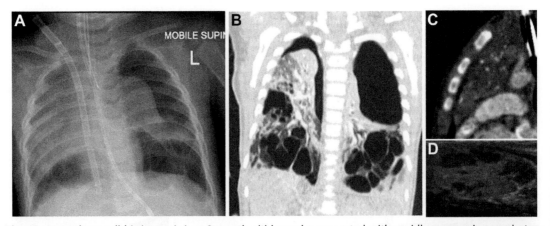

Fig. 18. Langerhans cell histiocytosis in a 9-month-old boy who presented with rapidly progressing respiratory distress. (*A*) Frontal chest radiograph shows large basal pulmonary cystic air spaces and a large left pneumothorax. Also note venovenous (VV) extracorporeal membrane oxygenation (ECMO) cannulae, endotracheal tube, nasogastric tube, and esophageal temperature probe. (*B*) Coronal lung window CT image demonstrates numerous large pulmonary cysts, ground glass opacification, and pneumothoraces on both sides. (*C*) Sagittal soft tissue window CT image shows thymic calcification. (*D*) Longitudinal ultrasonographic image demonstrates multiple hypoechogenic lesions within the thyroid gland.

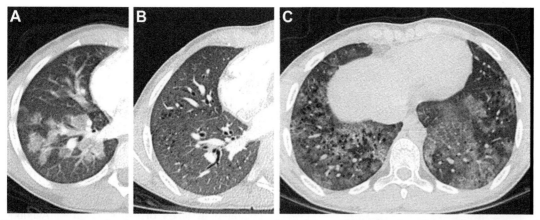

Fig. 19. Progression of pulmonary hemorrhage to hemosiderosis in a male pediatric patient with antineutrophil cytoplasmic antibody-positive vasculitis presenting with hemoptysis. (*A*) Axial lung window CT image obtained at 10 years of age shows multiple round areas of ground glass opacification in keeping with acute pulmonary hemorrhage. (*B*) Axial lung window CT image obtained at 12 years of age demonstrates progressive ground glass opacification and formation of multiple cysts. (*C*) Axial lung window CT image obtained at 15 years of age shows further progression of ground glass opacification and cyst formation along with interlobular septal thickening (best seen in the left lower lobe) in keeping with repeated hemorrhage and the development of pulmonary hemosiderosis.

ematosus, cow's milk allergy (Heiner syndrome), and idiopathic pulmonary hemorrhage.[142,143] Pulmonary hemorrhage varies in appearance on imaging from subtle "smoke-like" centrilobular ground glass opacification to dense consolidation with peripheral ground glass opacification. Repeated episodes of hemorrhage may result in hemosiderin deposition with a mild interstitial fibrosis appearing as additional fine interlobular septal thickening.[144]

Collagen vascular disease The collagen vascular diseases are also associated with ILD in children, with 50% of children with systemic sclerosis reported as having ILD (often NSIP pattern) at presentation and up to 19% of children with juvenile dermatomyositis and expression of the now well-recognized anti-MDA5 antibody having ILD (predominantly NSIP and/or organizing pneumonia pattern disease)[142,145,146] (Fig. 20).

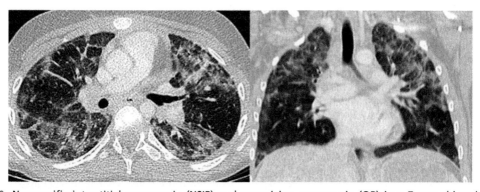

Fig. 20. Nonspecific interstitial pneumonia (NSIP) and organizing pneumonia (OP) in a 7-year-old male with collagen vascular disease and autoimmune hepatitis; this was confirmed on lung biopsy with subsequent pathologic evaluation. Axial (left) and coronal (right) lung window CT images show extensive ground glass consolidation in a perilobular and peribronchovascular distribution, in keeping with organizing pneumonia and/or NSIP pattern disease, both patterns associated with autoimmune/connective tissue diseases.

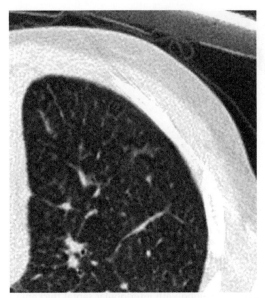

Fig. 21. Depositional lung disease due to Niemann-Pick disease in an 8-year-old female who presented with respiratory distress. Axial lung window CT image shows fine interlobular septal thickening in keeping with pulmonary interstitial deposition of sphingomyelin.

Storage disorders The lysosomal storage disorders may result in deposition of material within the pulmonary interstitium and resulting respiratory disease. Gaucher disease is the most common of the so-called depositional lung diseases and is caused by deficiency of glucocerebrosidase. Glucosylceramide is deposited within macrophages in the spleen and liver, resulting in hepatosplenomegaly, and within the bone marrow, neural tissue, lungs, skin, kidneys, conjunctivae, and heart.[147] Pulmonary involvement is most common in type I Gaucher disease following splenectomy and in type III disease and has been reported to cause sufficient interstitial infiltration to result in pulmonary hypertension.[148] The CT appearance of glucoceramide deposition is generally thin, potentially nodular-appearing, interlobular septal thickening. Niemann-Pick disease causes a very similar-appearing depositional lung disease, caused by sphingomyelinase deficiency and deposition of sphingomyelin[149] (**Fig. 21**).

Disorders of the immunocompromised host
ILD is a relatively common feature of immunodeficiency and may be the presenting feature. Lung involvement in immunodeficiency may be infection mediated, immune mediated, or malignant disease.

The most commonly encountered ILD pattern in patients with immunodeficiency is GLILD, a term encompassing LIP, follicular bronchiolitis, nodular lymphoid hyperplasia, and granulomatous disease. Although rare, when encountered, GLILD is a strong sign of underlying immune dysfunction, present in up to 40% of children with AIDS.[150]

Imaging in GLILD typically demonstrates pulmonary nodules varying from 2 to 30 mm in diameter with a mid to lower lobe predominance and a perilymphatic distribution, often surrounding airways[151] (**Fig. 22**). "Tree-in-bud," interlobular septal thickening and prominent mediastinal lymph nodes may also be demonstrated. Additional lesions and extensive ground glass opacification may be demonstrated at times of exacerbation.[152] Although presentations with extensive severe disease are encountered, most patients with common variable immunodeficiency-related ILD are asymptomatic and CT screening for lung disease is highly recommended at the time of diagnosis.[153]

As described previously, following lung or HSCT transplantation, patients frequently develop COB as an allograft dysfunction or graft-versus-host phenomenon. An additional entity related to complications of transplantation (and also encountered following high-dose chemotherapy and in certain telomeropathies such as dyskeratosis congenita), is pleuroparenchymal fibroelastosis (PPFE). Clinical presentation is often with increasing dyspnea and/or spontaneous pneumothorax. Imaging typically demonstrates a characteristic apical-predominant pleural and subpleural thickening/consolidation, evidence of fibrosis (adjacent bronchial traction dilatation and distortion), and subpleural emphysema–like blebs, often in association with marked reduction in anteroroposterior thoracic diameter (platythorax) and prominence of the suprasternal notch[154–156] (**Fig. 23**).

SUMMARY

Imaging plays a central role in ChILD diagnosis, providing confirmation of ChILD, sometimes a specific ChILD entity, guidance of surgical biopsy and informing interpretation of histopathology. In many cases, accurate diagnosis may be reached with an entirely noninvasive approach. The advancement of networks of ChILD experts, via organizations such as ChILD-EU (within the European Union) and ChILDRN has already enabled multicenter international collaboration. The addition of imaging experts to these groups and specific ChILD imaging research programs is likely to substantially advance the fields of imaging-based diagnosis, prognostication, and assessment of treatment success.

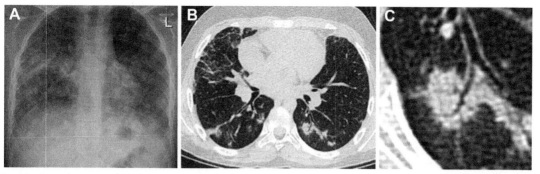

Fig. 22. Granulomatous lymphocytic interstitial lung disease (GLILD) in an 11-year-old male who presented with fevers and cough not responsive to antibiotics. The child was later found to have a complex partial immunodeficiency. (*A*) Frontal chest radiograph shows bilateral nodular consolidations with a mid and lower lung zone predominance. (*B, C*) Axial lung window CT images demonstrate interlobular septal thickening and multiple nodules with peribronchovascular distribution, with at least one nodular consolidation in the left lower lobe appearing centered on an airway (magnified in *C*). This later finding likely represents disease centered on the bronchus-associated lymphoid tissue and is relatively specific for GLILD disorders.

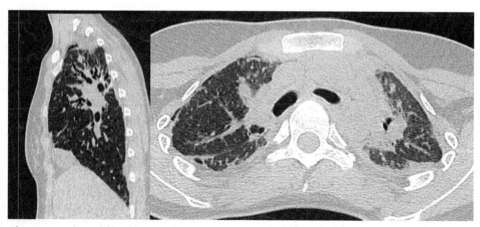

Fig. 23. Pleuroparenchymal fibroelastosis (PPFE) in a 14-year-old male who presented with sudden chest pain and shortness of breath due to pneumothorax after bone marrow transplantation. Sagittal (*left*) and axial (*right*) lung window CT images show bilateral apical pleural and subpleural thickening and consolidation with bronchial distortion and a tiny pneumothorax. Also note the short anteroposterior diameter of the thorax (referred to as *platythorax*), a common feature of PPFE.

CLINICS CARE POINTS

- Owing to its high sensitivity and increased likelihood of providing a specific diagnosis, CT remains the gold-standard imaging modality for the confirmation and characterization of suspected ChILD after chest radiography.

- Centers providing CT imaging of infants and children with suspected ChILD should be familiar with the optimal CT image technique required for evaluation of ChILD (as opposed to use of generic low-dose CT protocols, which are adequate for airways imaging but may be suboptimal for ChILD investigation).

- ChILD CT protocols should be designed with the input of medical physics experts, alongside radiologists and radiologic technicians, with a regular image quality check and dose audit program to ensure adequate image quality at an appropriate dose.

- Imaging for the assessment of possible ChILD should be avoided in times of acute infection, particularly adenovirus infection, to ensure accurate assessment of ILD extent and appearance without acute infection mimicking COB.

- When possible, interpretation of a possible ChILD should involve a radiologist with specific expertise in ChILD imaging. Although adult ILD experts are able to give useful insight into some ChILD entities, ILD has differing imaging appearances in children compared with adults and many ChILD entities are unique to childhood.

- The final diagnosis of ChILD can be optimally reached by expert multidisciplinary team discussion with integration of all available information from clinical history, spirometry, laboratory test results, imaging, and genetics. When a specific ChILD diagnosis cannot confidently be made without invasive testing, lung biopsy should be strongly considered as specific treatments are increasingly emerging for specific disease entities.

DISCLOSURE

For T. Semple: Consultancy: Parexel, Boehringer Ingelheim. Educational fees: Vertex Phamaceuticals. Research grants: Chiesi Pharmaceuticals. (This article does not influence any of the aforementioned projects). No other disclosure or conflict of interest for other 2 authors (E.Y. Lee and A.J. Winant).

REFERENCES

1. Wells AU, Hirani N. Interstitial lung disease guideline: the British Thoracic Society in collaboration with the Thoracic Society of Australia and New Zealand and the Irish Thoracic Society. Thorax 2008; 63:v1–58.

2. Antoniou KM, Margaritopoulos GA, Tomassetti S, et al. Interstitial lung disease. Eur Respir Rev 2014;23:40–54.

3. Travis WD, Costabel U, Hansell DM, et al. An official American Thoracic Society/European Respiratory Society statement: update of the international multidisciplinary classification of the idiopathic interstitial pneumonias. Am J Respir Crit Care Med 2013;188:733–48.

4. Nicholson AG, Colby TV, du Bois RM, et al. The prognostic significance of the histologic pattern of interstitial pneumonia in patients presenting with the clinical entity of cryptogenic fibrosing alveolitis. Am J Respir Crit Care Med 2000;162: 2213–7.

5. Deterding RR. Children's interstitial and diffuse lung disease. Progress and future horizons. Ann Am Thorac Soc 2015;12:1451–7.

6. Coultas DB, Zumwalt RE, Black WC, et al. The epidemiology of interstitial lung diseases. Am J Respir Crit Care Med 1994;150:967–72.

7. Bush A, Cunningham S, De Blic J, et al. European protocols for the diagnosis and initial treatment of interstitial lung disease in children. Thorax 2015; 70:1078–84.

8. Deutsch GH, Young LR, Deterding RR, et al. Diffuse lung disease in young children: Application of a novel classification scheme. Am J Respir Crit Care Med 2007;176:1120–8.

9. Kurland G, Deterding RR, Hagood JS, et al. An official american thoracic society clinical practice guideline: classification, evaluation, and management of childhood interstitial lung disease in infancy. Am J Respir Crit Care Med 2013;188:376–94.

10. Griese M, Irnstetter A, Hengst M, et al. Categorizing diffuse parenchymal lung disease in children Rare pulmonary diseases. Orphanet J Rare Dis 2015;10:1–6.

11. Jacob J, Owens CM, Brody AS, et al. Evaluation of inter-observer variation for computed tomography identification of childhood interstitial lung disease. ERJ Open Res 2019;5:00100–2019.

12. Wambach JA, Young LR. New clinical practice guidelines on the classification, evaluation and management of childhood interstitial lung disease in infants: what do they mean? Expert Rev Respir Med 2014;8:653–5.

13. Clement A, Allen J, Corrin B, et al. Task force on chronic interstitial lung disease in immunocompetent children. Eur Respir J 2004;24:686–97.

14. Deterding RR, DeBoer EM, Cidon MJ, et al. Approaching clinical trials in childhood interstitial lung disease and pediatric pulmonary fibrosis. Am J Respir Crit Care Med 2019;200:1219–27.

15. Padley SPG, Hansell DM, Flower CDR, et al. Comparative accuracy of high resolution computed tomography and chest radiography in the diagnosis of chronic diffuse infiltrative lung disease. Clin Radiol 1991;44:222–6.

16. Copley SJ, Coren M, Nicholson AG, et al. Diagnostic accuracy of thin-section CT and chest radiography of pediatric interstitial lung disease. AJR Am J Roentgenol 2000;174:549–54.

17. Semple T, Akhtar MR, Owens CM. Imaging bronchopulmonary dysplasia-a multimodality update. Front Med 2017;4:88.

18. Gilbert C, Bush A, Cunningham S. Childhood interstitial lung disease: Family experiences. Pediatr Pulmonol 2015;50:1301–3.

19. Long FR, Castile RG, Brody a S, et al. Lungs in infants and young children: improved thin-section CT with a noninvasive controlled-ventilation technique–initial experience. Radiology 1999;212:588–93.

20. Bridoux A, Hutt A, Faivre J-B, et al. Coronary artery visibility in free-breathing young children on non-gated chest CT: impact of temporal resolution. Pediatr Radiol 2015;45:1761–70.

21. Brody AS. Imaging considerations: interstitial lung disease in children. Radiologic Clin North America 2005;43:391–403.

22. Lucaya J, García-Peña P, Herrera L, et al. Expiratory chest CT in children. AJR Am J Roentgenol 2000;174:235–41.

23. Salamon E, Lever S, Kuo W, et al. Spirometer guided chest imaging in children: it is worth the effort! Pediatr Pulmonol 2017;52:48–56.

24. Hansell DM, Goldin JG, King TEJ, et al. CT staging and monitoring of fibrotic interstitial lung diseases in clinical practice and treatment trials: a position paper from the Fleischner Society. Lancet Respir Med 2015;3:483–96.

25. Hansell DM, Bankier AA, MacMahon H, et al. glossary of terms for thoracic imaging. Radiology 2008;246:697–722.

26. Mechri M, Epaud R, Emond S, et al. Surfactant protein C gene (SFTPC) mutation-associated lung disease: high-resolution computed tomography (HRCT) findings and its relation to histological analysis. Pediatr Pulmonol 2010;45:1021–9.

27. Stadler JAM, Andronikou S, Zar HJ. Lung ultrasound for the diagnosis of community-acquired pneumonia in children. Pediatr Radiol 2017;47:1412–9.

28. Yokoyama S, Nakaoka T, Fukao D, et al. Pulmonary Langerhans cell histiocytosis with thyroid involvement manifesting as recurrent bilateral pneumothorax and tension bullae in a 3-year-old child. Int J Surg Case Rep 2019;60:239–43.

29. Usui N, Kamiyama M, Kamata S, et al. A novel association of alveolar capillary dysplasia and duodenal atresia with paradoxical dilatation of the duodenum. J Pediatr Surg 2004;39:1808–11.

30. Adar T, Ilan Y, Elstein D, et al. Liver involvement in Gaucher disease - REVIEW and clinical approach. Blood Cells Mol Dis 2018;68:66–73.

31. Serai SD, Rapp JB, States LJ, et al. Pediatric lung MRI: currently available and emerging techniques. AJR Am J Roentgenol 2021;216:781–90.

32. Liszewski MC, Ciet P, Lee EY. MR imaging of lungs and airways in children:: past and present. Magn Reson Imaging Clin N Am 2019;27:201–25.

33. Sodhi KS, Sharma M, Lee EY, et al. Diagnostic utility of 3T lung MRI in children with interstitial lung disease. Acad Radiol 2017;25(3):380–6.

34. Liszewski MC, Görkem S, Sodhi KS, et al. Lung magnetic resonance imaging for pneumonia in children. Pediatr Radiol 2017;47:1420–30.

35. Sodhi KS, Khandelwal N, Saxena AK, et al. Rapid lung MRI in children with pulmonary infections: Time to change our diagnostic algorithms. J Magn Reson Imaging 2016;43:1196–206.

36. Ciet P, Tiddens HAWM, Wielopolski PA, et al. Magnetic resonance imaging in children: common problems and possible solutions for lung and airways imaging. Pediatr Radiol 2015;45:1901–15.

37. Baez JC, Ciet P, Mulkern R, et al. Pediatric Chest MR Imaging: Lung and Airways. Magn Reson Imaging Clin N Am 2015;23:337–49.

38. Campbell-Washburn AE, Ramasawmy R, Restivo MC, et al. Opportunities in interventional and diagnostic imaging by using high-performance low-field-strength MRI. Radiology 2019;293:384–93.

39. Kern AL, Vogel-Claussen J. Hyperpolarized gas MRI in pulmonology. Br J Radiol 2018;20170647. https://doi.org/10.1259/bjr.20170647.

40. Schreiber WG, Eberle B, Laukemper-Ostendorf S, et al. Dynamic 19F-MRI of pulmonary ventilation using sulfur hexafluoride (SF6) gas. Magn Reson Med 2001. https://doi.org/10.1002/mrm.1082.

41. Halaweish AF, Moon RE, Foster WM, et al. Perfluoropropane gas as a magnetic resonance lung imaging contrast agent in humans. Chest 2013. https://doi.org/10.1378/chest.12-2597.

42. Wolf U, Scholz A, Heussel CP, et al. Subsecond fluorine-19 MRI of the lung. Magn Reson Med 2006. https://doi.org/10.1002/mrm.20859.

43. Wen WY, Muccitelli JA. Thermodynamics of some perfluorocarbon gases in water. J Solution Chem 1979. https://doi.org/10.1007/BF00648882.

44. Friedman HL. The solubilities of sulfur hexafluoride in water and of the rare gases, sulfur hexafluoride and osmium tetroxide in nitromethane. J Am Chem Soc 1954. https://doi.org/10.1021/ja01641a065.

45. Martini K, Gygax CM, Benden C, et al. Volumetric dynamic oxygen-enhanced MRI (OE-MRI): comparison with CT Brody score and lung function in cystic fibrosis patients. Eur Radiol 2018. https://doi.org/10.1007/s00330-018-5383-5.

46. Zhang WJ, Niven RM, Young SS, et al. Dynamic oxygen-enhanced magnetic resonance imaging of the lung in asthma - Initial experience. Eur J Radiol 2015;84:318–26.

47. Flors L, Altes TA, Mugler JP, et al. New insights into lung diseases using hyperpolarized gas MRI. Radiol (English Ed) 2015. https://doi.org/10.1016/j.rxeng.2014.12.003.

48. Qing K, Mugler JP, Altes TA, et al. Assessment of lung function in asthma and COPD using hyperpolarized 129Xe chemical shift saturation recovery spectroscopy and dissolved-phase MRI. NMR Biomed 2014. https://doi.org/10.1002/nbm.3179.

49. Wang JM, Robertson SH, Wang Z, et al. Using hyperpolarized 129Xe MRI to quantify regional gas transfer in idiopathic pulmonary fibrosis. Thorax 2018. https://doi.org/10.1136/thoraxjnl-2017-210070.

50. Doganay O, Chen M, Matin T, et al. Magnetic resonance imaging of the time course of hyperpolarized 129 Xe gas exchange in the human lungs and heart. Eur Radiol 2019. https://doi.org/10.1007/s00330-018-5853-9.

51. Nyilas S, Bauman G, Pusterla O, et al. Ventilation and perfusion assessed by functional MRI in children with CF: reproducibility in comparison to lung function. J Cyst Fibros 2019;18:543–50.

52. Voskrebenzev A, Vogel-Claussen J. Proton MRI of the lung: how to tame scarce protons and fast signal decay. J Magn Reson Imaging 2021;53:1344–57.

53. Biko DM, Johnstone JA, Dori Y, et al. Recognition of neonatal lymphatic flow disorder: fetal MR findings and postnatal MR lymphangiogram correlation. Acad Radiol 2018;25:1446–50.

54. Chavhan GB, Amaral JG, Temple M, et al. MR lymphangiography in children: technique and potential applications. Radiogr A Rev Publ Radiol Soc North Am Inc 2017;37:1775–90.

55. Shaikh R, Biko DM, Lee EY. MR imaging evaluation of pediatric lymphatics:: overview of techniques and imaging findings. Magn Reson Imaging Clin N Am 2019;27:373–85.

56. Keijsers RGM, Grutters JC. In which patients with sarcoidosis is FDG PET/CT indicated? J Clin Med 2020;9:890.

57. Agarwal KK, Seth R, Behra A, et al. 18F-Fluorodeoxyglucose PET/CT in Langerhans cell histiocytosis: spectrum of manifestations. Jpn J Radiol 2016;34:267–76.

58. Yu S, Shao L, Kilbride H, et al. Haploinsufficiencies of FOXF1 and FOXC2 genes associated with lethal alveolar capillary dysplasia and

59. Zufferey F, Martinet D, Osterheld M-C, et al. 16q24.1 microdeletion in a premature newborn: Usefulness of array-based comparative genomic hybridization in persistent pulmonary hypertension of the newborn. Pediatr Crit Care Med 2011;12:e427–32.

60. Stankiewicz P, Sen P, Bhatt SS, et al. Genomic and genic deletions of the FOX gene cluster on 16q24.1 and inactivating mutations of FOXF1 cause alveolar capillary dysplasia and other malformations. Am J Hum Genet 2009;84:780–91.

61. Bush A, Griese M, Seidl E, et al. Early onset children's interstitial lung diseases: discrete entities or manifestations of pulmonary dysmaturity? Paediatr Respir Rev 2019;30:65–71.

62. Dishop MK. Diagnostic pathology of diffuse lung disease in children. Pediatr Allergy Immunol Pulmonol 2010;23:69–85.

63. Cherukupalli K, Larson JE, Rotschild A, et al. Biochemical, clinical, and morphologic studies on lungs of infants with bronchopulmonary dysplasia. Pediatr Pulmonol 1996;22:215–29.

64. Coalson J. in Bland and Coalson: chronic lung disease in early infancy. Boca Raton (FL): CRC Press, Taylor & Francis; 1999. p. 85–124.

65. Northway WJ. Bronchopulmonary dysplasia: twenty-five years later. Pediatrics 1992;89:969–73.

66. Jobe A. The new BPD: an arrest of lung development. Pediatr Res 1999;46:641.

67. Griscom NT, Wheeler WB, Sweezey NB, et al. Bronchopulmonary dysplasia: radiographic appearance in middle childhood. Radiology 1989;171:811–4.

68. Biyyam DR, Chapman T, Ferguson MR, et al. Congenital lung abnormalities: embryologic features , prenatal diagnosis , and postnatal. Radiographics 2010;30:1721–39.

69. Cooney TP, Thurlbeck WM. Pulmonary hypoplasia in down's syndrome. N Engl J Med 1982;307:1170–3.

70. Biko DM, Schwartz M, Anupindi SA, et al. Subpleural lung cysts in down syndrome: Prevalence and association with coexisting diagnoses. Pediatr Radiol 2008;38:280–4.

71. Radhakrishnan R, Towbin AJ. Imaging findings in down syndrome. Pediatr Radiol 2014;44:506–21.

72. Deterding RR, Pye C, Fan LL, et al. Persistent tachypnea of infancy is associated with neuroendocrine cell hyperplasia. Pediatr Pulmonol 2005;40:157–65.

73. Deterding RR, Fan LL, Morton R, et al. Persistent tachypnea of infancy (PTI)–a new entity. Pediatr Pulmonol 2001;(Suppl 23):72–3.

74. Young LR, Brody AS, Inge TH, et al. Neuroendocrine cell distribution and frequency distinguish neuroendocrine cell hyperplasia of infancy from other pulmonary disorders. Chest 2011;139:1060–71.

75. Brody AS, Guillerman RP, Hay TC, et al. Neuroendocrine cell hyperplasia of infancy: diagnosis with high-resolution CT. Am J Roentgenol 2010;194: 238–44.

76. Spielberg DR, Brody AS, Baker ML, et al. Ground-glass burden as a biomarker in neuroendocrine cell hyperplasia of infancy. Pediatr Pulmonol 2019;54:822–7.

77. Rauch D, Wetzke M, Reu S, et al. Persistent tachypnea of infancy: usual and aberrant. Am J Respir Crit Care Med 2016;193:438–47.

78. Nevel RJ, Garnett ET, Worrell JA, et al. Persistent lung disease in adults with NKX2.1 mutation and familial neuroendocrine cell hyperplasia of infancy. Ann Am Thorac Soc 2016;13:1299–304.

79. Weinman JP, White CJ, Liptzin DR, et al. High-resolution CT findings of pulmonary interstitial glycogenosis. Pediatr Radiol 2018;48:1066–72.

80. Lanfranchi M, Allbery SM, Wheelock L, et al. Pulmonary interstitial glycogenosis. Pediatr Radiol 2010;40:361–5.

81. Ross MK, Ellis LS, Bird LM, et al. Pulmonary interstitial glycogenosis in a patient ultimately diagnosed with Noonan syndrome. Pediatr Pulmonol 2014;49:508–11.

82. Cutz E, Chami R, Dell S, et al. Pulmonary interstitial glycogenosis associated with a spectrum of neonatal pulmonary disorders. Hum Pathol 2017; 68:154–65.

83. Deutsch GH, Young LR. Lipofibroblast phenotype in pulmonary interstitial glycogenosis. Am J Respir Crit Care Med 2016;193:694–6.

84. Bernhard W. Lung surfactant: Function and composition in the context of development and respiratory physiology. Ann Anat 2016;208:146–50.

85. Han SH, Mallampalli RK. The role of surfactant in lung disease and host defense against pulmonary infections. Ann Am Thorac Soc 2015;12:765–74.

86. Doan ML, Guillerman RP, Dishop MK, et al. Clinical, radiological and pathological features of ABCA3 mutations in children. Thorax 2008;63:366–73.

87. Bullard JE, Nogee LM. Heterozygosity for ABCA3 mutations modifies the severity of lung disease associated with a surfactant protein C gene (SFTPC) mutation. Pediatr Res 2007;62:176–9.

88. Bullard JE, Wert SE, Whitsett JA, et al. ABCA3 mutations associated with pediatric interstitial lung disease. Am J Respir Crit Care Med 2005;172: 1026–31.

89. Turcu S, Ashton E, Jenkins L, et al. Genetic testing in children with surfactant dysfunction. Arch Dis Child 2013;98:490–5.

90. LeMoine BD, Browne LP, Liptzin DR, et al. High-resolution computed tomography findings of thyroid transcription factor 1 deficiency (NKX2–1 mutations). Pediatr Radiol 2019;869–75.

91. Breedveld GJ, Percy a K, MacDonald ME, et al. Clinical and genetic heterogeneity in benign hereditary chorea. Neurology 2002;59:579–84.

92. Breedveld GJ, van Dongen JWF, Danesino C, et al. Mutations in TITF-1 are associated with benign hereditary chorea. Hum Mol Genet 2002; 11:971–9.

93. Carré A, Szinnai G, Castanet M, et al. Five new TTF1/NKX2.1 mutations in brain-lung-thyroid syndrome: rescue by PAX8 synergism in one case. Hum Mol Genet 2009;18:2266–76.

94. Cavaliere E, Gortan AJ, Passon N, et al. NKX2.1 run-on mutation associated to familial brain–lung–thyroid syndrome. Clin Genet 2021;100(1):114–6.

95. Martinez-Moczygemba M, Doan ML, Elidemir O, et al. Pulmonary alveolar proteinosis caused by deletion of the GM-CSFRalpha gene in the X chromosome pseudoautosomal region 1. J Exp Med 2008;205:2711–6.

96. Bush A, gilbert C, Gregory Jo, et al. Pediatric interstitial lung disease. J Pan African Thorac Soc 2021; 2:18–32.

97. Cho K, Yamada M, Agematsu K, et al. Heterozygous mutations in OAS1 cause infantile-onset pulmonary alveolar proteinosis with hypogammaglobulinemia. Am J Hum Genet 2018;102:480–6.

98. Tanaka-Kubota M, Shinozaki K, Miyamoto S, et al. Hematopoietic stem cell transplantation for pulmonary alveolar proteinosis associated with primary immunodeficiency disease. Int J Hematol 2018; 107:610–4.

99. Griese M, Zarbock R, Costabel U, et al. GATA2 deficiency in children and adults with severe pulmonary alveolar proteinosis and hematologic disorders. BMC Pulm Med 2015;15:87.

100. Spinner MA, Sanchez LA, Hsu AP, et al. GATA2 deficiency: a protean disorder of hematopoiesis, lymphatics, and immunity. Blood 2014;123:809–21.

101. Comisso M, Hadchouel A, de Blic J, et al. Mutations in MARS identified in a specific type of pulmonary alveolar proteinosis alter methionyl-tRNA synthetase activity. FEBS J 2018;285:2654–61.

102. Revenu C, Athman R, Robine S, et al. The co-workers of actin filaments: from cell structures to signals. Nat Rev Mol Cell Biol 2004;5:635–46.

103. Shelmerdine SC, Semple T, Wallis C, et al. Filamin A (FLNA) mutation-A newcomer to the childhood interstitial lung disease (ChILD) classification. Pediatr Pulmonol 2017;52(10):1306–15.

104. Masurel-Paulet A, Haan E, Thompson EM, et al. Lung disease associated with periventricular nodular heterotopia and an FLNA mutation. Eur J Med Genet 2011;54:25–8.

105. Has C, Spartà G, Kiritsi D, et al. Integrin α3 mutations with kidney, lung, and skin disease. N Engl J Med 2012;366:1508–14.

106. Rani MRS, Shrock J, Appachi S, et al. Novel interferon-beta-induced gene expression in peripheral blood cells. J Leukoc Biol 2007;82:1353–60.

107. de Jesus AA, Hou Y, Brooks S, et al. Distinct interferon signatures and cytokine patterns define additional systemic autoinflammatory diseases. J Clin Invest 2020;130:1669–82.

108. Liu Y, Jesus AA, Marrero B, et al. Activated STING in a vascular and pulmonary syndrome. N Engl J Med 2014;371:507–18.

109. Vece TJ, Watkin LB, Nicholas S, et al. Copa syndrome: a novel autosomal dominant immune dysregulatory disease. J Clin Immunol 2016;36:377–87.

110. Frémond M-L, Legendre M, Fayon M, et al. Use of ruxolitinib in COPA syndrome manifesting as life-threatening alveolar haemorrhage. Thorax 2020; 75:92–5.

111. Frémond M-L, Nathan N. COPA syndrome, 5 years after: where are we? Jt Bone Spine 2021;88:105070.

112. Kavaliunaite E, Aurora P. Diagnosing and managing bronchiolitis obliterans in children. Expert Rev Respir Med 2019;13:481–8.

113. Myers JL, Colby TV. Pathologic manifestations of bronchiolitis, constrictive bronchiolitis, cryptogenic organizing pneumonia, and diffuse panbronchiolitis. Clin Chest Med 1993;14:611–22.

114. Teper AM, Marcos CY, Theiler G. Association between HLA and the incidence of bronchiolitis obliterans (BO) in Argentina. Am J 2004;169:382.

115. Meyer KC, Raghu G, Verleden GM, et al. An international ISHLT/ATS/ERS clinical practice guideline: diagnosis and management of bronchiolitis obliterans syndrome. Eur Respir J 2014;44:1479–503.

116. Versluys B, Bierings M, Murk JL, et al. Infection with a respiratory virus before hematopoietic cell transplantation is associated with alloimmune-mediated lung syndromes. J Allergy Clin Immunol 2018;141: 697–703.e8.

117. Versluys AB, Rossen JWA, van Ewijk B, et al. Strong association between respiratory viral infection early after hematopoietic stem cell transplantation and the development of life-threatening acute and chronic alloimmune lung syndromes. Biol Blood Marrow Transpl J Am Soc Blood Marrow Transpl 2010;16:782–91.

118. Copley SJ, Padley SPG. High-resolution CT of paediatric lung disease. Eur Radiol 2001;11:2564–75.

119. Colom AJ, Teper AM. Clinical prediction rule to diagnose post-infectious bronchiolitis obliterans in children. Pediatr Pulmonol 2009;44:1065–9.

120. Vece TJ, Fan LL. Interstitial lung disease in children older than 2 years. Pediatr Allergy Immunol Pulmonol 2010;23:33–41.

121. Griese M, Haug M, Hartl D, et al. Hypersensitivity pneumonitis: lessons for diagnosis and treatment of a rare entity in children. Orphanet J Rare Dis 2013;8:121.

122. Chung JH, Zhan X, Cao M, et al. Presence of air trapping and mosaic attenuation on chest computed tomography predicts survival in chronic hypersensitivity pneumonitis. Ann Am Thorac Soc 2017;14:1533–8.

123. Walsh SLF, Sverzellati N, Devaraj A, et al. Chronic hypersensitivity pneumonitis: high resolution computed tomography patterns and pulmonary function indices as prognostic determinants. Eur Radiol 2012;22:1672–9.

124. Ley B, Torgerson DG, Oldham JM, et al. Rare protein-altering telomere-related gene variants in patients with chronic hypersensitivity pneumonitis. Am J Respir Crit Care Med 2019;200:1154–63.

125. Bouros D, Tzouvelekis A. Telomeropathy in chronic hypersensitivity pneumonitis. Am J Respir Crit Care Med 2019;200:1086–7.

126. Kim KW, Ahn K, Yang HJ, et al. Humidifier disinfectant-associated children's interstitial lung disease. Am J Respir Crit Care Med 2014;189: 48–56.

127. Yoon HM, Lee E, Lee JS, et al. Humidifier disinfectant-associated children's interstitial lung disease: computed tomographic features, histopathologic correlation and comparison between survivors and non-survivors. Eur Radiol 2016;26: 235–43.

128. Marangu D, Gray D, Vanker A, et al. Exogenous lipoid pneumonia in children: a systematic review. Paediatr Respir Rev 2020;33:45–51.

129. Marangu D, Pillay K, Banderker E, et al. Exogenous lipoid pneumonia: an important cause of interstitial lung disease in infants. Respirology case Rep 2018;6:e00356.

130. Odame I, Li P, Lau L, et al. Pulmonary Langerhans cell histiocytosis: a variable disease in childhood. Pediatr Blood Cancer 2006;47:889–93.

131. Kambouchner M, Emile J-F, Copin M-C, et al. Childhood pulmonary Langerhans cell histiocytosis: a comprehensive clinical-histopathological and BRAF(V600E) mutation study from the French national cohort. Hum Pathol 2019;89:51–61.

132. Sharma S, Dey P. Childhood pulmonary langerhans cell histiocytosis in bronchoalveolar lavage. a case report along with review of literature. Diagn Cytopathol 2016;44:1102–6.

133. Bano S, Chaudhary V, Narula MK, et al. Pulmonary Langerhans cell histiocytosis in children: a spectrum of radiologic findings. Eur J Radiol 2014;83: 47–56.

134. Allen CE, Ladisch S, McClain KL. How I treat Langerhans cell histiocytosis. Blood 2015;126:26–35.

135. Jariwala M, Laxer RM. Childhood GPA, EGPA, and MPA. Clin Immunol 2020;211:108325.

136. Jariwala MP, Laxer RM. Primary vasculitis in childhood: GPA and MPA in childhood. Front Pediatr 2018;6:226.

137. Filocamo G, Torreggiani S, Agostoni C, et al. Lung involvement in childhood onset granulomatosis with polyangiitis. Pediatr Rheumatol Online J 2017;15:28.

138. Feragalli B, Mantini C, Sperandeo M, et al. The lung in systemic vasculitis: radiological patterns and differential diagnosis. Br J Radiol 2016;89:20150992.

139. Eleftheriou D, Gale H, Pilkington C, et al. Eosinophilic granulomatosis with polyangiitis in childhood: retrospective experience from a tertiary referral centre in the UK. Rheumatology (Oxford) 2016;55:1263–72.

140. Zwerina J, Eger G, Englbrecht M, et al. Churg-Strauss syndrome in childhood: a systematic literature review and clinical comparison with adult patients. Semin Arthritis Rheum 2009;39:108–15.

141. Razenberg FGEM, Heynens JWCM, Jan de Vries G, et al. Clinical presentation of Churg-Strauss syndrome in children. A 12-year-old-boy with ANCA-negative Churg-Strauss syndrome. Respir Med Case Rep 2012;7:4–7.

142. Semple TR, Ashworth MT, Owens CM. Interstitial lung disease in children made easier...well, almost. Radiographics 2017;37:1679–703.

143. Susarla SC, Fan LL. Diffuse alveolar hemorrhage syndromes in children. Curr Opin Pediatr 2007; 19:314–20.

144. Guillerman RP, Brody AS. Contemporary perspectives on pediatric diffuse lung disease. Radiologic Clin North Am 2011;49:847–68.

145. Tansley SL, Betteridge ZE, Gunawardena H, et al. Anti-MDA5 autoantibodies in juvenile dermatomyositis identify a distinct clinical phenotype: a prospective cohort study. Arthritis Res Ther 2014;16: R138.

146. Koh DM, Hansell DM. Computed tomography of diffuse interstitial lung disease in children. Clin Radiol 2000;55:659–67.

147. Hill SC, Damaska BM, Tsokos M, et al. Radiographic findings in type 3b Gaucher disease. Pediatr Radiol 1996;26:852–60.

148. Nagral A. Gaucher disease. J Clin Exp Hepatol 2014;4:37–50.

149. Dinwidie R, Sonnappa S. Systemic disease and the lung. Paediatr Respir Rev 2005;6:181–9.

150. Becciolini V, Gudinchet F, Cheseaux JJ, et al. Lymphocytic interstitial pneumonia in children with AIDS: High-resolution CT findings. Eur Radiol 2001;11:1015–20.

151. Tanaka N, Kim JS, Bates CA, et al. Lung diseases in patients with common variable immunodeficiency: chest radiographic, and computed tomographic findings. J Comput Assist Tomogr 2006; 30:828–38.

152. Pac M, Bielecka T, Grzela K, et al. Interstitial lung disease in children with selected primary immunodeficiency disorders—a multicenter observational study. Front Immunol 2020;11:1–13.

153. Hurst JR, Verma N, Lowe D, et al. British Lung Foundation/United Kingdom primary immunodeficiency network consensus statement on the definition, diagnosis, and management of granulomatous-lymphocytic interstitial lung disease in common variable immunodeficiency disorders. J Allergy Clin Immunol Pract 2017;5:938–45.

154. Von Der Thüsen JH. Pleuroparenchymal fibroelastosis: its pathological characteristics. Curr Respir Med Rev 2013;9:238–47.

155. von der Thüsen JH, Hansell DM, Tominaga M, et al. Pleuroparenchymal fibroelastosis in patients with pulmonary disease secondary to bone marrow transplantation. Mod Pathol 2011;24:1633–9.

156. Nguyen HN, Das S, Gazzaneo MC, et al. Clinicoradiologic features of pleuroparenchymal fibroelastosis in children. Pediatr Radiol 2019;49:1163–70.

Pediatric Abdominal Masses
Imaging Guidelines and Recommendations

Helen H.R. Kim, MD[a,*], Nathan C. Hull, MD[b], Edward Y. Lee, MD, MPH[c],
Grace S. Phillips, MD[a]

KEYWORDS

- Pediatric • Abdominal • Mass • Imaging guidelines • Imaging recommendations • Congenital
- Neoplasm • Pseudomass

KEY POINTS

- The primary role of abdominal imaging in the setting of a suspected pediatric abdominal mass is to establish its presence and to identify salient imaging features that can narrow the differential diagnosis.
- Abdominal radiography may help assess the mass effect on bowel loops and detect calcifications associated with abnormal masses.
- Abdominal ultrasound is the preferred initial imaging modality to determine the origin of the mass and evaluate its vascular supply with Doppler imaging.
- If a neoplasm is suspected on ultrasound, cross-sectional imaging, such as computed tomography (CT) or magnetic resonance imaging (MRI), is indicated to further characterize the mass, stage extent of disease, and assist in presurgical planning.

INTRODUCTION

Pediatric abdominal masses are commonly encountered in the pediatric population with a broad differential diagnosis that encompasses benign and malignant entities. Although there are American College of Radiology (ACR) appropriateness imaging guidelines for abdominal masses in adults, the ACR appropriateness criteria do not specifically address pediatric abdominal masses. Therefore, the purpose of this article is to discuss an evidence-based practical imaging algorithm for pediatric abdominal masses. In addition, the characteristic imaging appearances of the most commonly encountered abdominal masses in infants and children are reviewed with an emphasis on reaching an accurate diagnosis which, in turn, can lead to optimal pediatric patient management.

EVIDENCE-BASED IMAGING ALGORITHM

The primary role of abdominal imaging in the setting of a suspected pediatric abdominal mass is to establish its presence, as nonneoplastic entities can mimic an abdominal mass, and to further characterize the mass location as well as other salient imaging features that might help narrow the differential diagnosis. Abdominal radiographs may help with determining the mass effect on bowel loops and with the detection of tumoral calcifications. Abdominal ultrasound is the preferred initial imaging modality to determine the origin of the mass and to evaluate the vascular supply with Doppler imaging.[1] If a tumor is confirmed on ultrasound, then cross-sectional imaging [computed tomography (CT) and/or magnetic resonance imaging (MRI)] is indicated to further characterize the

[a] Department of Radiology, Seattle Children's Hospital and University of Washington, 4800 Sand Point Way Northeast, Seattle, WA 98105, USA; [b] Department of Radiology, Mayo Clinic, 200 First Street Southwest, Rochester, MN 55905, USA; [c] Department of Radiology, Boston Children's Hospital, Harvard Medical School, 330 Longwood Avenue, Boston, MA 02115, USA
* Corresponding author.
E-mail address: Helenhr.kim@seattlechildrens.org

mass, stage extent of disease, and assist in presurgical planning.

The 3 most common abdominal malignancies in children are neuroblastoma, Wilms tumor, and hepatoblastoma, and therefore, we discuss the specific evidence-based imaging recommendations for these entities; clinical features and imaging characteristics for these 3 malignancies are further discussed in the subsequent section entitled, "Spectrum of Neonatal and Pediatric Abdominal Masses." Additionally, currently recommended imaging protocols that exist to screen pediatric patients with certain syndromes and conditions such as Beckwith–Wiedemann and Wilms–aniridia–genitourinary–mental retardation (WAGR) syndromes who have an increased risk of abdominal malignancy are summarized in **Table 1**.

Table 1
Screening imaging protocols for syndromic abdominal malignancies

Genetic Syndrome	Associated Abdominal Masses	Surveillance Imaging Recommendations
Beckwith–Wiedemann Syndrome[58]	Wilms tumor, nephroblastomatosis, hepatoblastoma, neuroblastoma, rhabdomyosarcoma, adrenal carcinoma	Abdominal US every 3–4 mo
Wilms–Aniridia–Genitourinary–mental Retardation (WAGR)[59]	Wilms tumor	Abdominal US every 3–4 mo
Denys–Drash syndrome (DDS) and Frasier Syndrome[59]	Wilms tumor, gonadoblastoma	Abdominal US every 3–4 mo
DICER1 Syndrome[60]	Renal lesions (cystic nephroma and Wilms tumor), ovarian sex cord-stromal tumors, genitourinary rhabdomyosarcomas	Abdominal US every 6 mo until age 8 y and then every year until age 12 y. For women: abdominal and pelvic US every 6–12 mo from age 8–10 y to age 40 y.
Von Hippel–Lindau Syndrome[61]	Clear cell renal cell carcinoma, pheochromocytoma, pancreatic neuroendocrine tumors, epididymal and broad ligament cystadenoma, and renal and pancreatic cysts	Variable recommendations based on expert consensus, with annual screening with either abdominal US or MRI starting as early as 10 y of age.
Tuberous Sclerosis Complex[62]	Renal angiomyolipomas, renal cell carcinoma	Surveillance for renal lesions (interval not specified).
Multiple Endocrine Neoplasia Syndrome 1[63,64]	Pancreatic neuroendocrine tumors, adrenal lesions	Annual imaging surveillance for pancreatic neuroendocrine tumors and adrenal lesions with CT, MRI, or US before the age of 10 y.
Multiple Endocrine Neoplasia Syndrome 2[65]	Pheochromocytoma	Variable screening guidelines, with some favoring imaging in the setting of biochemical abnormalities, and others suggesting abdominal imaging for pheochromocytoma every 3 y.
Li-Fraumeni Syndrome[66]	Rhabdomyosarcoma, adrenal cortical tumors	Abdominal US every 4 mo

Abbreviations: CT, computed tomography; MRI, magnetic resonance imaging; US, ultrasound.

Neuroblastoma

Although neuroblastoma may initially be detected by abdominal radiographs or ultrasound, further evaluation with CT or MRI is necessary for tumor staging and clinical management. Both CT and MRI have various advantages and disadvantages, without a clear consensus favoring one modality over the other for initial staging.[1–3] CT is more sensitive than MRI for detecting calcifications.[3] MRI is superior to CT for the characterization of intraspinal extension, bone marrow disease, and liver metastasis.[2–6] Nuclear medicine metaiodobenzylguanidine (MIBG) imaging is also indicated at initial staging, because 90% of neuroblastoma tumors demonstrate MIBG avidity.[7] For MIBG-avid neuroblastoma tumors, MIBG imaging complements CT or MRI for treatment planning and monitoring tumor response. Data are still emerging regarding the use of fluorodeoxyglucose/positron emission tomography (FDG/PET) for the 10% of neuroblastoma lacking MIBG avidity.[8]

Wilms Tumor

Similar to neuroblastoma, Wilms tumor is typically initially diagnosed by ultrasound but requires CT or MRI for staging.[9] CT and MRI have similar accuracy with respect to staging,[10] and therefore, the institutional preference often dictates the choice of modality.[9] Contrast-enhanced chest CT is indicated for diagnosing pulmonary metastatic disease, including nodal involvement of the mediastinum and hilum, as well as potential tumor thrombus within the inferior vena cava and heart.[9]

Hepatoblastoma

As with neuroblastoma and Wilms tumor, the diagnosis of hepatoblastoma is often suspected by ultrasound findings.[1] MRI is preferred over CT for staging due to its superior contrast resolution, use of hepatobiliary-specific contrast agents, and potential for multiphase, dynamic contrast-enhanced imaging in the absence of ionizing radiation that is inherent to CT.[11] Given the propensity for hepatoblastoma to involve the hepatic vessels, a thorough evaluation for vessel involvement with tumor is mandatory for staging.[1] In the absence of MRI, CT may also be used for staging hepatoblastoma.[1]

PRACTICAL IMAGING APPROACH TO PEDIATRIC ABDOMINAL MASSES

Various imaging modalities are currently available for evaluating pediatric abdominal masses. A clear understanding of their advantages and disadvantages as well as specific situations for certain imaging modalities is essential for the practical imaging approach to pediatric abdominal masses.

Radiography

Conventional radiographs of the abdomen are often requested by clinicians as the initial imaging modality for the evaluation of a possible abdominal mass in children based on the clinical history and physical examination. The results of radiography are often nonspecific, but can be helpful, especially if an abdominal mass is large enough to cause local mass effect on adjacent organs such as the bowel. For example, a large hepatic mass can displace bowel loops inferiorly to the lower abdomen or pelvis, whereas a pelvic mass such as an ovarian tumor tends to displace the bowel loops superiorly. A large kidney or adrenal mass can displace the bowel loops to the contralateral side of the abdomen. Additionally, the presence of abnormal calcifications can provide clues to diagnosis.[12] When a pediatric patient presents with abdominal pain, at least 2 radiographs of the abdomen are needed. These should include a frontal supine view, and either a decubitus, upright, or cross-table lateral view to assess for bowel obstruction and pneumoperitoneum.

Ultrasound

Abdominal ultrasound is the preferred initial imaging modality in children with a suspected abdominal mass mainly due to its accessibility, flexibility, lack of ionizing radiation, lack of sedation, and relatively low cost compared to CT and MRI. Ultrasound has the potential to determine the anatomic origin and borders of the mass, as well as to characterize internal characteristics such as solid, cystic, and vascular components. Specifically, the vascularity and vascular supply of the mass can be evaluated by Doppler imaging. Local and distant abdominal metastasis in the abdomen can be assessed as well, but may lack sensitivity compared with CT and MRI. A potential pitfall of ultrasound is operator dependency; an inexperienced sonographer may completely fail to image a mass. Furthermore, the acoustic windows for visualizing structures in the abdomen may be limited by bowel gas. When successful, however, ultrasound characteristics of the abdominal mass narrow the differential diagnosis and thus help to guide management.

Computed Tomography

CT of the abdomen and pelvis with contrast is recommended if abdominal ultrasound is inconclusive or if further characterization of a mass or extent of disease is needed. The clinical setting and suspected diagnosis dictate the exact CT protocol. For instance, hepatic tumors such as hepatoblastoma, require identifying which hepatic se-gments are involved as well as the relationship of the mass to the hepatic vessels for surgical planning. Therefore, a dual-phase CT with both arterial and venous phases may be needed. Additionally, given the propensity for hepatoblastoma to metastasize to the lungs, a chest CT is typically also simultaneously performed. Advantages of CT include its wide availability and rapid acquisition, particularly with the newer generation CT machines, which may avoid the need for sedation in many pediatric patients. CT also excels in characterizing abdominal masses and provides a more global view of anatomy than ultrasound, and therefore, can assist in problem-solving and staging. An important disadvantage of CT is the inherent use of radiation, and therefore, it is important to routinely apply the as low as reasonably achievable (ALARA) principle with respect to radiation dose and technique.

Magnetic Resonance Imaging

MRI has been steadily gaining popularity in pediatric imaging due to advances in technology. Faster imaging acquisition, specialized pediatric coils, and dynamic contrast imaging allow superior contrast resolution than other imaging modalities to aid in accurately diagnosing an abdominal mass. Newer techniques, such as excretory MRI, can provide functional and quantitative information for obstructive processes involving the kidney. Although neonates can be imaged using the "wrap-and-feed" technique, most infants and young children may still require sedation for diagnostic quality MRI. Thus, the risks of anesthesia should be carefully considered when deciding MRI as an imaging modality for the evaluation of abdominal masses in infants and children.

Nuclear Medicine

Nuclear medicine is a helpful adjunct imaging modality in select clinical scenarios in the pediatric population. For instance, MIBG scans can help to differentiate neuroblastoma from other adrenal lesions, including adrenal tumors and adrenal hemorrhage. MAG3 (mercaptoacetyltriglycine) diuretic renal scans can help to differentiate ureteropelvic junction (UPJ) obstruction from other congenital kidney conditions. It is important to note, however, that there is both inherent risks of radiation and limited spatial resolution with nuclear medicine.

Interventional Radiology

Interventional radiology (IR) is an integral component of radiology that facilitates the diagnosis and treatment of abdominal masses. Minimally invasive image-guided procedures performed by interventional radiologists may provide both diagnosis and treatment in lieu of open surgery. For example, some lesions may be amenable to image-guided percutaneous biopsy. Additionally, therapeutic procedures such as fluid drainage, embolization of tumors, and sclerotherapy may also be provided by IR. Unfortunately, pediatric IR service is currently not universally available and is often limited to tertiary children's hospitals.

THE SPECTRUM OF NEONATAL AND PEDIATRIC ABDOMINAL MASSES

The differential diagnosis of pediatric abdominal masses is broad and includes congenital and acquired lesions that may be benign or malignant (Tables 2 and 3). The most common entities that comprise the differential diagnosis, with a focus on the characteristic imaging appearance and optimal imaging strategies for each condition, are reviewed in the following section.

Congenital Disorders

Enteric duplication cysts
Enteric duplication cysts (EDCs) are a subtype of foregut duplication cysts that result from the defective development of the ventral foregut. EDCs can occur anywhere along the gastrointestinal tract from the mouth to the rectum.[13] Clinical presentation depends on the location and histologic type of the EDCs. Gastric and intestinal duplication cysts can cause abdominal pain, nausea, and bloating due to the local mass effect on the adjacent bowel. Intussusception and bowel obstruction with EDCs acting as lead points can also occur.[14] The most serious complications typically present when EDCs are lined with gastric mucosa, which may result in mucosal ulceration and even bowel perforation.[15]

With technological advances in prenatal ultrasound, there has been increased detection of EDCs in prenatal imaging. Ultrasound is the imaging modality of choice for the diagnosis of EDCs. On ultrasound imaging, EDCs are known for a characteristic "gut signature" or a "double wall" sign corresponding to alternating bands of the bowel wall layers. When complications of EDCs occur, CT and MRI can further aid in surgical planning (Fig. 1). With symptomatic EDCs, surgical resection is needed for treatment.

Subdiaphragmatic extralobar pulmonary sequestration
Subdiaphragmatic extralobar pulmonary sequestration (EPS) consists of malformed pulmonary

Table 2
Underlying causes of abdominal masses in infants and children

Congenital	Infectious/Inflammatory	Neoplasm	Miscellaneous
Enteric duplication cysts	Abscess	See Table 3	Adrenal hemorrhage
Subdiaphragmatic extralobar pulmonary sequestration	Pancreatic pseudocyst		Constipation
Congenital kidney disorders Abdominal lymphatic malformation	Meconium pseudocyst		

parenchyma that lacks a normal connection to the bronchial tree and receives direct arterial supply from the aorta or its branches. EPS is believed to develop from the abnormal budding of the foregut, often associated with bronchial atresia.[16] Subdiaphragmatic EPS is uncommon and accounts for approximately 10% of EPS; 90% of EPS occur within the chest, between the lower lobe and diaphragm.[17] EPS is associated with other congenital anomalies such as diaphragmatic hernia, vertebral body anomalies, and congenital heart disease.[18] Affected pediatric patients with EPS often present in infancy with a respiratory illness.

EPS is typically first evaluated with abdominal ultrasound and is characterized by a homogenous round or triangular-shaped mass that is inferior to the diaphragm (**Fig. 2**A, B). Occasionally, arterial supply arising from the aorta can be appreciated on Doppler ultrasound. Multidetector CT (MDCT) can accurately detect the arterial supply from the aorta as well as determine venous drainage, and therefore, MDCT is often chosen as the next imaging step (**Fig. 2**C, D). The management of EPS is surgical resection if the patient is symptomatic with recurrent infections. Some cases of EPS may regress spontaneously within 4 years without treatment, particularly when the affected pediatric patient is asymptomatic and systemic arterial supply is diminutive on initial imaging,.[19]

Congenital kidney disorders
A variety of congenital kidney disorders such as hydronephrosis, UPJ obstruction, ureterovesical

junction (UVJ) obstruction, multicystic dysplastic kidney (MCDK), and autosomal recessive polycystic kidney disease (ARPCKD) can present in children as an abdominal mass by the virtue of either the degree of dilation of the collecting system or the extent of nephromegaly related to the pathologic parenchymal process.[20] Although a detailed description of these various entities is beyond the scope of this article, many of these entities are either suspected or diagnosed in utero on screening ultrasound, and are further evaluated with postnatal ultrasound (**Fig. 3**A). In the case of suspected UPJ or UVJ obstruction, functional imaging can be further accomplished by either nuclear medicine scintigraphy or MR urography (**Fig. 3**B).

Infectious and Inflammatory Disorders

Several inflammatory and infectious entities, including abscess, pancreatic pseudocyst, and meconium pseudocyst, can simulate an intraabdominal mass on imaging, leading to a diagnostic dilemma in the pediatric population. Often, the correct diagnosis is made by correlating imaging findings with additional clinical data. The clinical and imaging features of these 3 entities are discussed in the following sections.

Abscess and phlegmon
An intraabdominal abscess implies an infected fluid collection, which can involve parenchymal organs such as the liver and spleen, or peritoneal or retroperitoneal spaces. The term phlegmon refers to an inflammatory mass and implies a lack of a

Table 3
Most commonly encountered abdominal neoplasm by organ of origin

Origin	Neoplasm
Liver	Infantile hepatic hemangioma, hepatoblastoma
Pancreas	Pancreatoblastoma, solid pseudopapillary epithelial neoplasm (SPEN)
Kidney	Wilms tumor
Adrenal Gland	Neuroblastoma
Blood Cells	Lymphoma

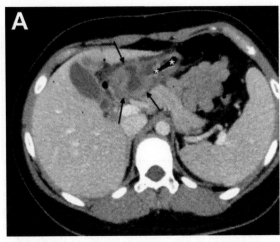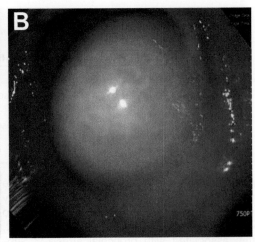

Fig. 1. Enteric duplication cysts in a 16-year-old girl who presented with abdominal pain. (*A*) Contrast-enhanced axial CT image of the abdomen demonstrates a bilobed, thick-wall cystic structure (*arrows*) in the expected location of the gastric antrum. The gas-filled adjacent gastric lumen (*asterisks*) is seen proximally. (*B*) Endoscopic image reveals an extrinsic mass compressing the gastric antrum, which caused a gastric outlet obstruction. This mass was surgically excised. Pathologic diagnosis confirmed enteric duplication cysts lined with gastric mucosa, with resultant mucosal ulceration.

substantial, drainable fluid component. Although abscess and phlegmon involving the peritoneal spaces can occur in children in a variety of clinical scenarios, they are most frequently seen with perforated appendicitis. Appendicitis is the most common surgical emergency in children.[21] Typical presenting clinical signs and symptoms include right lower quadrant abdominal pain, fever, and leukocytosis. Perforation markedly increases the risk of abscess formation from 0.8% in nonperforated appendicitis to 20% in patients with perforated appendicitis.[21]

The typical ultrasound findings of intraabdominal abscess after appendicitis include solitary or multiple loculated complex intraperitoneal fluid collections, often with surrounding hyperemia. CT and MRI similarly demonstrate rim-enhancing intraperitoneal fluid collections, with increased density on CT, and signal intensity on MRI reflective of proteinaceous content. A dislodged fecalith may be apparent on cross-sectional imaging either within or near the fluid collection. A phlegmon typically manifests as mass-like, heterogeneous, solid tissue which demonstrates internal color Doppler flow on ultrasound and variable internal enhancement by CT and MRI (**Fig. 4**). Both abscess and phlegmon associated with appendicitis can have substantial mass effects on surrounding structures, for example, obstruction of the right distal ureter. Despite the nonspecific imaging features of intraabdominal abscess, the diagnosis is well-supported in the clinical context of known or suspected perforated ap-

pendicitis. Phlegmon may pose a greater diagnostic dilemma due to the predominantly solid appearance (see **Fig. 4**), but the diagnosis can be favored in children with a compatible clinical course.

Pancreatic and peripancreatic fluid collections

Acute pancreatitis refers to inflammatory changes in the pancreas caused by acinar cell injury and subsequent pancreatic tissue damage. The incidence of acute pancreatitis in children is approximately 1/10,000, which is nearly that of adults.[22] The 3 most common causes of pancreatitis in children are biliary obstruction, medications, and various underlying systemic diseases, although it may be idiopathic in 15% to 30% of cases.[22] Diagnostic criteria include abdominal pain, an elevated serum lipase, and typical imaging features such as pancreatic enlargement and edema. Pancreatic and peripancreatic fluid collections are well-described complications of acute pancreatitis.

On imaging, pancreatic and peripancreatic fluid collections may occur in the intrapancreatic or extrapancreatic locations, and they have variable internal complexity with cross-sectional imaging. With time, pancreatic and peripancreatic fluid collections typically become more loculated and well-defined (**Fig. 5**), with an enhancing rim demonstrated by CT or MRI.[23]

Meconium pseudocyst

Meconium pseudocyst is a meconium-containing intraperitoneal fluid collection that typically occurs

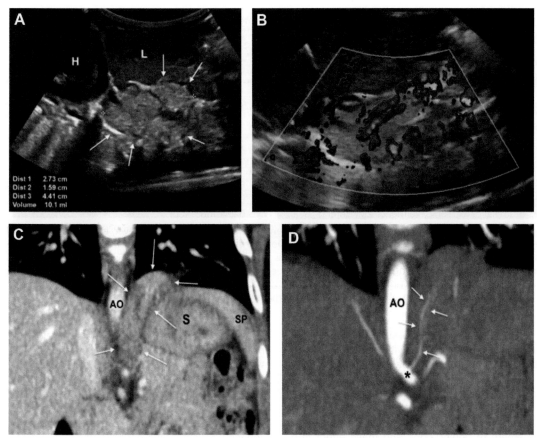

Fig. 2. Extralobar pulmonary sequestration in a 4-month-old boy with prenatal diagnosis of abdominal mass. (*A*) Longitudinal grayscale ultrasound of the abdomen demonstrates a relatively homogenous echogenic mass (*arrows*) inferior to the diaphragm and heart (H) and posterior to the left hepatic lobe (L). (*B*) Longitudinal color Doppler ultrasound demonstrates hypervascularity within the mass. (*C*) Contrast-enhanced coronal CT image re-demonstrates a triangular-shaped oblong mass (*arrows*) in between the aorta (AO) and stomach (S). The spleen (SP) is seen within the left upper quadrant. (*D*) Contrast-enhanced arterial phase coronal CT image delineates an aberrant feeding artery (*arrows*) arising from the celiac axis (*asterisk*) of the abdominal aorta (AO).

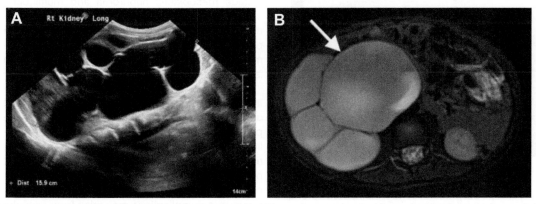

Fig. 3. Ureteropelvic junction obstruction in a 3-year-old boy who presented with a palpable abdominal mass. (*A*) Longitudinal grayscale ultrasound of the right kidney shows severe dilation of the right renal collecting system (between cursors). (*B*) Axial T2-weighted MR image confirms severe right pelvicaliectasis with mass-like enlargement of the right kidney (*arrow*).

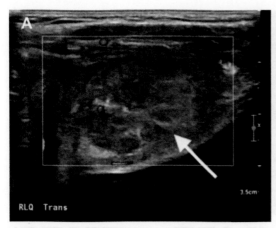
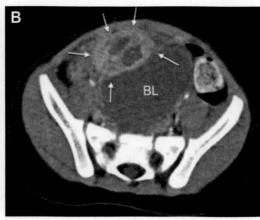

Fig. 4. Abscess in a 3-year-old girl with perforated appendicitis who presented with fever, elevated white blood cell count, and abdominal pain. (*A*) Transverse color Doppler ultrasound of the right lower quadrant demonstrates pseudomass (*arrow*) appearance of early abscess formation with both complex, septated cystic areas as well as vascular, solid-appearing structures. (*B*) Contrast-enhanced axial CT image demonstrates a fluid collection with an irregularly thickened rim of enhancement (*arrows*), causing mass effect on the urinary bladder (BL). The interventional radiologist was able to aspirate approximately 6 mL of frank pus the next day.

in utero in the setting of intestinal volvulus, intussusception, or obstruction, with resultant intestinal perforation. Although the diagnosis is sometimes suspected on prenatal ultrasound, presenting clinical signs and symptoms in the neonate include progressive abdominal distention and feeding intolerance. Abdominal radiographs may show displacement of bowel loops and mass effect from the meconium pseudocyst. Coarse, peripheral rim calcifications are a well-described radiographic

feature (**Fig. 6**A).[24] Typical ultrasound features of meconium pseudocyst include a complex cyst with peripheral echogenic foci corresponding to the rim calcifications (**Fig. 6**B), that can be in continuity with the intestine. The imaging features and clinical scenario typically help to narrow the differential diagnosis and exclude the considerations of malignancy. Symptomatic pediatric patients with meconium pseudocyst are typically treated surgically.

Neoplastic Disorders

Benign tumors
There are multiple benign tumors that can arise in the liver, kidneys, and other abdominal organs. Although not described in detail in this article, some of the benign, congenital renal tumors include mesoblastic nephroma and multilocular cystic nephroma, and benign congenital liver tumors include mesenchymal hamartoma. For the purposes of this article, the most common liver tumor of infancy, infantile hepatic hemangioma (IHH) is discussed.

Infantile hepatic hemangioma IHH is the most common liver tumor in infancy. IHH is a benign, hepatic vascular tumor composed of endothelial-lined vascular channels. IHH is classified as focal, multifocal, or diffuse based on distribution. Most pediatric patients with IHH are asymptomatic or present with associated cutaneous hemangiomas. Some rare complications may arise from vascular shunting with resultant high-output congestive heart failure, Kasabach–Merritt syndrome, liver failure, or hypothyroidism.[25]

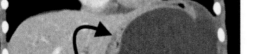
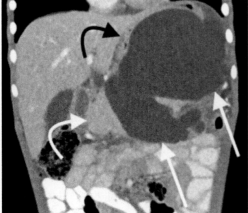

Fig. 5. Peripancreatic fluid collection in an 8-year-old boy with pancreatitis who presented with epigastric pain and palpable mass. Contrast-enhanced coronal CT image shows a bilobed peripancreatic fluid collection (*white straight arrows*) that displaces the pancreatic head (*white curved arrow*) and stomach (*black curved arrow*).

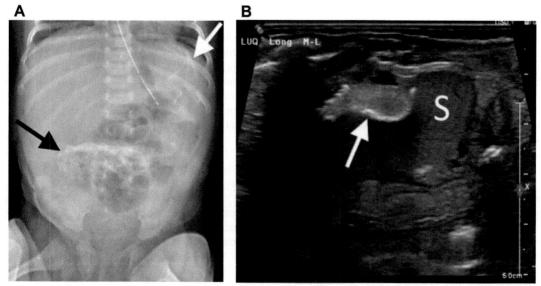

Fig. 6. Meconium pseudocyst in a 1-month-old girl who presented with abdominal distension. (*A*) Frontal supine abdominal radiograph shows amorphous calcifications in the central lower abdomen (*black arrow*) as well as within the left upper quadrant (*white arrow*). (*B*) Longitudinal grayscale ultrasound of the left upper quadrant shows a complex fluid collection (*arrow*) with a hyperechoic rim corresponding to the calcifications seen on the radiograph, adjacent to the spleen (*S*).

Ultrasound is the favored imaging modality to screen for IHH. MRI can further characterize IHH; hepatic lesions are particularly conspicuous on T2-weighted sequences with pronounced hyperintensity relative to hepatic parenchyma (**Fig. 7**). IHH is considered benign and generally has a favorable prognosis. For asymptomatic pediatric patients, abdominal ultrasound can be used to follow lesion size. In symptomatic pediatric patients, propranolol can be considered to promote regression.[26] In severe symptomatic cases, more aggressive treatment measures may include partial resection, embolization, or liver transplant.[26]

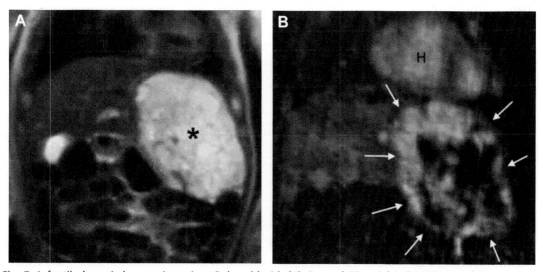

Fig. 7. Infantile hepatic hemangioma in a 2-day-old girl. (*A*) Coronal T2-weighted MR image demonstrates a large, hyperintense mass (*asterisk*) occupying the left hepatic lobe. (*B*) Contrast-enhanced coronal T1-weighted MR image demonstrates early peripheral enhancement (*arrows*) with subsequent marked gradual central filling of the left hepatic mass (not shown), characteristic of infantile hepatic hemangioma. Intravascular contrast within the heart (*H*) is also seen.

Malignant tumors

Neuroblastoma Neuroblastoma is the most aggressive malignant tumor of neural crest cells, which can arise anywhere along the sympathetic chain but most often originates in the adrenal glands (30%–40%).[27] Neuroblastoma is the most common extracranial solid tumor in the pediatric population, particularly in infancy.[28] The clinical presentation of neuroblastoma varies from an asymptomatic abdominal mass to neurologic symptoms related to spinal involvement to opsoclonus–myoclonus syndrome.[29]

The imaging features of neuroblastoma vary as well, but the most frequent appearance is a retroperitoneal mass arising from the adrenal gland that extends and surrounds the adjacent organs without substantial displacement or vascular invasion, for example, a retroperitoneal mass surrounding and displacing the abdominal aorta anteriorly from the vertebral body (**Fig. 8**A). As with other abdominal masses, abdominal ultrasound is the initial imaging modality of choice to confirm a solid mass and quantify the degree of mass effect on adjacent organs, such as the ipsilateral kidney. CT or MRI is needed for the evaluation of metastatic disease because roughly 50% of affected pediatric patients have metastatic disease at the time of diagnosis (**Fig. 8**B).[30] Common metastatic sites from neuroblastoma are liver, bone, and regional lymph nodes. CT can readily and accurately assess the extent of the disease and clearly demonstrate calcifications. MRI is especially helpful when evaluating for intraspinal extension and bone marrow involvement of the tumor.

Recently, whole-body MRI has been gaining popularity to detect distant osseous metastases in pediatric patients with neuroblastoma.[31] Nuclear medicine MIBG also plays a role in the initial imaging of neuroblastoma as well as to document treatment response. MIBG scintigraphy can help to characterize the primary tumor as well as extent of metastatic disease in MIBG-avid tumors.[32] Dotatate imaging, which links a newer somatostatin receptor agent with [68]gallium for use in PET/CT and PET/MRI, has shown potential recently for increased sensitivity than MIBG scintigraphy for the detection of metastatic neuroblastoma.[33] Treatment of neuroblastoma involves chemotherapy followed by resection for surgically amenable tumors. I-131 MIBG therapy can be considered in advanced neuroblastoma.[34]

Wilms tumor Wilms tumor is the most common solid abdominal tumor in children less than 10 years old and represents about 90% of all pediatric renal tumors.[35] Although the majority or approximately 75% of Wilms tumor occurs sporadically, 15% of cases are associated with underlying syndromes, most commonly Beckwith–Wiedmann, WAGR, and Denys–Drash syndromes.[36] The clinical presentation varies but may include a palpable abdominal mass, abdominal pain, and hematuria.

Ultrasound of Wilms tumor often reveals a large solid mass with vascular supply arising from the ipsilateral kidney. Doppler ultrasound can assess for the tumoral invasion of the renal vein or inferior vena cava. CT or MRI with contrast is indicated for further characterization. Both cross-sectional modalities can accurately demonstrate a large

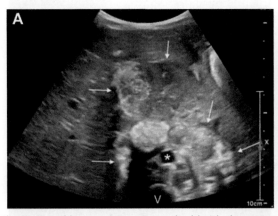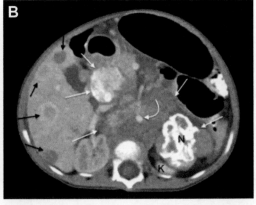

Fig. 8. Neuroblastoma in an 18-month-old girl who presented with weight loss, increased irritability, and abdominal distension. (*A*) Transverse grayscale ultrasound of the abdomen demonstrates a conglomerate of retroperitoneal masses (*arrows*) encasing and displacing the aorta (*asterisk*) anteriorly from the vertebral body (V). (*B*) Contrast-enhanced axial CT image demonstrates a large partially calcified left suprarenal mass (N), large retroperitoneal and intraperitoneal masses (*white arrows*) encasing the abdominal aorta (*curved arrow*), and multiple hepatic metastatic lesions (*black arrows*). Upper pole of the left kidney (K) is partially seen.

heterogeneously enhancing mass originating from the kidney with a characteristic "claw" sign (**Fig. 9**A, B) that refers to a thin margin of renal parenchyma partially surrounding the lesion. CT or MRI is excellent for the evaluation of local spread and metastatic disease involving lymph nodes or, less commonly, the liver. To evaluate for lung metastases, CT remains the preferred imaging tool compared to MRI due to its superior spatial resolution and lesser degree of motion artifact. Treatment for Wilms tumor is generally surgical resection either with or without chemotherapy or radiation. Children with predisposing syndromes, such as those described above, require abdominal ultrasound surveillance every 3 months until 8 years of age.

Hepatoblastoma Hepatoblastoma is the most common primary liver malignancy seen in younger children. Predisposing factors include certain syndromes such as Beckwith–Wiedemann and familial adenomatous polyposis, as well as low birth weight and prematurity.[37] The vast majority (90%–95%) of affected patients present before 4 years of age.[38] Presenting symptoms vary but may include a palpable abdominal mass, weight loss, or, rarely, precocious puberty due to the tumoral secretion of human chorionic gonadotropin.[39]

Typical ultrasound features of hepatoblastoma are a large, heterogenous solid mass arising from the liver (**Fig. 10**). Once a large neoplastic process in the liver is seen on abdominal ultrasound, cross-sectional imaging with MRI or CT is needed to further stage extent of disease and to assist with presurgical planning. Calcifications can be seen in up to 50% of hepatoblastoma cases.[40] The use of either a dynamic contrast-enhanced MRI or a dual-phase CT may assist in determining the relationship of tumor to hepatic vessels, including vascular invasion. Chest CT is indicated for staging because the lungs are the most common site of metastasis.[40] Treatment options include surgical resection, chemotherapy with subsequent surgical resection, and liver transplantation.[41]

Lymphoma Lymphoma ranks third in frequency after brain tumors and leukemia as one of the most common pediatric cancers.[42] There are many subtypes of lymphoma which comprise the 2 main categories of Hodgkin (HL) and non–Hodgkin lymphomas (NHL). Although HL is known for nodal diseases, such as in the form of cervical lymphadenopathy, NHL is often extranodal within the chest or abdomen. Therefore, NHL involving the abdomen is highlighted in this article. Although NHL can arise in any organ in the abdomen, it most often involves the bowels and kidneys. For instance, Burkitt's lymphoma, a type of B-cell NHL, is known for tumoral spread within the mucosal layer of bowel with resultant bowel wall thickening, mural mass, or dilatation.[43] Presenting symptoms vary and may include an asymptomatic palpable mass, intussusception with a pathologic lead point, bowel obstruction, or urinary obstruction.

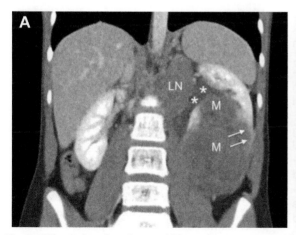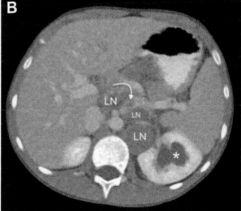

Fig. 9. Wilms tumor in a 9-year-old boy who presented with hematuria and a palpable left abdominal mass. (*A*) Contrast-enhanced coronal CT image of the abdomen demonstrates a large, solid, hypodense mass (M) arising from the left kidney with a characteristic "claw" sign (*arrows*), with associated obstructive hydronephrosis (*asterisks*). Multiple large conglomerates of retroperitoneal lymph nodes (LN) are also seen. (*B*) Contrast-enhanced axial CT image shows multiple retroperitoneal lymph nodes (LN) and tumoral invasion of the renal vein (*curved arrow*). Hydronephrosis (*asterisk*) is again seen.

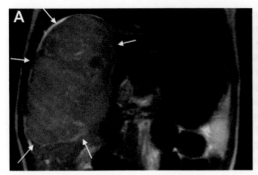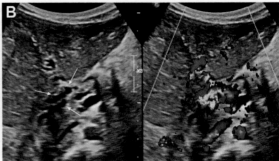

Fig. 10. Hepatoblastoma in a 3-year-old boy who presented with abdominal pain and a palpable mass. (A) Coronal T2-weighted MR image of the abdomen demonstrates a large, heterogenous mass (arrows) within the right hepatic lobe. (B) Dual-screen grayscale (left) and color Doppler (right) transverse ultrasound images of the porta hepatis demonstrate cavernous transformation (arrows, left) of the portal vein due to tumoral thrombus involving the main portal vein.

Abdominal ultrasound remains the primary initial imaging tool to assess for bowel, abdominal nodal, or intraabdominal organ involvement. Contrast-enhanced abdominal CT is effective in evaluating the extent of lymphomatous involvement of intraperitoneal organs, including bowel (Fig. 11). Unlike ultrasound, CT is not limited by bowel gas. MRI is typically not indicated unless there is a concern for central nervous system (CNS) involvement, in which case MRI is the preferred modality. PET/CT also plays a major role in documenting residual disease and guiding further therapy, including radiation therapy.[44] Chemotherapy is typically the primary treatment.

Pancreatoblastoma Pancreatoblastoma is a rare entity, yet is the most common primary pancreatic malignancy that occurs in children less than 10 years old.[45] There is an increased risk with Beckwith–Wiedemann syndrome.[46] Given the retroperitoneal location of the pancreas, affected pediatric patients with pancreatoblastoma often present at an advanced stage, with symptoms of pain or a large, palpable abdominal mass.

Ultrasound remains the favored initial imaging modality and demonstrates a large retroperitoneal mass with central hypoechogenic areas due to necrosis.[47] Contrast-enhanced CT or MRI is indicated to further characterize and stage pancreatoblastoma (Fig. 12). Pancreatoblastoma often replaces either a segment of or the entire pancreas, and when large, can be exophytic with mass effect on adjacent bowel loops. Local spread can occur among regional lymph nodes. Distant metastases from pancreatoblastoma typically primarily involve liver and lungs.[45] Treatment commonly involves both surgery and chemotherapy.

Vascular Disorders

Abdominal lymphatic malformation

Abdominal lymphatic malformations (LMs), which are often mistakenly referred to by the misnomers lymphangiomas or cystic hygromas, consist of a group of abnormally formed and dilated lymphatic channels. LMs are a subtype of vascular malformations and are considered a benign entity. The vast majority (95%) of LMs occur in the head and neck, and the remaining 5% occur in the chest and abdomen, specifically in the mesentery, omentum,

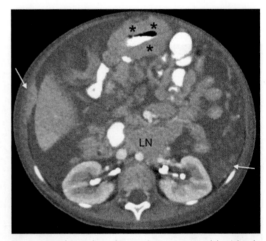

Fig. 11. Burkitt's lymphoma in a 4-year-old girl who presented with diffuse abdominal pain and distension. Contrast-enhanced axial CT image of the abdomen demonstrates fusiform dilatation and bowel wall thickening (asterisks) of a small bowel loop. There are multiple conglomerates of mesenteric and retroperitoneal lymph nodes (LNs) and peritoneal carcinomatosis (arrows) causing ascites.

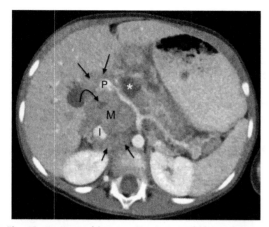

Fig. 12. Pancreatoblastoma in a 4-year-old boy who presented with vomiting and abdominal pain. Contrast-enhanced axial CT image of the abdomen demonstrates a large hypodense mass (*M*) arising from the pancreatic head with an area of central hypoattenuation due to necrosis (*asterisk*). There are regional lymph nodes (*straight arrows*) within the retroperitoneum and porta hepatis. The mass encases portal vein (*P*), IVC (*I*), and common bile duct (*curved arrow*).

mesocolon, and retroperitoneum.[48] Abdominal LMs are, therefore, rare and usually present indolently with a palpable abdominal mass in childhood unless complications occur, such as bowel obstruction, volvulus, or hemorrhage.[49]

Abdominal ultrasound demonstrates well-defined cysts with and without septations (**Fig. 13**A). The wall of the cysts may demonstrate color Doppler flow. Once multiloculated cysts in the abdomen are identified by ultrasound, contrast-enhanced MRI is preferred over CT for further evaluation, owing to the superior contrast resolution of MRI, particularly in the case of retroperitoneal involvement (**Fig. 13**B). It is crucial to accurately define the anatomic relationship of LMs to adjacent vessels and organs in advance of the often arduous surgical resection, which is also associated with a high recurrence rate.[50] Despite the high recurrence rate, surgical resection remains the primary treatment for LMs. Sclerotherapy is sometimes considered for smaller LMs as an alternative and less invasive treatment option.[51]

Miscellaneous

Adrenal hemorrhage

In the newborn, the adrenal glands are 10 to 20 times larger in proportion to their body size than adults.[52] Therefore, the adrenal glands are readily visualized with a linear, high-frequency transducer on ultrasound. The unique vascular supply of the adrenal glands, which consists of generous arterial supply and comparatively fewer draining venous structures, causes blood to pool in the adrenal glands, and thus, predisposes the gland to hemorrhage.[53] Adrenal hemorrhage can be traumatic or nontraumatic. In a newborn, for which adrenal hemorrhage may be palpable on physical examination, adrenal hemorrhage is most often related to the physiologic stress of birth.[54] The hemorrhage itself has no clinical significance, but the clinical dilemma stems from the potential difficulty in differentiating adrenal hemorrhage from congenital neuroblastoma.

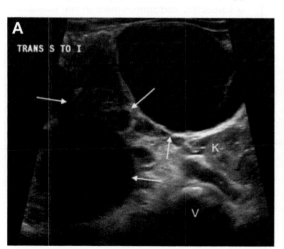

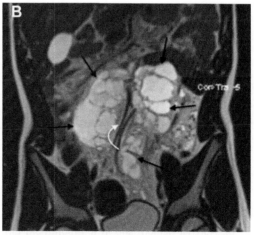

Fig. 13. Lymphatic malformation in a 5-year-old girl who presented with diffuse abdominal distension. (*A*) Transverse grayscale ultrasound of the midabdomen demonstrates cysts of varying sizes (*white arrows*) in the retroperitoneal and intraperitoneal spaces. Left kidney (K) and vertebral body (V) are partially visualized. (*B*) Coronal T2-weighted fast turbo spin-echo MR image demonstrates the extent of the mesenteric lymphatic malformation (*black arrows*) which is centered around the superior mesenteric artery and superior mesenteric vein (*curved arrow*).

Initial ultrasound of adrenal hemorrhage demonstrates an avascular, complex cyst, or mass (Fig. 14), which may be large enough to cause local mass effect on the adjacent kidney. CT or MRI may assist in detecting blood products associated with a hemorrhage. The clinical course of adrenal hemorrhage and congenital neuroblastoma may overlap, as both entities often involute over time. Given the benign nature of adrenal hemorrhage, serial ultrasound is used to confirm the involution of the hemorrhage and to further exclude the possibility of refractory congenital neuroblastoma. Urine catecholamines can aid in the distinction between the 2 entities, as they are absent with adrenal hemorrhage and elevated in the setting of congenital neuroblastoma.[55]

Constipation

Constipation is one of the most common chronic disorders in children, comprising 3% pediatrician visits and 10% to 15% of pediatric gastroenterologist visits.[56] With limited medical history, vague symptoms, and nonspecific physical examination, functional constipation can be difficult to distinguish from constipation caused by organic causes, including an underlying abdominal mass.

Although abdominal radiography has limited value in diagnosing constipation due to a lack of interobserver reliability and accuracy,[57] abdominal radiography can assess the amount of stool present throughout the colon which may be reassuring to the clinicians and parents. If there is a large abdominal mass, abdominal radiography may show abnormal calcifications or local mass effects on adjacent organs. If clinical suspicion for a mass persists by either radiographs or other clinical data, abdominal ultrasound can be pursued to further assess for an underlying mass. However, most cases of constipation require no imaging, and treatment generally involves supportive management with diet, medication, and behavioral modification in the pediatric population.

SUMMARY

The differential diagnosis and clinical presentation of pediatric abdominal masses are wide-ranging, and include benign and malignant entities, both of which may present with indolent to life-threatening symptoms. It is important to be familiar with the most common entities that constitute the differential diagnosis of a pediatric abdominal mass. A systematic imaging approach facilitates the detection and characterization of a pediatric abdominal mass. The optimal use of various imaging modalities allows for narrowing the differential diagnosis and guiding timely, appropriate treatment for this population.

CLINICS CARE POINTS

- Abdominal ultrasound is recommended as the initial imaging modality to evaluate for a suspected abdominal mass in the pediatric population.
- CT is used to further characterize a mass if a neoplasm is suspected on ultrasound.
- MRI provides superior contrast resolution than CT, which is of benefit in the further characterization of a mass, but typically requires anesthesia for most infants and young children.
- The optimal use of various imaging modalities to evaluate a pediatric abdominal mass expedites diagnosis and treatment.

DISCLOSURES

The authors have nothing to disclose.

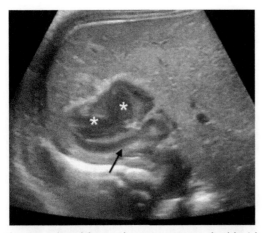

Fig. 14. Adrenal hemorrhage in a 1-month-old girl. Transverse grayscale ultrasound shows a heterogeneous avascular complex cyst (*asterisks*) abutting the right adrenal gland (*arrow*). Serum homovanillic acid (HVA) and vanillylmandelic acid (VMA) were negative. Follow-up serial ultrasound demonstrated subsequent interval resolution (not shown).

REFERENCES

1. Morin CE, Artunduaga M, Schooler GR, et al. Imaging for staging of pediatric abdominal tumors: an update, from the *AJR* Special Series on Cancer

Staging. AJR Am J Roentgenol 2021;217(4):786–99. https://doi.org/10.2214/AJR.20.25310.

2. Sarioglu FC, Salman M, Guleryuz H, et al. Radiological staging in neuroblastoma: computed tomography or magnetic resonance imaging? Pol J Radiol 2019;84:e46–53.

3. Mehta K, Haller JO, Legasto AC. Imaging neuroblastoma in children. Crit Rev Comput Tomogr 2003;44(1):47–61.

4. Maris JM, Hogarty MD, Bagatell R, et al. Neuroblastoma. Lancet 2007;369(9579):2106–20.

5. Tanabe M, Ohnuma N, Iwai J, et al. Bone marrow metastasis of neuroblastoma analyzed by MRI and its influence on prognosis. Med Pediatr Oncol 1995;24(5):292–9.

6. Sofka CM, Semelka RC, Kelekis NL, et al. Magnetic resonance imaging of neuroblastoma using current techniques. Magn Reson Imaging 1999;17(2):193–8.

7. Bar-Sever Z, Biassoni L, Shulkin B, et al. Guidelines on nuclear medicine imaging in neuroblastoma. Eur J Nucl Med Mol Imaging 2018;45(11):2009–24.

8. Bleeker G, Tytgat GAM, Adam JA, et al. 123I-MIBG scintigraphy and 18F-FDG-PET imaging for diagnosing neuroblastoma. Cochrane Database Syst Rev 2015;(9):CD009263.

9. Servaes SE, Hoffer FA, Smith EA, et al. Imaging of Wilms tumor: an update. Pediatr Radiol 2019; 49(11):1441–52.

10. Servaes S, Khanna G, Naranjo A, et al. Comparison of diagnostic performance of CT and MRI for abdominal staging of pediatric renal tumors: a report from the Children's Oncology Group. Pediatr Radiol 2015;45(2):166–72.

11. Schooler GR, Squires JH, Alazraki A, et al. Pediatric hepatoblastoma, hepatocellular carcinoma, and other hepatic neoplasms: consensus imaging recommendations from American College of Radiology Pediatric Liver Reporting and Data System (LI-RADS) Working Group. Radiology 2020;296(3): 493–7.

12. Dickson PV, Sims TL, Streck CJ, et al. Avoiding misdiagnosing neuroblastoma as Wilms tumor. J Pediatr Surg 2008;43(6):1159–63.

13. Macpherson RI. Gastrointestinal tract duplications: clinical, pathologic, etiologic, and radiologic considerations. Radiographics 1993;13(5):1063–80.

14. Khan RA, Wahab S, Ghani I. Neonatal Intestinal Obstruction: when to suspect duplication cyst of bowel as the cause. J Neonatal Surg 2016;5(4):52.

15. Puligandla PS, Nguyen LT, St-Vil D, et al. Gastrointestinal duplications. J Pediatr Surg 2003;38(5): 740–4.

16. Riedlinger WFJ, Vargas SO, Jennings RW, et al. Bronchial atresia is common to extralobar sequestration, intralobar sequestration, congenital cystic adenomatoid malformation, and lobar emphysema. Pediatr Dev Pathol 2006;9(5):361–73.

17. Savic B, Birtel FJ, Tholen W, et al. Lung sequestration: report of seven cases and review of 540 published cases. Thorax 1979;34(1):96–101.

18. Lee EY, Chu WC, Dillman JR, et al. Pediatric radiology practical imaging evaluation of infants and children 2018. Available at: http://ovidsp.ovid.com/ovidweb.cgi?T=JS&PAGE=booktext&NEWS=N&DF=bookdb&CSC=Y&AN=01938979/1st_Edition&XPATH=/PG(0). Accessed March 8, 2021.

19. Yoon HM, Kim EA-R, Chung S-H, et al. Extralobar pulmonary sequestration in neonates: the natural course and predictive factors associated with spontaneous regression. Eur Radiol 2017;27(6):2489–96.

20. Chung EM, Soderlund KA, Fagen KE. Imaging of the pediatric urinary system. Radiologic Clin North America 2017;55(2):337–57.

21. Rentea RM, St. Peter SD. Pediatric appendicitis. Surg Clin North Am 2017;97(1):93–112.

22. Pohl JF, Uc A. Paediatric pancreatitis. Curr Opin Gastroenterol 2015;31(5):380–6.

23. Foster BR, Jensen KK, Bakis G, et al. Revised atlanta classification for acute pancreatitis: a pictorial essay. Radiographics 2016;36(3):675–87.

24. Minato M, Okada T, Miyagi H, et al. Meconium pseudocyst with particular pathologic findings: a case report and review of the literature. J Pediatr Surg 2012;47(4):e9–12.

25. Chung EM, Cube R, Lewis RB, et al. From the archives of the AFIP: Pediatric liver masses: radiologic-pathologic correlation part 1. Benign tumors. Radiographics 2010;30(3):801–26.

26. Christison-Lagay ER, Burrows PE, Alomari A, et al. Hepatic hemangiomas: subtype classification and development of a clinical practice algorithm and registry. J Pediatr Surg 2007;42(1):62–7 [discussion 67–8].

27. Brisse HJ, McCarville MB, Granata C, et al. Guidelines for imaging and staging of neuroblastic tumors: consensus report from the International Neuroblastoma Risk Group Project. Radiology 2011;261(1): 243–57.

28. McHugh K. Renal and adrenal tumours in children. Cancer Imaging 2007;7:41–51.

29. Brunklaus A, Pohl K, Zuberi SM, et al. Investigating neuroblastoma in childhood opsoclonus-myoclonus syndrome. Arch Dis Child 2012;97(5):461–3.

30. McCarville MB. Imaging neuroblastoma: what the radiologist needs to know. Cancer Imaging 2011; 11(Spec No A):S44–7.

31. Siegel MJ, Acharyya S, Hoffer FA, et al. Whole-body MR imaging for staging of malignant tumors in pediatric patients: results of the American College of Radiology Imaging Network 6660 Trial. Radiology 2013;266(2):599–609.

32. Sharp SE, Gelfand MJ, Shulkin BL. Pediatrics: diagnosis of neuroblastoma. Semin Nucl Med 2011; 41(5):345–53.

33. McElroy KM, Binkovitz LA, Trout AT, et al. Pediatric applications of Dotatate: early diagnostic and therapeutic experience. Pediatr Radiol 2020;50(7):882–97.

34. DuBois SG, Matthay KK. 131I-Metaiodobenzylguanidine therapy in children with advanced neuroblastoma. Q J Nucl Med Mol Imaging 2013;57(1):53–65.

35. Howlader N, Noone AM, Krapcho M, et al, editorss. SEER Cancer Statistics Review, 1975-2017. SEER. Available at: https://seer.cancer.gov/csr/1975_2017/index.html. Accessed March 18, 2021.

36. Lowe LH, Isuani BH, Heller RM, et al. Pediatric renal masses: Wilms tumor and beyond. Radiographics 2000;20(6):1585–603.

37. Tomlinson GE, Kappler R. Genetics and epigenetics of hepatoblastoma: genetics and epigenetics of hepatoblastoma. Pediatr Blood Cancer 2012;59(5):785–92.

38. Meyers RL. Tumors of the liver in children. Surg Oncol 2007;16(3):195–203.

39. Khanna R, Verma SK. Pediatric hepatocellular carcinoma. World J Gastroenterol 2018;24(35):3980–99.

40. McCarville MB, Roebuck DJ. Diagnosis and staging of hepatoblastoma: imaging aspects. Pediatr Blood Cancer 2012;59(5):793–9.

41. Meyers RL, Tiao GM, Dunn SP, et al. Liver transplantation in the management of unresectable hepatoblastoma in children. Front Biosci (Elite Ed) 2012;4:1293–302.

42. Toma P, Granata C, Rossi A, et al. Multimodality imaging of hodgkin disease and non-hodgkin lymphomas in children. Radiographics 2007;27(5):1335–54.

43. Chung EM, Pavio M. Pediatric extranodal lymphoma. Radiologic Clin North America 2016;54(4):727–46.

44. Riad R, Omar W, Kotb M, et al. Role of PET/CT in malignant pediatric lymphoma. Eur J Nucl Med Mol Imaging 2010;37(2):319–29.

45. Bien E, Godzinski J, Dall'igna P, et al. Pancreatoblastoma: a report from the European cooperative study group for paediatric rare tumours (EXPeRT). Eur J Cancer 2011;47(15):2347–52.

46. Chung EM, Travis MD, Conran RM. Pancreatic tumors in children: radiologic-pathologic correlation. Radiographics 2006;26(4):1211–38.

47. Nijs E, Callahan MJ, Taylor GA. Disorders of the pediatric pancreas: imaging features. Pediatr Radiol 2005;35(4):358–73 [quiz 457].

48. Lugo-Olivieri CH, Taylor GA. CT differentiation of large abdominal lymphangioma from ascites. Pediatr Radiol 1993;23(2):129–30.

49. Levy AD, Cantisani V, Miettinen M. Abdominal lymphangiomas: imaging features with pathologic correlation. AJR Am J Roentgenol 2004;182(6):1485–91.

50. Lal A, Gupta P, Singhal M, et al. Abdominal lymphatic malformation: spectrum of imaging findings. Indian J Radiol Imaging 2016;26(4):423–8.

51. Stein M, Hsu RK, Schneider PD, et al. Alcohol ablation of a mesenteric lymphangioma. J Vasc Interv Radiol 2000;11(2):247–50.

52. Barwick TD, Malhotra A, Webb JW, et al. Embryology of the adrenal glands and its relevance to diagnostic imaging. Clin Radiol 2005;60(9):953–9.

53. Kawashima A, Sandler CM, Ernst RD, et al. Imaging of nontraumatic hemorrhage of the adrenal gland. Radiographics 1999;19(4):949–63.

54. Lee E. Pediatric radiology: practical imaging evaluation of infants and children. Philadelphia: Lippincott Williams & Wilkins; 2017.

55. Hwang SM, Yoo S-Y, Kim JH, et al. Congenital adrenal neuroblastoma with and without cystic change: differentiating features with an emphasis on the of value of ultrasound. AJR Am J Roentgenol 2016;207(5):1105–11.

56. Tabbers MM, DiLorenzo C, Berger MY, et al. Evaluation and treatment of functional constipation in infants and children: evidence-based recommendations from ESPGHAN and NASPGHAN. J Pediatr Gastroenterol Nutr 2014;58(2):258–74.

57. Nurko S, Zimmerman LA. Evaluation and treatment of constipation in children and adolescents. Am Fam Physician 2014;90(2):82–90.

58. Brioude F, Kalish JM, Mussa A, et al. Expert consensus document: Clinical and molecular diagnosis, screening and management of Beckwith-Wiedemann syndrome: an international consensus statement. Nat Rev Endocrinol 2018;14(4):229–49.

59. Liu EK, Suson KD. Syndromic Wilms tumor: a review of predisposing conditions, surveillance and treatment. Transl Androl Urol 2020;9(5):2370–81.

60. Schultz KAP, Williams GM, Kamihara J, et al. DICER1 and associated conditions: identification of at-risk individuals and recommended surveillance strategies. Clin Cancer Res 2018;24(10):2251–61.

61. Rednam SP, Erez A, Druker H, et al. Von hippel-lindau and hereditary pheochromocytoma/paraganglioma syndromes: clinical features, genetics, and surveillance recommendations in childhood. Clin Cancer Res 2017;23(12):e68–75.

62. Krueger DA, Northrup H, International Tuberous Sclerosis Complex Consensus Group. Tuberous sclerosis complex surveillance and management: recommendations of the 2012 International Tuberous Sclerosis Complex Consensus Conference. Pediatr Neurol 2013;49(4):255–65.

63. Kamilaris CDC, Stratakis CA. Multiple endocrine neoplasia Type 1 (MEN1): an update and the significance of early genetic and clinical diagnosis. Front Endocrinol 2019;10:339.

64. Thakker RV, Newey PJ, Walls GV, et al. Clinical practice guidelines for multiple endocrine neoplasia Type 1 (MEN1). J Clin Endocrinol Metab 2012; 97(9):2990–3011.

65. Scarsbrook AF, Thakker RV, Wass JAH, et al. Multiple endocrine neoplasia: spectrum of radiologic appearances and discussion of a multitechnique imaging approach. Radiographics 2006;26(2):433–51.

66. Mai PL, Khincha PP, Loud JT, et al. Prevalence of cancer at baseline screening in the National Cancer Institute Li-Fraumeni Syndrome Cohort. JAMA Oncol 2017;3(12):1640–5.

Neonatal and Pediatric Bowel Obstruction
Imaging Guidelines and Recommendations

Nathan C. Hull, MD[a],*, Helen H.R. Kim, MD[b], Grace S. Phillips, MD[b],
Edward Y. Lee, MD, MPH[c]

KEYWORDS

- Child • Neonate • Pediatric • Bowel • Obstruction • Radiograph • Ultrasound • Fluoroscopy

KEY POINTS

- The age of the patient and suspected location of an obstruction can help determine which imaging modality to use when imaging bowel obstructions in the pediatric population.
- Plain radiography is a first-line imaging modality to evaluate for signs and location of bowel obstruction.
- In neonates, fluoroscopic upper gastrointestinal series are helpful in evaluating upper intestinal obstruction, whereas a fluoroscopic enema may determine the cause and location of a lower intestinal obstruction.
- Ultrasound is an excellent noninvasive imaging modality in cases of pediatric bowel obstruction that are caused by acute appendicitis, ileocolic intussusception, and abdominal or inguinal hernias.
- Computed tomography often is used as a second-line modality to better localize an obstruction or characterize its cause.

INTRODUCTION

Pediatric bowel obstructions are one of the most common surgical emergencies in children, and imaging plays a vital role in the evaluation and diagnosis (Tables 1 and 2). The main purposes of this article are to (1) discuss up-to-date evidence-based imaging algorithms; (2) describe a practical approach to pediatric bowel obstructions using imaging; (3) present the imaging spectrum of pediatric bowel obstructions and discuss their underlying causes; and (4) link imaging findings to management recommendations for practicing radiologists and physicians.

EVIDENCE-BASED IMAGING ALGORITHM

Imaging is highly useful in diagnosing and localizing pediatric bowel obstructions. In almost every case of suspected obstruction, abdominal radiographs are helpful as a first-line imaging examination in children of any age to determine (1) if there are signs of obstruction; (2) if the obstruction is in the upper or lower gastrointestinal (GI) tract; and (3) if there is evidence of bowel perforation, such as pneumoperitoneum. If perforation is suspected, obtaining subsequent upright or left lateral decubitus views is important and increases sensitivity for detecting free air to 85%

[a] Department of Radiology, Mayo Clinic, 200 First Street Southwest, Rochester, MN 55905, USA; [b] Department of Radiology, Seattle Children's Hospital and University of Washington, 4800 Sand Point Way Northeast, Seattle, WA 98105, USA; [c] Department of Radiology, Boston Children's Hospital, Harvard Medical School, 330 Longwood Avenue, Boston, MA 02115, USA
* Corresponding author.
E-mail address: hull.nathan@mayo.edu

Radiol Clin N Am 60 (2022) 131–148
https://doi.org/10.1016/j.rcl.2021.08.006
0033-8389/22/© 2021 Elsevier Inc. All rights reserved.

Table 1
Underlying causes of high versus low intestinal obstruction in neonates

High Intestinal Obstructions	Low Intestinal Obstructions
Esophageal atresia	Ileal atresia
Duodenal atresia	Meconium ileus
Duodenal web	Functional immaturity of the left colon
Duodenal stenosis/annular pancreas	Hirschsprung disease
Malrotation with midgut volvulus	Colonic atresia
Jejunal atresia/stenosis	Megacystis microcolon intestinal hypoperistalsis
	Anal atresia/anorectal malformations

and 96%, respectively.[1–3] Although radiographs are an appropriate first step, their sensitivity for diagnosing a specific etiology often is lacking; therefore, additional imaging modalities may be necessary for a definitive diagnosis. A practical and evidence-based imaging algorithm (**Figs. 1** and **2**) based on the age of the patients (neonate vs older child) can be used to help guide management.

Neonate

Following initial radiographs, if an upper tract obstruction is suspected in a neonate, a fluoroscopic upper GI imaging (UGI) series is performed next to localize and delineate the obstruction. UGI adequately characterizes duodenal stenosis, duodenal web, and jejunal atresia and can suggest a diagnosis of annular pancreas, although a proximal jejunal atresia usually is a radiographic diagnosis with a triple bubble sign. Although sensitivity and specificity are not abundant in the literature for these,[4] UGI generally is the most appropriate and widely accepted imaging study for these diagnoses.[5] UGI is the imaging study used most commonly for the detection of malrotation and midgut volvulus, with approximate sensitivity of 96% and 79%, respectively.[4] The use of ultrasound (US) for diagnosis of malrotation with

midgut volvulus has more variable degrees of accuracy reported in the literature.[6,7] Radiographs typically are adequate for establishing a diagnosis of esophageal or duodenal atresia due to their characteristic and nearly pathognomonic findings (discussed later).

If a lower obstruction is suspected in a neonate, fluoroscopic contrast enema is the most widely used and appropriate imaging test to evaluate for etiologies including: ileal atresia, meconium ileus, functional immaturity of the colon, colonic atresia, and Hirschsprung disease.[5] Contrast enema has sensitivity and specificity of 70% and 83%, respectively, for Hirschsprung disease and can help with a clinical decision to perform rectal wall biopsy.[4] When anorectal malformations are suspected, inverted or prone radiographs can suggest a distance to a rectal pouch but with relatively low sensitivity (27%).[4] Perineal US, however, improves sensitivity to 86%[4] and contrast colostography has a reported sensitivity of up to 100%.[8]

Older Child

Typically, radiographs are a useful first choice to evaluate for signs of bowel obstruction and possible bowel perforation. If bilious vomiting is present and malrotation with midgut volvulus is

Table 2
Underlying causes of bowel obstruction in older children

Congenital	Infectious/Inflammatory	Iatrogenic	Other
Malrotation w/midgut volvulus	Appendicitis	Adhesions	Ingested foreign body
Meckel's diverticulum	Ileocolic intussusception	Acquired hernia	Distal intestinal obstruction syndrome
Congenital inguinal hernia	Inflammatory bowel disease		

The mnemonic AIM can be used to remember the causes of bowel obstructions in children: A, appendicitis and adhesions; I, intussusception, inguinal hernia, inflammatory bowel disease, ingested foreign body, and iatrogenic; and M, Meckel's diverticulum and malrotation with midgut volvulus.

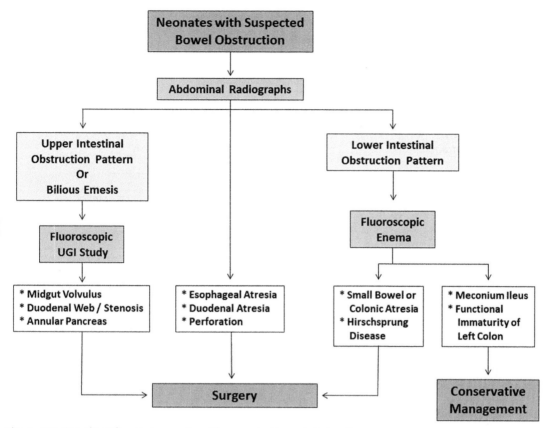

Fig. 1. Imaging algorithm in a neonate with suspected bowel obstruction.

suspected, an emergent UGI should be performed, as discussed previously.

Many other etiologies for bowel obstruction in older children, including acute appendicitis, ileocolic intussusception, and inguinal or acquired abdominal wall hernia, can be evaluated with US. US for diagnosis of acute appendicitis has reported sensitivity and specificity of 88% and 94%, respectively,[9–14] and is highly specific in cases of perforated appendicitis.[15,16] If US is equivocal, further evaluation with CT (sensitivity 96%/specificity 95%) or MR imaging (sensitivity 97%/specificity 97%) can be considered.[17] US for diagnosis of ileocolic intussusception has a high sensitivity of 98% to 100% and specificity of 88% to 100%.[18–21] Focused US of the groin can supplement physical examination and radiographs in detecting inguinal hernias, with high degrees of accuracy (95%), sensitivity (95%), and specificity (86%).[22] Meckel's diverticulum is diagnosed most often with imaging using a technetium pertechnetate abdominal scintigram, with reported sensitivity of 80% to 90% and specificity of 95% in pediatric patients.[23,24]

In the setting of acute obstruction, however, US or CT may be helpful for detecting an inflamed Meckel's diverticulum causing the obstruction.[25]

Abdominal adhesions are not often seen on imaging but signs that they may be present can be seen with US and CT with abrupt transition points or swirling of the bowel around a fixed point.

PRACTICAL IMAGING APPROACH TO PEDIATRIC BOWEL OBSTRUCTIONS
Plain Radiography

Radiographs of the abdomen typically are the initial imaging test in children who present with abdominal pain and possible bowel obstruction. They generally are the most available, least expensive, and simplest imaging examination. Although radiographs often are not sensitive or specific as to the underlying cause of a bowel obstruction, they are excellent at showing signs of obstruction (dilated bowel loops with air-fluid levels), can help localize to an upper or lower intestinal obstruction, and show complications, such as perforation with pneumoperitoneum. Although standard supine views are helpful, decubitus, cross-table lateral, or upright views are much more sensitive for detecting pneumoperitoneum and can demonstrate air-fluid levels better.

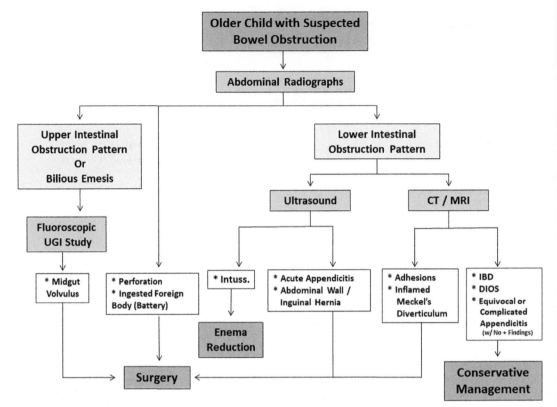

Fig. 2. Imaging algorithm in an older child with suspected bowel obstruction. DIOS, distal intestinal obstruction syndrome; IBD, inflammatory bowel disease; Intuss, intussusception; UGI, upper gastrointestinal series; w/No + findings, without positive findings.

Fluoroscopy

Contrast fluoroscopy frequently is used to diagnose and localize sites of bowel obstructions, especially in neonates and young children. UGI examinations can show causes of upper obstructions, including malrotation with midgut volvulus and duodenal stenosis, atresia, or web. Fluoroscopic enemas often reveal the cause of lower intestinal obstructions in neonates who have failed to pass meconium or in children with chronic constipation. It also is used during pneumatic reductions of ileocolic intussusceptions.

Ultrasound

US is an essential tool in the work-up of pediatric bowel obstructions. US has wide availability and a lack of ionizing radiation; offers high-resolution, real-time capability at a relatively low cost; and rarely requires sedation. It frequently is used for targeted evaluation of suspected acute appendicitis, abdominal wall and inguinal hernias, and ileocolic intussusceptions.

Computed Tomography

Computed tomography (CT) generally allows for a more comprehensive evaluation of abdominopelvic anatomy. Due to use of ionizing radiation and increased cost, however, it generally is reserved for the setting of pediatric bowel obstruction for troubleshooting when other imaging tools (such as radiographs or US) are not definitive. CT can be highly valuable in identifying specific locations and causes of bowel obstructions, such as with luminal masses; and secondary imaging findings, such as focal bowel dilatation due to abdominal adhesions.

MR Imaging

MR imaging rarely is used in the imaging work-up of bowel obstruction in the pediatric population. Although it does not use ionizing radiation, MR imaging generally is less available than other modalities, is more expensive, and usually requires sedation in infants and young children. MR imaging, however, does provide excellent soft tissue contrast resolution and may be helpful in the evaluation of bowel obstruction if a cause cannot be identified with other modalities or if more detailed imaging is needed for presurgical planning in the setting of an abdominal mass or chronic obstruction.

Nuclear Medicine

Nuclear medicine imaging is not used routinely for the work-up of acute bowel obstruction because it is relatively time-intensive, uses ionizing radiation, is less available than many other modalities (especially after normal business hours), and may not provide a specific answer in most cases. It can be useful, however, in selected clinical scenarios in the pediatric population, such as a suspected Meckel's diverticulum.

SPECTRUM OF BOWEL OBSTRUCTION IN INFANTS AND CHILDREN

Bowel obstruction in the pediatric population can be evaluated best when a patient is categorized into either neonatal or older children groups based on the age of the patient, because the typical underlying causes and types of imaging used for the evaluation often are different.

Neonatal Bowel Obstruction

Neonatal bowel obstruction can be high or low in location depending on the underlying causes.

High intestinal obstruction

Six congenital anomalies (including esophageal atresia, duodenal atresia, duodenal web, duodenal stenosis/annual pancreas, malrotation with midgut volvulus, and jejunal atresia/stenosis) account for a majority of high intestinal obstruction in neonates.

Esophageal atresia Esophageal atresia classically is a clinical diagnosis, with affected patients presenting with symptoms of choking, sialorrhea, or respiratory distress within the first hours of life. This disorder represents a spectrum and is usually classified based on if and where a fistulous connection between the esophagus and the trachea exists. Associated VACTERL anomalies (vertebral anomaly, anorectal atresia, cardiac lesion, tracheoesophageal fistula, renal anomaly, and limb defect) also may be present. Prenatal US or MR imaging may detect an esophageal pouch, small stomach, and polyhydramnios.[26–28]

After birth, radiographs often show failure to pass an enteric tube beyond the upper esophagus to midesophagus (Figs. 3 and 4). Bowel gas may be absent if there is no tracheoesophageal fistula, whereas the presence of bowel gas suggests a fistulous communication with the airway.[29] Although

timing of surgical repair often depends on the length of the gap between the proximal and distal limbs as well as other concomitant congenital anomalies, surgical repair typically occurs in the first 2 days of life. Contrast esophagram can be used to assess for recurrent fistulae and narrowing at the surgical site after surgical repair.

Duodenal atresia Duodenal atresia is thought to occur due to complete failure of recanalization of the duodenal lumen and often presents with vomiting. Trisomy 21 can be associated and be present in up to 40% of cases.[30,31] The double bubble sign with absence of distal bowel gas classically is seen on radiographs, representing the dilated stomach and proximal duodenum, and is diagnostic (Fig. 5).

Duodenal web Duodenal web is similar to atresia but there is only partial failure of recanalization of the lumen with a residual membrane with a central pinhole, which can lead to partial or intermittent obstruction.[30] Radiographically, it can appear similar to duodenal atresia, but distal bowel gas usually is present. Classically, a diagnosis is made on contrast fluoroscopic UGI examination, which shows partial obstruction and ballooned, windsock deformity (Fig. 6) with a faint radiolucent membrane from barium filling around the membrane.

Duodenal stenosis/annular pancreas As in duodenal atresia, duodenal stenosis, with or without annular pancreas, often shows gastroduodenal distention, but distal bowel gas is present (Figs. 7 and 8). There is partial duodenal obstruction due to a stenotic duodenal segment from partial atresia or from an anomalous congenital ring of pancreatic tissue surrounding the second portion of the duodenum, or annular pancreas. UGI examination can be suggestive of a diagnosis with narrowing of the descending duodenum. CT or MR imaging may be needed to confirm the diagnosis and can demonstrate a ring of pancreatic tissue surrounding the descending duodenum.

Malrotation with midgut volvulus In normal embryonic development, the bowel rotates counterclockwise 270° to form a broad mesenteric attachment, with the duodenojejunal junction in the left upper quadrant and the ileocecal junction in the right lower quadrant. This broad attachment prevents the bowel from twisting around its mesentery. Conversely, in malrotation, the bowel has a narrower mesenteric attachment and may twist around its vascular pedicle and cause vascular obstruction and luminal narrowing of the proximal small bowel, a surgical emergency, called *midgut volvulus*.

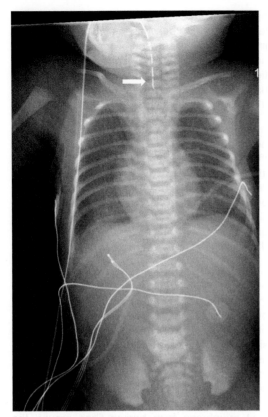

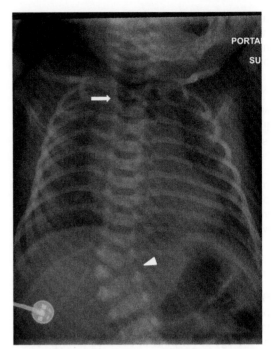

Fig. 4. Esophageal atresia in a newborn boy who presented with respiratory distress. Frontal supine radiograph shows a distended air-filled esophageal pouch (*arrow*) and vertebral anomalies (*arrowhead*).

Fig. 3. Esophageal atresia in a newborn boy who presented with difficulty passing a nasogastric tube. Frontal supine radiograph shows a gasless abdomen and nasogastric tube (*arrow*) terminating in the cervical esophagus.

Additionally, anomalous peritoneal fibrous bands, termed *Ladd bands*, may be present and contribute to duodenal narrowing/obstruction. Pediatric patients with malrotation may be asymptomatic but typically develop bilious emesis when midgut volvulus is present.

Abdominal radiographs often are nonspecific and may appear normal or show signs of upper intestinal obstruction. If midgut volvulus is suspected, regardless of the radiographic findings, an emergent UGI study should be performed. The classic fluoroscopic findings show a duodenum that fails to cross the midline, with twisting, or corkscrew configuration of the duodenum (Fig. 9). Although typically not the modality of choice, CT and US can show evidence of midgut volvulus with abnormal relationship of the superior mesenteric artery and vein or swirling of the mesenteric vessels in the so-called whirlpool sign. Treatment is urgent surgical decompression and correction, called a *Ladd procedure*.

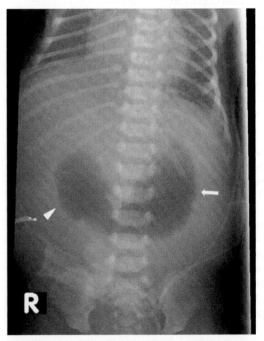

Fig. 5. Duodenal atresia in a newborn boy who presented with feeding intolerance. Frontal supine radiograph shows the double bubble sign with air distended stomach (*arrow*) and a dilated proximal duodenum (*arrowhead*) with absent distal bowel gas.

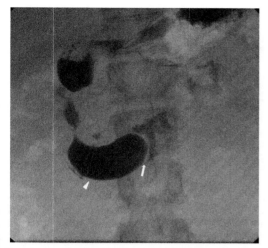

Fig. 6. Duodenal web in a 2-year-old boy who presented with chronic vomiting and feeding intolerance. Frontal image from fluoroscopic UGI shows distended transverse duodenum (*arrowhead*) and a thin, curvilinear filling defect representing a web (*arrow*).

Jejunal atresia/stenosis Jejunal obstruction in neonates often is caused by a congenital atresia or stenosis. It is thought to be due to in utero vascular insults, and multiple atresias may coexist. Affected pediatric patients usually present with abdominal distention and bilious vomiting. Abdominal radiographs often show dilated bowel loops, fewer than seen with a lower obstruction pattern but more than the double bubble that is pathognomonic for duodenal atresia.[30] A triple bubble sign may be present (**Fig. 10**) with proximal jejunal atresia. An UGI is not necessarily needed prior to surgical repair but may show a contrast-filled and dilated duodenum and jejunum. A contrast enema typically is performed, which may show a diffuse microcolon (**Fig. 11**) in the setting of additional distal bowel atresias.

Low intestinal obstruction
Low intestinal obstruction in neonates can involve either small bowel or large bowel, discussed in the following section.

Small bowel involvement
Ileal atresia Similar to jejunal atresia, ileal atresia is thought to occur from intrauterine ischemic insult and reported to have an incidence of 1 in 5000 live births.[30] It less commonly has associated congenital anomalies than is seen with duodenal or jejunal atresia. Affected pediatric patients often present with abdominal distension, failure to pass meconium, and/or vomiting. Abdominal radiographs show multiple dilated bowel loops suggesting a lower tract obstruction. Contrast enema shows a diffuse microcolon (see **Fig. 11**), and contrast may not be able to be refluxed into the atretic ileum (unlike meconium ileus).

Meconium ileus Meconium ileus often is the earliest manifestation of cystic fibrosis and accounts for an estimated 20% of neonatal bowel obstructions.[30] It occurs when impaction of desiccated meconium pellets obstructs the distal small bowel, often the terminal ileum, and causes a mechanical obstruction.[31] Due to the obstruction, abdominal radiographs show dilated upstream bowel loops, suggesting a lower tract obstruction. Contrast enema typically shows an unused microcolon; several small filling defects can be seen in the colon and terminal ileum representing meconium concretions (**Fig. 12**).

Large bowel involvement
Functional immaturity of the colon Functional immaturity of the colon (sometimes called small left colon syndrome or meconium plug) generally is a transient and self-limited functional colonic obstruction in neonates. It is thought to be related to immaturity of the ganglion cells from the myenteric nerve plexus of the colon. Functional immaturity of

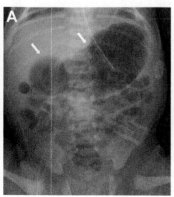

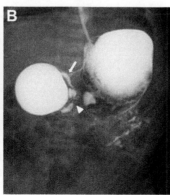

Fig. 7. Annular pancreas in a newborn boy who presented with feeding intolerance. (*A*) Frontal supine radiograph shows dilated, air-filled stomach and proximal duodenum (*arrows*) with distal bowel gas. (*B*) Frontal view from a contrast fluoroscopic UGI shows narrowing of the descending duodenum (*arrowhead*) with reflux of contrast into the biliary tree (*arrow*). Note very little contrast passed distally to the descending duodenum.

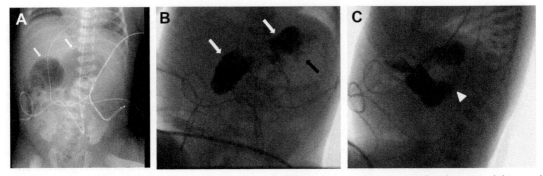

Fig. 8. Duodenal stenosis in a newborn girl with congenital heart disease who presented with emesis. (*A*) Frontal supine radiograph shows dilated, air-filled stomach and proximal duodenum (*arrows*) with some distal bowel gas present. Frontal (*B*) and lateral (*C*) images from fluoroscopic UGI show contrast filling the stomach and proximal duodenum (*white arrows*) with an abrupt cutoff of contrast (*arrowhead*), and only trace amounts of contrast passing distally (*black arrow*). Surgery revealed duodenal stenosis.

the colon is seen more frequently in neonates whose mothers are diabetic or received magnesium sulfate during pregnancy for preeclampsia. It is the most common diagnosis in infants who fail to pass meconium within 48 hours.[30]

Similar to other causes of colonic obstruction, abdominal radiographs usually show multiple dilated bowel loops. Contrast enema typically demonstrates a normal-sized rectum with a relatively small caliber colon from the sigmoid to the splenic flexure of the colon, with variable meconium plugs, seen as filling defects in the left colon (**Fig. 13**). The ascending and transverse colon often are normal caliber or slightly dilated. Contrast enema is diagnostic and often therapeutic in helping a neonate dispel the meconium plugs and relieve the obstruction. Although this entity has a characteristic appearance on contrast enema, if symptoms do not resolve with time, Hirschsprung disease (discussed below) should be considered and colonic wall biopsy may be warranted.[32]

Hirschsprung disease Hirschsprung disease is a low intestinal obstruction caused by absence of colonic ganglion cells and accounts for approximately 15% to 20% of bowel obstructions in neonates.[31] Approximately 2% of affected patients also have trisomy 21. During development, colonic ganglion cells migrate from proximal to distal colon. If this migration is arrested prematurely, the remaining distal colon cannot relax and causes a functional obstruction. Due to the craniocaudad cell migration, the aganglionic segment usually is continuous and extends proximally from the anus.[29] The aganglionic segment can vary in length from an ultrashort segment involving the region near the anal sphincter (rare), the rectosigmoid region (most common, approximately 75%), longer segments, or even the entire colon (8%).[33,34] A majority of cases present with clinical symptoms of lower obstruction with delayed passage of meconium and abdominal distention.

Radiographs in Hirschsprung disease show nonspecific findings of a lower obstruction with multiple

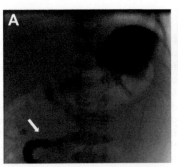
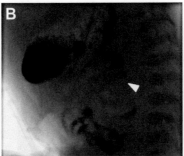
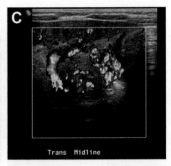

Fig. 9. Newborn boy with malrotation with midgut volvulus who presented with bilious emesis. Frontal supine (*A*) and lateral decubitus (*B*) views from fluoroscopic UGI show failure of the duodenum (*arrow*) to cross the midline on the frontal view, and a corkscrew appearance (*arrowhead*) of the proximal small bowel on the lateral view. (*C*) Transverse color Doppler US image near the midline of the upper abdomen shows the swirl sign of the superior mesenteric artery and vein concerning for midgut volvulus.

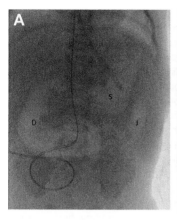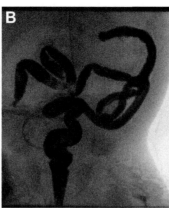

Fig. 10. Newborn girl with jejunal atresia who presented with abdominal distension and vomiting. (*A*) Frontal supine fluoroscopic image prior to instillation of contrast on an UGI examination shows the triple bubble sign with 3 distended air-filled bubbles, including the stomach (S), duodenum (D), and proximal jejunum (J) with lack of distal bowel gas. (*B*) Frontal image from fluoroscopic contrast enema shows a diffuse microcolon, in keeping with an upstream atresia.

dilated bowel loops. Although the gold standard for diagnosis is rectal wall suction biopsy to evaluate for the presence of ganglion cells, contrast enema is helpful to look for findings of Hirschsprung disease, which include rectosigmoid ratio less than 1, transition zone of relative narrowing, and irregular sawtooth rectal contractions (**Fig. 14**). Very short segment disease near the anus can be difficult to see on enema. Total colonic Hirschsprung disease involving the entire colon can show a microcolon or question-mark shaped colon on enema study. If a diagnosis still is suspected after an unremarkable enema, rectal biopsy should be considered for definitive diagnosis.

Colonic atresia Colonic atresia is less common than small bowel atresias, accounting for approximately 5% to 15% of all intestinal atresias.[30,35] It typically affects the colon proximal to the splenic flexure. Abdominal radiographs show multiple dilated bowel loops and an absence of distal colonic and rectal gas. Contrast enema usually shows a distal microcolon with failure to reflux contrast to the more proximal colon (**Fig. 15**).

Megacystis-microcolon-intestinal hypoperistalsis syndrome Megacystis-microcolon-intestinal hypoperistalsis syndrome is a relatively rare and severe form of functional intestinal obstruction in the newborn and can be fatal.[36,37] It can be associated with malrotation.[38] The cause of this condition is uncertain but may have an autosomal-recessive inheritance.[39] Abnormalities in the ganglion cells that control smooth muscle as well as in smooth muscles themselves have been reported[37] in histologic findings and likely lead to the clinical manifestations of abdominal distention and a dilated urinary bladder. Abdominal radiographs tend to show abdominal distention with paucity of bowel gas and a distended urinary bladder displacing bowel loops.[39] Contrast enema shows a microcolon. UGI examination shows diminished or absent peristalsis. US or CT may show a distended urinary bladder.

Anal atresia and anorectal malformations Anorectal malformations are a spectrum of abnormalities, which include imperforate anus, anal stenosis and atresia,

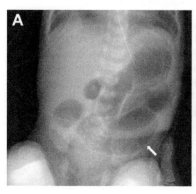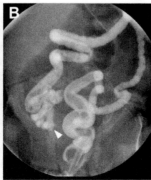

Fig. 11. Newborn girl with jejunal and ileal atresia who presented with abdominal distension. (*A*) Frontal supine radiograph shows dilated air-filled proximal bowel loops compatible with an upper obstruction beyond the duodenum (*arrow*). (*B*) Frontal supine image from contrast enema demonstrates a diffuse microcolon with reflux of contrast into narrow-caliber distal ileal loops (*arrowhead*).

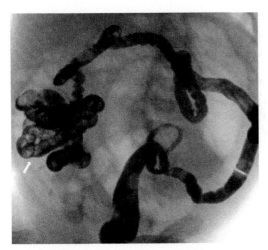

Fig. 12. A 2-day-old newborn girl with meconium ileus who presented with abdominal distension. Frontal supine view from a contrast enema shows a diffuse microcolon with multiple small filling defects in the terminal ileum representing inspissated meconium (*arrow*).

and rectal atresia. Affected newborns often present with signs and symptoms of a lower tract obstruction, including abdominal distention and failure to pass meconium. The incidence is estimated to be 1 in 5000 live births and both genders are affected

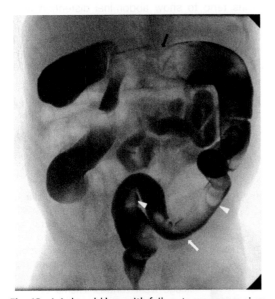

Fig. 13. A 1-day-old boy with failure to pass meconium from functional immaturity of the colon who presented with abdominal distension. Smaller caliber sigmoid and descending colon (*arrow*) with multiple meconium filling defects (*arrowheads*). Note mild proximal dilation of the transverse colon (*black arrow*).

equally.[30] Anal atresia and anorectal malformations can be seen in the setting of VACTERL syndrome, as well as Currarino syndrome (anorectal malformation, presacral mass, and malformed sacrum). They typically are classified as either high or low lesions, depending on the position of the blind ending rectum relative to the levator ani muscles.[39] In low lesions, the blind ending rectum is close to the skin and typically can be treated with anoplasty, pull-through, or dilation. Conversely, in high lesions, the rectal pouch is located higher in the pelvis and can be seen with fistulous connections to the vagina, bladder, or urethra. This often requires a temporary colostomy with subsequent surgical repair.

Abdominal radiographs often show findings of a distal bowel obstruction and also may demonstrate sacral anomalies. Cross-table lateral radiographs in a prone position may show the air-filled rectal pouch and the distance to the skin can be estimated. US of the perineum or via transanal approach also can be used to visualize the abnormality and help classify the lesion as high or low (**Fig. 16**). Additional imaging, including voiding cystourethrogram and MR imaging, should be considered to identify any fistulae and help characterize associated abnormalities and pelvic anatomy.

Older Children with Bowel Obstruction

Bowel obstruction in older children can be due to underlying congenital or acquired causes, including infectious or inflammatory, and iatrogenic etiologies, discussed in the following section.

Congenital causes

Malrotation with midgut volvulus Although a majority of cases are seen in children during the first year of life, older children also can present with malrotation with midgut volvulus. Typical clinical symptoms include acute onset of abdominal pain and bilious vomiting from acute obstruction as well as less severe intermittent symptoms if the midgut is only intermittently twisting and untwisting.[40] The imaging features of this entity are the same as those described previously.

Meckel's diverticulum Meckel's diverticula result from abnormal remnants of the omphalomesenteric duct and are located along the antimesenteric border of the distal ileum.[40] Most are asymptomatic, but affected children may present with painless GI tract bleeding from ectopic gastric or pancreatic tissue within the diverticulum or with symptoms related to inflammation of the diverticulum. Approximately 40% of symptomatic Meckel's diverticula present with bowel obstruction[41] either due to torsion of the distal ileum around an omphalomesenteric band or from inflammation of the diverticulum,

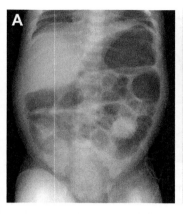
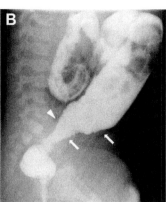

Fig. 14. A 5-day-old boy with Hirschsprung disease who presented with abdominal distension and vomiting. (*A*) Frontal supine radiograph shows multiple dilated air-filled bowel loops with paucity of gas in the pelvis suggesting a lower tract obstruction. (*B*) Lateral view from contrast enema demonstrates greater luminal distension of the sigmoid compared with the rectum (*arrows*). Note spasmodic sawtooth contractions about the rectum (*arrowhead*).

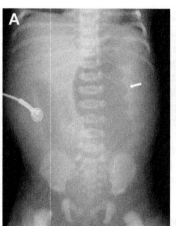
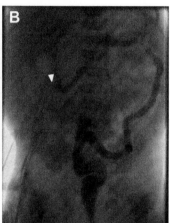

Fig. 15. Newborn girl with colonic atresia who presented with abdominal distension and failure to pass meconium. (*A*) Frontal supine radiograph shows markedly dilated air-filled bowel (*arrow*) with paucity of other bowel gas. (*B*) Frontal view from contrast enema shows a microcolon with abrupt cutoff of the colon near the hepatic flexure (*arrowhead*). Surgery confirmed focal atresia of the right colon.

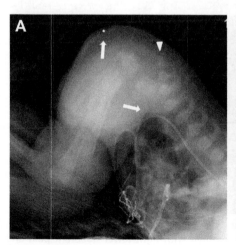
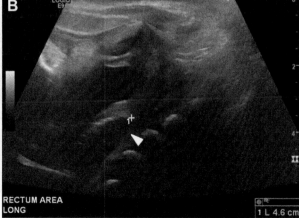

Fig. 16. Newborn boy with anal atresia and sacral dysplasia. (*A*) Lateral, prone abdominopelvic radiograph with a metallic pellet on the skin marking the expected anal opening shows an approximate 5 cm to 6 cm gap from the skin to the rectal gas (*arrows*). Note associated sacral dysplasia (*arrowhead*). (*B*) Longitudinal grayscale US image shows the estimated distance (between cursors) from the blind-ending, fluid-filled rectal pouch (*arrowhead*) to the skin surface.

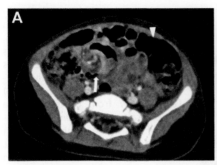 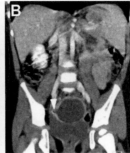 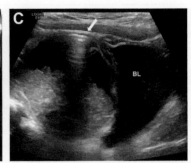

Fig. 17. A 2-year-old boy with torsed Meckel's diverticulum who presented with acute abdominal pain. (*A*) Axial contrast-enhanced CT image shows swirling (*arrow*) of the right lower mesentery and vessels. There are air-filled proximal small bowel loops (*arrowhead*). (*B*) Coronal contrast-enhanced CT image shows a peripherally enhancing and fluid-filled structure in the central pelvis with a small neck (*arrowhead*). (*C*) Longitudinal grayscale US image shows the same fluid-filled structure (*arrow*) from the CT with some internal debris centered superior to the bladder (BL).

which can cause luminal obstruction and act as a lead point for bowel intussusception.[42]

Meckel's diverticula typically are not seen on radiographs, but signs of bowel obstruction may be present. Cross-sectional imaging, including US, CT, or MR imaging, may show an inflamed blind ending structure in the right lower abdomen and can have an appearance similar to the appendix (**Fig. 17**). A nuclear medicine Meckel's scan (99mTc-pertechnetate scintigraphy) can show increased focal radiotracer and confirm diagnosis if the lesion contains gastric mucosa (**Fig. 18**).

Congenital inguinal hernia Congenital inguinal hernias generally affect a small percentage of children (approximately 1%–2%), but 10% can be complicated by bowel obstruction and incarceration.[41] Although these often are diagnosed clinically by physical examination, imaging may be helpful in finding the cause of obstruction when not clinically apparent. For example, abdominal radiographs may show gas within the inguinal canal or scrotum (**Fig. 19**). Radiographs also can show signs of bowel obstruction, if present, with dilated air-filled bowel loops. US can be especially helpful if a hernia is suspected as visualization of bowel loops in the inguinal canal or scrotum is diagnostic. Hernias in symptomatic pediatric patients usually are treated urgently with an open or closed reduction to relieve a bowel obstruction, if present, or to prevent one from occurring. Surgical herniorrhaphy may be performed to repair the fascial defect.

Infectious or inflammatory causes
Appendicitis The most common atraumatic emergent surgical indication in children is acute appendicitis.[29,43] Secondary bowel obstruction is a well-known complication of acute appendicitis (**Fig. 20**)

and usually it occurs in the setting of complicated or perforated appendicitis. With complicated/perforated appendicitis, marked inflammation and adhesive bands can develop, which may cause a mechanical and functional bowel obstruction.

Abdominal radiographs may show a calcified appendicolith and/or dilated bowel loops with relative paucity of bowel loops in the right lower abdomen. US is the modality of choice for suspected appendicitis in pediatrics due to availability, low cost, and lack of ionizing radiation. CT may be helpful to further delineate related complications

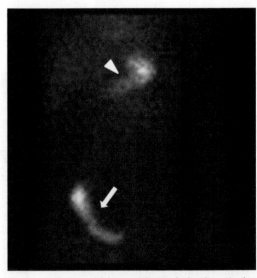

Fig. 18. A 9-year-old boy with Meckel's diverticulum who presented with right lower quadrant pain and abdominal distension. Frontal planar image from a pertechnetate-99m Meckel's scan shows a persistent focus (*arrow*) of uptake confirming the presence of a Meckel's diverticulum with ectopic gastric mucosa. Note the normal uptake in the stomach (*arrowhead*).

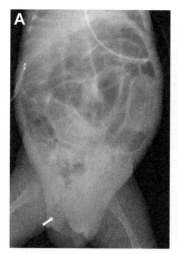 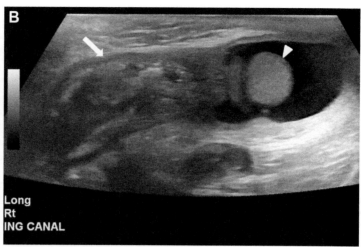

Fig. 19. Newborn boy with congenital inguinal hernia who presented with abdominal distension. (*A*) Frontal radiograph shows multiple dilated bowel loops with air-filled loops (*arrow*) in the right inguinal canal. (*B*). Longitudinal grayscale US image demonstrates loops of bowel in the right inguinal canal (*arrow*) extending to the right scrotum adjacent the testicle (*arrowhead*). A small hydrocele also is seen.

including secondary bowel obstruction and abscesses that may need image-guided drainage. MR imaging also can be used to diagnose or troubleshoot cases of suspected acute appendicitis with comparable accuracy to CT.[44] Treatment often is dependent on imaging findings, ranging from urgent appendectomy for uncomplicated cases, or antibiotics and subsequent appendectomy when the inflammation has diminished, as well as image-guided drainage if an abscess is present.

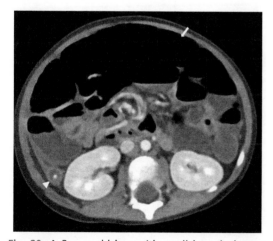

Fig. 20. A 3-year-old boy with small bowel obstruction secondary to acute appendicitis who presented with fever, right lower quadrant pain, and abdominal distension. Axial contrast-enhanced CT image shows a dilated retrocecal appendix (*arrowhead*) containing an appendicolith. Note multiple air-filled proximal bowel loops (*arrow*).

Intussusception Ileocolic intussusception is the most common cause of small bowel obstructions in children.[45,46] It occurs when a portion of distal small bowel telescopes into colon and causes a luminal obstruction, most frequently along the course of the right colon.[47] This occurs most commonly in children 3 months to 36 months of age, with a peak between 5 months and 9 months.[46] Most often the cause is idiopathic and thought to be due to hypertrophy of lymphoid tissue (Peyer patches) in the wall of the terminal ileum from viral infection.[18,46] Pathologic lead points, including Meckel's diverticulum, intestinal duplication cyst or polyp, or lymphoma, also can cause intussusception. Pathologic lead points are more common in older children and the likelihood increases with age, particularly over age 5 years.[46] Affected pediatric patients may present with the classic triad of crampy abdominal pain, red currant jelly stool, and a palpable abdominal mass, although this triad is present in less than 50% of children.[48] Alternatively, pediatric patients with intussusception can present with signs of a bowel obstruction with a distended abdomen and pain.

Abdominal radiographs may show findings of bowel obstruction but are not sensitive or specific for intussusception.[49] A curvilinear soft tissue mass partly surrounded by bowel gas along the course of the colon, the so-called crescent sign, can suggest a diagnosis. US is the modality of choice and approaches 100% sensitivity and specificity.[19–21] US typically shows a 3-cm to 5-cm mass along the expected course of the colon with a characteristic targetoid or donut appearance in transverse images, or a pseudokidney appearance

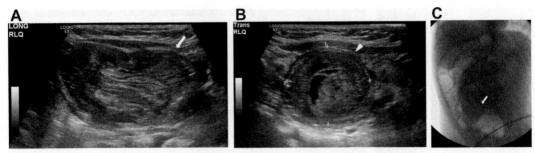

Fig. 21. A 2-year boy with ileocolic intussusception who presented with worsening abdominal pain, abdominal distension and bloody stool. Longitudinal (*A*) and transverse (*B*) grayscale US images show the pseudokidney (*arrow*) and target (*arrowhead*) signs of ileocolic intussusception with alternating layers of bowel. (*C*) Frontal image from a fluoroscopic pneumatic reduction of an intussusception shows a soft tissue density (*arrow*) near the ileocecal valve.

on longitudinal images (**Fig. 21**). Small bowel-small bowel intussusceptions typically are transient, incidental, and measure 2 cm or smaller on US and should not be mistaken for an ileocolic intussusception.[50] Treatment is performed with fluoroscopically or US-guided air or contrast/hydrostatic enema with a reduction rate of approximately 80%.[41] Surgical reduction typically is performed only if image-guided enema is unsuccessful or if there are signs of bowel perforation.

Inflammatory bowel disease Inflammatory bowel disease can be a cause of bowel obstruction in children due to acute inflammation of the bowel or from chronic wall thickening and strictures. In the acute setting, symptoms and imaging features may overlap with more common causes, including acute appendicitis; special attention should be paid to where the nidus of inflammation is located to ensure proper care. Treatment usually is nonsurgical with immunotherapies and bowel rest.

Abdominal radiographs typically are not specific or sensitive. A fluoroscopic small bowel follow-through rarely is indicated when signs of bowel obstruction are present. CT and MR imaging are best at delineating the location of the inflammation and obstruction and can show the length of bowel involved, luminal narrowing and wall thickening, strictures, and fistulae (**Figs. 22** and **23**).

Iatrogenic causes
Adhesions Adhesions result as part of the healing process after abdominal surgery in up to 95% of patients after laparotomy[51] and usually are more abundant in children with a history of perforated appendicitis or multiple surgeries.[52,53] Approximately 5% of children with adhesions eventually develop secondary bowel obstructions[41] and should be suspected in children with a history of prior surgery. Symptomatic pediatric patients

usually present with abdominal distention, pain, and emesis. Treatment can include bowel rest and conservative management in hopes of spontaneous resolution of the obstruction; approximately

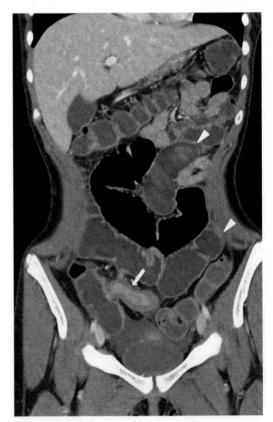

Fig. 22. A 17-year-old girl with Crohn disease who presented with abdominal pain and distension. Coronal contrast-enhanced CT image shows an active inflammatory stricture of the terminal ileum (*arrow*) causing obstruction of proximal loops (*arrowheads*).

85% of patients, however, eventually may require surgical intervention.[41]

Abdominal radiographs show typical findings of small bowel obstruction, including multiple dilated loops of bowel with air-fluid levels and areas with a paucity of bowel gas. This may be sufficient for diagnosis; however, CT often is performed subsequently to localize the point of bowel obstruction and help guide management. Usually, discrete adhesions cannot be seen on CT.[53]

Acquired hernia Children who have undergone prior surgeries or procedures may be at risk of an acquired or iatrogenic hernia and secondary bowel obstruction. These acquired hernias can include abdominal wall incisional defects or diaphragmatic hernias after cardiothoracic surgeries. Imaging studies can show herniated loops of bowel through a fascial defect. Treatment includes surgical reduction and repair.

Other etiologies

Ingested foreign body In the pediatric population, ingested foreign bodies are relatively common,

with more than 100,000 ingestions each year in the United States.[41] Fortunately, surgical intervention is needed in fewer than 1% of cases. Magnets are especially worrisome when multiple have been ingested because they may be located in different bowel loops and become attracted to one another resulting in pressure necrosis (**Fig. 24**). This can lead to complications, such as obstruction, perforation, or fistula formation.[54] Radiographs can be helpful to determine what was ingested and its current location, track its course through the GI tract, and monitor for developing obstruction or complication.

Bezoars are a conglomeration of ingested indigestible foreign material in the GI tract and most commonly include hair (trichobezoar), portions of vegetables/fruits (phytobezoar), undigested milk products (lactobezoar), or medications (pharmacobezoar).[55] Bezoars may be suspected clinically or

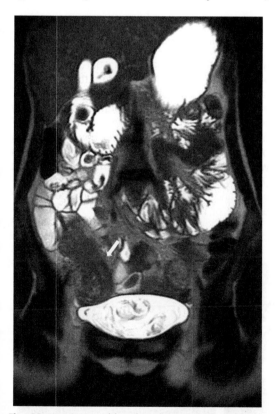

Fig. 23. A 14-year-old girl with Crohn disease who presented with vomiting, abdominal pain and distension. Coronal fat-saturated T2 weighted MR imaging (fast imaging employing steady-state acquisition) shows marked thickening of the terminal ileum with luminal narrowing (*arrow*).

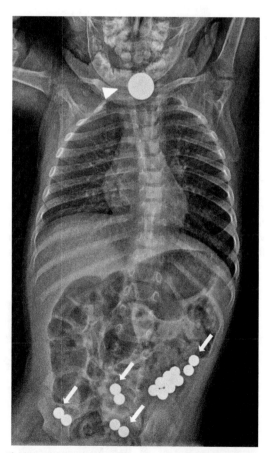

Fig. 24. A 14-month-old boy with swallowed foreign bodies who presented with drooling, abdominal pain and distension. Frontal radiograph shows a coin (*arrowhead*) in the cervical esophagus and multiple metallic objects (*arrows*) in the abdomen, which are clustered, concerning for multiple magnets.

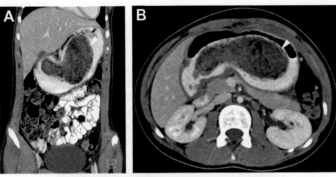

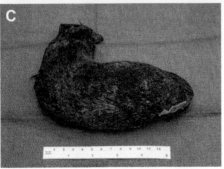

Fig. 25. A 1-year old boy with tricho-bezoar who presented with abdominal distension. Coronal (A) and axial (B) contrast-enhanced CT images show a large club-shaped mixed density struc-ture (*arrowheads*) in the gastric lumen outlined by enteric contrast. (C) Spec-imen photo of the large trichobezoar, which had to be removed surgically due to partial gastric outlet obstruc-tion.

from abnormal intraluminal structures or densities on imaging. These often appear as filling defects on fluoroscopic studies or have a mixed attenuation layered appearance and contain internal gas on CT (**Fig. 25**).[42] Treatment usually requires endoscopic or surgical removal.

Distal intestinal obstruction syndrome Distal in-testinal obstruction syndrome occurs in children with cystic fibrosis and is similar to meconium ileus seen in newborns. Inspissated secretions accrue in the terminal ileum near the ileocecal valve and create viscous fecal matter with resul-tant upstream obstruction. Radiographs may show dilated small bowel loops with a paucity of bowel gas in the right lower abdomen. CT often is most helpful and can show fecalization of contents within the lumen of the terminal ileum with upstream dilation of small bowel loops (**Fig. 26**). Primary treatment methods include en-emas and laxatives, with surgery reserved for extreme or refractory cases.

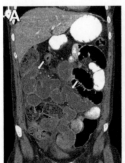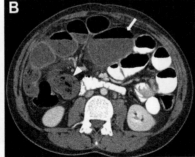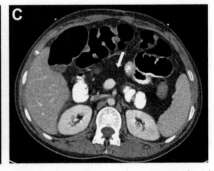

Fig. 26. A 20-year-old woman with cystic fibrosis and distal intestinal obstruction syndrome who presented with abdominal pain and distension. Coronal (A) and axial (B) contrast-enhanced CT images show multiple dilated bowel loops (*arrows*) with air-fluid levels apparent on axial image. There is inspissated enteric contents (*arrow-head*) in the distal ileum causing an obstruction. (C) Axial contrast-enhanced CT image demonstrates fatty replacement of the pancreas (*arrow*) consistent with cystic fibrosis.

SUMMARY

Initial evaluation of neonatal and pediatric bowel obstructions is based on age, clinical history, and detailed physical examination. Targeted imaging can be used to help identify both the bowel obstruction and the underlying cause. Appropriate choice of imaging facilitates timely and accurate diagnosis, which, in turn, can lead to optimal patient management.

CLINICS CARE POINTS

- Age of the patient and suspected diagnosis dictate which modality to use in diagnosis of bowel obstruction in the pediatric population.

- Plain radiography is a first-line imaging modality to evaluate for signs and location of bowel obstruction.

- Radiographs with an upright, decubitus, or cross-table lateral view can help in detecting signs and location of bowel obstruction.

- In neonates, fluoroscopic UGI is helpful in evaluating upper intestinal obstructions, whereas fluoroscopic enema may determine the cause and location of a lower intestinal obstruction.

- US is highly sensitive and specific for and should be used for diagnosis of acute appendicitis, ileocolic intussusception, and abdominal wall/inguinal hernias.

- CT should be considered when the etiology is not clear on initial imaging (radiographs, US, and contrast fluoroscopy studies).

- If there is a clinical concern for malrotation with midgut volvulus, emergent UGI should be performed irrespective of patient age.

REFERENCES

1. Marshall GB. The cupola sign. Radiology 2006; 241(2):623–4.

2. Chiu YH, Chen JD, Tiu CM, et al. Reappraisal of radiographic signs of pneumoperitoneum at emergency department. Am J Emerg Med 2009;27(3):320–7.

3. Menashe SJ, Iyer RS, Parisi MT, et al. Pediatric abdominal radiographs: common and less common errors. AJR Am J Roentgenol 2017;209(2):417–29.

4. Carroll AG, Kavanagh RG, Ni Leidhin C, et al. Comparative effectiveness of imaging modalities for the diagnosis of intestinal obstruction in neonates and infants. Acad Radiol 2016;23(5):559–68.

5. Alazraki AL, Rigsby CK, Iyer RS, et al. ACR appropriateness criteria® vomiting in infants. J Am Coll Radiol 2020;17(11):S505–15.

6. Chao HC, Kong MS, Chen JY, et al. Sonographic features related to volvulus in neonatal intestinal malrotation. J Ultrasound Med 2000;19(6):371–6.

7. Quail MA. Question 2 is Doppler ultrasound superior to upper gastrointestinal contrast study for the diagnosis of malrotation? Arch Dis Child 2011;96(3):317–8.

8. Niedzielski JK. Invertography versus ultrasonography and distal colostography for the determination of bowel-skin distance in children with anorectal malformations. Eur J Pediatr Surg 2005;15(4):262–7.

9. Doria AS, Moineddin R, Kellenberger CJ, et al. Us or CT for diagnosis of appendicitis in children and adults? A meta-analysis. Radiology 2006;241(1):83–94.

10. Kaiser S, Frenckner B, Jorulf HK. Suspected appendicitis in children: US and CT- a prospective randomized study. Radiology 2002;223(3):633–8.

11. Peletti AB, Baldisserotto M. Optimizing US examination to detect the normal and abnormal appendix in children. Pediatr Radiol 2006;36(11):1171–6.

12. Patriquin HB, Garcier JM, Lafortune M, et al. Appendicitis in children and young adults: Doppler sonographic-pathologic correlation. AJR Am J Roentgenol 1996;166(3):629–33.

13. Simonovsky V. Sonographic detection of normal and abnormal appendix. Clin Radiol 1999;54(8):533–9.

14. Wiersma F, Sramek A, Holscher HC. US features of the normal appendix and surrounding area in children. Radiology 2005;235(3):1018–22.

15. Carpenter JL, Orth RC, Zhang W, et al. Diagnostic performance of us for differentiating perforated from nonperforated pediatric appendicitis: a prospective cohort study. Radiology 2017;282(3):835–41.

16. Blumfield E, Nayak G, Srinivasan R, et al. Journal club: ultrasound for differentiation between perforated and nonperforated appendicitis in pediatric patients. AJR Am J Roentgenol 2013;200(5):957–62.

17. Eng KA, Abadeh A, Ligocki C, et al. Acute appendicitis: a meta-analysis of the diagnostic accuracy of US, CT, and MRI as second-line imaging tests after an initial us. Radiology 2018;288(3):717–27.

18. Applegate KE. Intussusception in children: evidence-based diagnosis and treatment. Pediatr Radiol 2009;39(S2):140–3.

19. Pracros JP, Tran-Minh VA, Morin de Finfe CH, et al. Acute intestinal intussusception in children. Contribution of ultrasonography (145 cases). Ann Radiol (Paris) 1987;30(7):525–30.

20. Verschelden P, Filiatrault D, Garel L, et al. Intussusception in children: reliability of US in diagnosis–a prospective study. Radiology 1992;184(3):741–4.

21. del-Pozo G, Albillos JC, Tejedor D, et al. Intussusception in children: current concepts in diagnosis and enema reduction. Radiographics 1999;19(2):299–319.

22. Kervancioglu R, Bayram MM, Ertaskin I, et al. Ultrasonographic evaluation of bilateral groins in children with unilateral inguinal hernia. Acta Radiol 2000; 41(6):653–7.

23. Sagar J, Kumar V, Shah DK. Meckel's diverticulum: a systematic review. J R Soc Med 2006;99(10): 501–5.

24. Kotecha M, Bellah R, Pena AH, et al. Multimodality imaging manifestations of the Meckel diverticulum in children. Pediatr Radiol 2012;42(1):95–103.

25. Won Y, Lee HW, Ku YM, et al. Multidetector-row computed tomography (MDCT) features of small bowel obstruction (SBO) caused by Meckel's diverticulum. Diagn Interv Imaging 2016;97(2):227–32.

26. Ethun CG, Fallon SC, Cassady CI, et al. Fetal MRI improves diagnostic accuracy in patients referred to a fetal center for suspected esophageal atresia. J Pediatr Surg 2014;49(5):712–5.

27. Shulman A, Mazkereth R, Zalel Y, et al. Prenatal identification of esophageal atresia: the role of ultrasonography for evaluation of functional anatomy. Prenat Diagn 2002;22(8):669–74.

28. Salomon LJ, Sonigo P, Ou P, et al. Real-time fetal magnetic resonance imaging for the dynamic visualization of the pouch in esophageal atresia. Ultrasound Obstet Gynecol 2009;34(4):471–4.

29. Dunn EA, Olsen OE, Huisman TAGM. The pediatric gastrointestinal tract: what every radiologist needs to know. In: Hodler J, Kubiak-Huch RA, von Schulthess GK, editors. Diseases of the Abdomen and pelvis 2018–2021: diagnostic imaging - IDKD Book. Springer; 2018. Available at: http://www.ncbi.nlm.nih.gov/books/NBK543791/. Accessed April 8, 2021.

30. Vinocur DN, Lee EY, Eisenberg RL. Neonatal intestinal obstruction. AJR Am J Roentgenol 2021;198(1):W1–10.

31. Berrocal T, Lamas M, Gutieerrez J, et al. Congenital anomalies of the small intestine, colon, and rectum. Radiographics 1999;19(5):1219–36.

32. Gillis DA, Grantmyre EB. The meconium-plug syndrome and hirschsprung's disease. Can Med Assoc J 1965;92:225–7.

33. Kleinhaus S, Boley SJ, Sheran M, et al. Hirschsprung's disease a survey of the members of the surgical section of the american academy of pediatrics. J Pediatr Surg 1979;14(5):588–97.

34. Buonomo C. Neonatal gastrointestinal emergencies. Radiol Clin North Am 1997;35(4):845–64.

35. Etensel B, Temir G, Karkiner A, et al. Atresia of the colon. J Pediatr Surg 2005;40(8):1258–68.

36. Puri P. Chapter 102 - Intestinal dysganglionosis and other disorders of intestinal motility. In: Coran AG, editor. Pediatric Surgery. Seventh Edition. Mosby; 2012. p. 1279-87. https://doi.org/10.1016/B978-0-323-07255-7.00102-1.

37. Puri P, Shinkai M. Megacystis microcolon intestinal hypoperistalsis syndrome. Semin Pediatr Surg 2005;14(1):58–63.

38. Berdon W, Baker D, Blanc W, et al. Megacystis-microcolon-intestinal hypoperistalsis syndrome: a new cause of intestinal obstruction in the newborn. Report of radiologic findings in five newborn girls. AJR Am J Roentgenol 1976;126(5):957–64.

39. Hernanz-Schulman M. Colon: congenital and neonatal disorders. In: Coley BD, editor. Caffey's pediatric diagnostic imaging. 12th edition. Philadelphia, PA: Saunders; 2013. p. 1107–21.

40. Hernanz-Schulman M. Duodenum and small intestine: congenital and neonatal disorders. In: Coley BD, editor. Caffey's pediatric diagnostic imaging. 12th edition. Philadelphia, PA: Saunders; 2013. p. 1057–80.

41. Hryhorczuk A, Lee EY, Eisenberg RL. Bowel obstructions in older children. AJR Am J Roentgenol 2013;201(1):W1–8.

42. Anupindi SA, Powers AM, Kannabiran S, et al. Gastrointestinal tract. In: Lee EY, editor. Pediatric radiology: practical imaging evaluation of infants and children. Philadelphia, PA: Wolters Kluwer; 2018. p. 807–80.

43. Rothrock SG, Pagane J. Acute appendicitis in children: emergency department diagnosis and management. Ann Emerg Med 2000;36(1):39–51.

44. Moore MM, Gustas CN, Choudhary AK, et al. MRI for clinically suspected pediatric appendicitis: an implemented program. Pediatr Radiol 2012;42(9):1056–63.

45. Plut D, Phillips GS, Johnston PR, et al. Practical imaging strategies for intussusception in children. AJR Am J Roentgenol 2020;215(6):1449–63.

46. Navarro O, Daneman A. Intussusception. Part 3: diagnosis and management of those with an identifiable or predisposing cause and those that reduce spontaneously. Pediatr Radiol 2004;34(4):305–12 [quiz 369].

47. Binkovitz LA, Kolbe AB, Orth RC, et al. Pediatric ileocolic intussusception: new observations and unexpected implications. Pediatr Radiol 2019;49(1):76–81.

48. Daneman A, Navarro O. Intussusception: Part 1: a review of diagnostic approaches. Ped Radiol 2003;33(2):79–85.

49. Sargent MA, Babyn P, Alton DJ. Plain abdominal radiography in suspected intussusception: a reassessment. Pediatr Radiol 1994;24(1):17–20.

50. Lioubashevsky N, Hiller N, Rozovsky K, et al. Ileocolic versus small-bowel intussusception in children: can us enable reliable differentiation? Radiology 2013;269(1):266–71.

51. Eeson GA, Wales P, Murphy JJ. Adhesive small bowel obstruction in children: should we still operate? J Pediatr Surg 2010;45(5):969–74.

52. Tsao KJ, St Peter SD, Valusek PA, et al. Adhesive small bowel obstruction after appendectomy in children: comparison between the laparoscopic and open approach. J Pediatr Surg 2007;42(6):939–42.

53. Delabrousse E, Lubrano J, Jehl J, et al. Small-bowel obstruction from adhesive bands and matted adhesions: ct differentiation. AJR Am J Roentgenol 2009;192(3):693–7.

54. Uchida K, Otake K, Iwata T, et al. Ingestion of multiple magnets: hazardous foreign bodies for children. Pediatr Radiol 2006;36(3):263–4.

55. Sanders MK. Bezoars: from mystical charms to medical and nutritional management. Pract Gastroenterol 2004;28:37–50.

Pediatric Hip Disorders
Imaging Guidelines and Recommendations

Lina Karout, MD[a], Lena Naffaa, MD[b],*

KEYWORDS

- Hip disorder • Pediatrics • Imaging • Developmental dysplasia of the hip
- Legg-Calves-Perthes disease • Slipped capital femoral epiphysis

KEY POINTS

- Ultrasound is the imaging modality of choice for the detection of joint effusion.
- Developmental dysplasia of the hip screening is recommended only to children older than 4–6 weeks with risk factors or abnormal physical examination.
- MR imaging is recommended when radiography and ultrasound fail to identify a specific disorder.

INTRODUCTION

Hip disorders are common in the pediatric population.[1] Affected children usually present with non-specific symptoms such as pain and/or limp. Establishing an early diagnosis and treatment is crucial to avoid long-term complications such as growth disturbance and degenerative disease.[1] Clinical history combined with physical examination and laboratory tests help in establishing a differential diagnosis. However, clinical and laboratory findings can overlap, making imaging evaluation crucial in the diagnosis.[2] To date, there is a lack of evidence-based imaging approach to pediatric hip disorders. Therefore, the main purpose of this article is to provide: (1) up-to-date evidence-based imaging algorithm for diagnosing pediatric hip disorders; and (2) overview of imaging spectrum of common pediatric hip disorders with an emphasis on imaging recommendations and guidelines for practicing radiologists and clinicians managing pediatric patients with various hip disorders in daily clinical practice.

IMAGING MODALITIES
Radiography

Radiography is the initial image modality used for the assessment of hip disorder in pediatric patients. It is preferred to be used by imaging the whole pelvis rather than the hip unilaterally. This allows the comparison between both hips and the detection of bilateral disease. Radiography is used in anteroposterior (AP) and frog-leg position views because of the great variability of the hip according to different ages. In patients with clinical examination demonstrating an absence of localized disease, bilateral lower extremities radiography is preferred, whereas when a localized disease is detected, AP and lateral unilateral radiography is indicated.

Ultrasound

Ultrasound (US) is the imaging modality of choice for the evaluation of hip disorders in infants because of the unossified nature of their bony structures. It is useful in screening and diagnosing developmental dysplasia of the hip (DDH) in infants, diagnosing

a Department of Radiology, Massachusetts General Hospital, 25 New Chardon Street, Boston, MA 02114, USA;
b Radiology Department, University of Central Florida, Nemours Children's Hospital, 6535 Nemours Parkway, Orlando, FL 32827, USA
* Corresponding author.
E-mail address: lena.naffaa@nemours.org

Radiol Clin N Am 60 (2022) 149–163
https://doi.org/10.1016/j.rcl.2021.08.007

bursal and periarticular fluid collections and hip joint effusion, and guiding hip aspiration and injections. If hip effusion is suspected, US is more sensitive than radiography and should be used first. In addition, US-guided aspiration should be performed if high clinical suspicion for septic arthritis (SA) is present.

MR Imaging

MR imaging is recommended when radiography and US fail to identify a specific disorder. MR imaging has a great sensitivity for the detection of early hip disorders in pediatric patients. Its greatest advantage is its ability to accurately demonstrate the presence of bone marrow edema, evaluate for acetabular cartilage and labral abnormalities, and to detect soft tissue inflammation and joint effusion. MR angiography (MRA) with intra-articular gadolinium injection provides a more accurate evaluation

of the joint anatomy and pathologies affecting the acetabular labrum and articular cartilage. It is mainly used for the assessment and follow-up of DDH, diagnosis of slipped capital femoral epiphysis (SCFE) and osteomyelitis, diagnosis and staging of LCPD, diagnosis of radiologically occult traumatic and stress-related bone injuries and tumor staging.

Bone Scintigraphy

Bone scintigraphy is indicated when US radiography failed to detect pathology and MR imaging is contra-indicated or not available. It is used for the evaluation of osteomyelitis, Legg-Calve-Perthes disease (LCPD), osteoid osteoma (OO), stress fractures, and metastatic disease. Its major disadvantage is the radiation exposure, poor anatomic details, and its nonspecific nature.

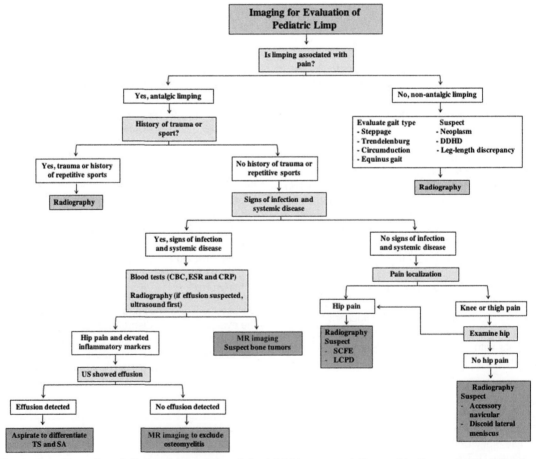

Fig. 1. An evidence-based diagnostic algorithm of the initial image modality used in the approach of limping children. CBC, Complete Blood Count; CRP, C-reactive protein; DDHD, Developmental Dysplasia of the Hip Disorder; ESR, erythrocyte sedimentation rate; LCPD, Legg-Calve-Perthes disease; SA, septic arthritis; SCFE, slipped capital femoral epiphysis; TS, transient synovitis.

EVIDENCE-BASED IMAGING ALGORITHM

A meta-analysis by the American Academy of Family Physicians (AAFP) provides key recommendations for imaging and management of limping children with a C evidence rating indicating consensus and disease-oriented evidence[3]:

1. Plain radiography is recommended in limping pediatric patients with no localized pathology on physical examination.
2. Anteroposterior and lateral radiography is recommended when localized pathology is detected on physical examination.
3. If joint effusion is suspected, ultrasound (US) is recommended because of its high sensitivity.
4. In patients with normal or equivocal physical examination, radiography, US and bone scintigraphy are recommneded.
5. The presence of elevated oral body temperature (>101.3°F), erythrocyte sedimentation rate (ESR; >40 mm/h), white blood cell (WBC) count (>12000/mm³), or C-reactive protein (>20 mg/L) raises the suspicion of septic arthritis (SA) over transient synovitis (TS).

A diagnostic algorithm with the first imaging modality recommended in limping children with and without pain is provided in **Fig. 1**.

THE SPECTRUM OF NEONATAL AND PEDIATRIC HIP DISORDERS
Congenital Pediatric Hip Disorders

Developmental dysplasia of the hip
Developmental dysplasia of the hip (DDH) consists of a wide spectrum of developmental abnormalities affecting the hip of infants and young children. It ranges in severity from abnormal acetabular morphology to hip dislocation.[4,5] Previously published studies have shown that female gender, third trimester breech position, positive family history,

and prolonged postnatal swaddling are 4 main factors associated with increased risk for DDH.[4,5] The prognosis of DDH is proportionate to the severity of hip disorder at the time of diagnosis and treatment. Physical examination is the main screening method for DDH.[4,5] Although imaging evaluation plays a fundamental role in screening, the American Academy of Pediatrics (AAP), American Academy of Orthopedics (AAOS), and American College of Radiology (ACR) recommend against universal imaging screening for DDH.[5]

Currently, selective imaging screening is recommended when an infant has risk factors or abnormal physical examination.[5,6] However, no screening imaging is recommended to neonates because studies have shown spontaneous resolution of radiological and physical abnormalities in the vast majority of cases.[4] To avoid overtreatment and iatrogenic complications, AAP recommends only starting imaging screening in patients older than 4 to 6 weeks.[4]

US is the initial imaging modality of choice for DDH evaluation in infants aged less than 6 months because, in contrary to radiography, it allows visualization of the nonossified femoral head (FH) and acetabulum.[5] According to the Graf system, classification is made by evaluating maturity of bony acetabulum, degree of FH coverage by corresponding acetabulum, and determination of alpha angle. A normal hip has angular or slightly rounded acetabulum, a FH coverage greater than 50%, and an alpha angle greater than 60° (**Fig. 2**A). Stress maneuver may induce instability of FH (**Fig. 2**B, C).

In infants older than 4 months, anteroposterior (AP) pelvis radiograph with hips in neutral position is the preferred image modality to diagnose DDH[4] complemented by frog-leg lateral view if any subluxation or dislocation is seen to determine reducibility. Radiographic evaluation includes measurement of acetabular index, size, and proper location of ossified FH.[5]

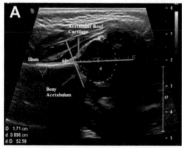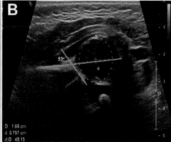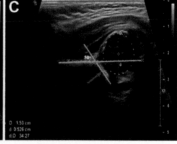

Fig. 2. A 2-month-old girl with left developmental dysplasia of the hip. (*A*) Coronal ultrasound image of normal right hip demonstrates normal alpha angle, angular appearance to bony acetabulum (*red arrow*), and 52.59% coverage of femoral head (FH) by acetabular roof cartilage (*green arrow*). (*B, C*) Coronal ultrasound images of left hip at rest (*B*) and following stress (*C*) demonstrate FH coverage decreasing from 48.15% to 34.27%, respectively, consistent with subluxation. Note abnormal flat bony acetabulum (*red arrow*) and abnormal alfa angles.

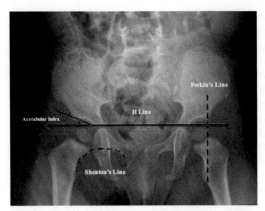

Fig. 3. A 15-month-old girl with normal hips. Frontal radiograph of the hips shows normal acetabular index, continuous Shenton line, and normal femoral head location.

Proper position of FH is assessed by Perkins's line and Shenton arc (**Fig. 3**). In normal hips, the FH is located in the inferomedial quadrant formed by the intersection of the Perkins and H lines and Shenton arc is continuous (see **Fig. 3**). Radiographic characteristics of DDH consist of increased acetabular index for age, and/or delayed appearance or small ossified FH, and/or lateral and superior position of FH (**Fig. 4**).

MR imaging has no role in screening or diagnosing DDH, as outlined by ACR.[7] It is a robust tool for confirming concentric reduction independent of ossific FH or hardware artifact following closed hip reduction and Spica cast placement or open reduction/osteotomy and hardware placement.[8] Concentric reduction is achieved when FH

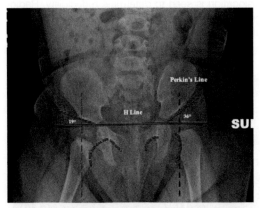

Fig. 4. A 7-month-old infant girl with left developmental dysplasia of the hip. Frontal radiograph shows increased acetabular index and disrupted Shenton arc on the left and smaller left femoral head located outside the inferomedial quadrant formed by the intersection of Perkins and H lines.

points toward corresponding triradiate cartilage in all planes (**Fig. 5**). MR imaging allows identification of obstacles to concentric reduction which can be extra-articular (tightening of iliopsoas tendon) or intra-articular (limbus, labral inversion, enlarged pulvinar, and ligament hypertrophy).[9] Following intravenous gadolinium, FH perfusion is assessed for geographic areas of hypoenhancement or global nonenhancement; only the latter has been associated with a high risk for osteonecrosis.[9] Sedation is generally not necessary for postreduction MR imaging because residual sedation following anesthesia administered during surgical reduction is sufficient for diagnostic imaging.

In pediatric patients with delayed diagnosis of DDH, MR imaging is advocated in presurgical evaluation because it delineates FH morphology, femoral acetabular coverage,[5] chondral surfaces, and labrum which help dictate timing for surgical intervention.[10] MR arthrography (MRA) following intra-articular administration of gadolinium is indicated in patients with DDH-induced femoroacetabular impingement.[11]

Similar to MR imaging, computed tomography (CT) plays no role in screening or diagnosis of DDH. Multidetector CT with 3-dimensional reconstruction can be used for preoperative planning and postoperative assessment of hip reduction.[10] Because of its ionizing radiation and poor soft tissue details and because repeat imaging may be required if unsuccessful initial reduction, it is only obtained when MR imaging is contraindicated or not available.[12]

Fluoroscopic arthrography is used intraoperatively to assess successful hip reduction[13] and detect obstacles for hip reduction (**Fig. 6**).[10] More precise intraoperative localization can be obtained with cone-beam CT (O-arm), which adds cross-sectional imaging to fluoroscopic evaluation.

Meyer dysplasia (dysplasia epiphysealis capitis femoris)

Meyer dysplasia (MD), also known as dysplasia epiphysealis capitis femoris, is an asymptomatic rare condition characterized by delayed and irregular ossification of FH. It commonly affects both hips, more often in boys, with a mean age of 2.5 years.[2] Although MD requires no treatment, its accurate diagnosis is crucial because it is commonly mistaken for Legg-Calve-Perthes disease (LCPD) potentially resulting in unnecessary intervention.[2]

In asymptomatic infants, MD is suggested radiographically by a small, irregular, or cystic FH, which resolves spontaneously after 2 to 4 years without subchondral fracture, collapse, or instability. MR imaging is used to differentiate MD from LCPD when a definitive diagnosis cannot be performed

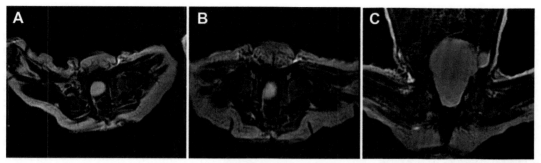

Fig. 5. A 1-month-old boy with bilateral developmental dysplasia of the hip, post closed reduction, and hip cast application (called SPICA). (A) Axial T2-weighted MR image of the hips demonstrates complete reduction on the left and posterior subluxation on the right. Femoral head (FH) points toward triradiate cartilage (red arrows). (B, C): Post right adductor tenotomy axial (B) and coronal (C) T2-weighted MR images show complete reduction of right FH and stable normal left FH. FH points toward triradiate cartilage (red arrows) in B and C.

by radiography. The absence of marrow signal abnormality is the main finding excluding LCPD.[2]

Proximal femoral focal deficiency

Proximal femoral focal deficiency (PFFD) is an uncommon congenital malformation characterized by partial or complete hypoplasia of proximal femur and abnormal development of the hip. PFFD occurs in 0.5 to 2 cases per 100,000 live births and is 90% unilateral.[14] PFFD is 50% associated with other congenital lower extremity abnormalities with ipsilateral fibular hemimelia being the most common[15] (Fig. 7A). Congenital short femur is related to PFFD,

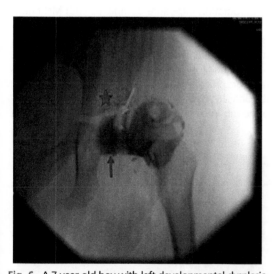

Fig. 6. A 7-year-old boy with left developmental dysplasia of the hip. Frontal view from intraoperative left hip arthrogram shows prominent contrast (blue arrow) in a widened left hip joint space and a filling defect superiorly (yellow arrow) suggesting inverted labrum interfering with complete relocation of femoral head (green oval) which remains partially outside the acetabulum (red star).

characterized by anterolateral bowing and shortening of the femur with valgus deformity of the knee. This condition is also associated with fibular hemimelia and foot deformities.[16]

Radiography is obtained in infants after antenatal US detection of femur abnormality. Radiography allows characterization of PFFD by the Aitken classification into 4 groups (A to D) depending on the degree of proximal femoral deficiency and acetabular dysplasia[17] (see Fig. 7A). However, radiographs are unable to show non-ossified FH or fibrocartilaginous connections between FH and shaft for accurate classification of PFFD. Therefore, MR imaging and US are indicated for the determination of type and prognosis of PFFD.[18]

MR imaging provides a more comprehensive evaluation for preoperative planning.[19] It allows to determine which portion of the acetabulum is deficient (posterior in PFFD vs anterior in DDH), size of cartilaginous acetabulum and FH, and detection of subtrochanteric pseudoarthrosis, femoroacetabular impingement, and labral hypertrophy[16,20] (Fig. 7B). In congenital short femur, MR imaging evaluates the extent of hamstring shortening and absence of anterior cruciate ligament.[16] Contrast-enhanced MRA is indicated to assess vascular anatomy when amputation or limb-salvage surgery is contemplated.

Developmental Pediatric Hip Disorders

Legg-Calve-Perthes disease

LCPD is idiopathic avascular necrosis of FH which results in cessation of growth. Boys are 5 times more likely affected than girls and 85% to 90% of cases are bilateral.[2] Affected pediatric patients typically present with hip pain and/or limp between 3 and 12 years of age with peak incidence at 5 to 7 years.[20] LCPD is a diagnosis of exclusion; other causes of osteonecrosis should be initially excluded.[2]

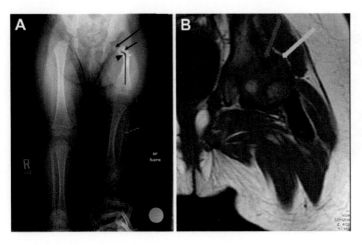

Fig. 7. A 16-month-old girl with type A left proximal femoral focal deficiency. (*A*) Scanogram shows smaller obliquely oriented left femoral head (*black long arrow*), foreshortened left femoral neck (*black short arrow*), coxa vara (*arrowhead*), and left fibular hemimelia (*orange arrow*). (*B*) Coronal T1-wei-ghted MR image of left hip demonstrates diminished distance between cartilaginous greater trochanter (*yellow arrow*) and hypertrophic labrum (*red arrow*) predisposing to impingement.

Radiography is the imaging modality of choice for diagnosis, classification, and follow-up of LCPD. In the initial stage of LCPD (first 6 months), radiography can be normal or equivocal (**Fig. 8**A).[21] AP radiograph with neutral and frog-leg lateral position of the hips are essential for the diagnosis and staging. Radiographic findings of early LCPD consist of apparent joint space widening and subchondral fracture, whereas the late radiographic findings consist of sclerosis, fragmentation, and subchondral collapse of the FH.[22]

US plays no role in the diagnosis of LCPD because all findings are nonspecific although should be suspected in recurrent or persistent hip joint effusion.[2]

Gadolinium-enhanced MR imaging is used in suspected LCPD with equivocal radiographs to confirm diagnosis. It is more sensitive than radiography because of its ability to detect bone marrow edema and diminished enhancement following intravenous gadolinium (**Fig. 8**B–D). The optimal protocol routine versus dynamic contrast-enhanced imaging with subtraction currently remains a source of debate in the literature. MR imaging provides added information regarding containment of FH within the acetabulum[23] and prognosis.[24] Enhancement of lateral column of FH and less than 50% of FH necrosis on MR imaging are associated with good prognosis.[24] Global FH hypoenhancement, transphyseal neovascularity, and bony bridging on MR imaging are associated with worse prognosis such as proximal femoral growth disturbance.[24] Besides its diagnostic and prognostic values, gadolinium-enhanced MR imaging can be used for staging of LCPD.[24] MRA helps assess LCPD complications such as femoroacetabular impingement.[24]

CT in LCPD is rarely performed because of its high radiation exposure compared with MR imaging. However, when obtained, it can allow early diagnosis of bone collapse, curvilinear sclerosis, and changes in bone trabecular patterns.[21]

Radionuclide bone scintigraphy (RBS) shows radiographically occult disease when MR imaging is contraindicated or not available and provides prognostic information. RBS shows a focal area of

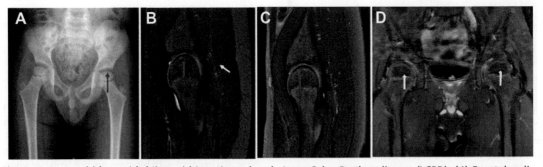

Fig. 8. A 5-year-old boy with bilateral hip pain and early Legg-Calve-Perthes disease (LCPD). (*A*) Frontal radiograph of the pelvis demonstrates tiny subchondral lucency in left femoral head (FH) (*red arrow*). (*B–D*) Sagittal T2-weighted fat-suppressed MR images of left hip (*B*) and right hip (*C*) and coronal postcontrast T1-weighted fat-suppressed MR image (*D*) confirm subchondral curvilinear fracture and marrow edema involving bilateral FH (*arrows* in *B*), subchondral fracture (*arrows* in *C*) and hypoenhancement (*arrows* in *D*) confirming LCPD.

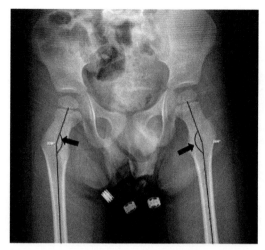

Fig. 9. A 4-year-old boy with spastic quadriplegia. Frontal radiograph shows abnormally increased femoral neck-shaft angle angles (*arrows*) consistent with bilateral coxa valga.

decreased uptake in the FH which correlates with the degree of FH ischemia.[23] Early lateral column formation (type A Conway classification pathway) is associated with good end result, whereas central activity at the base of the epiphysis or absent epiphyseal activity after 5 months (type B pathway) is predictive of poor outcome.[25]

Coxa vara

Coxa vara (CV) is an uncommon deformity of proximal femur characterized by abnormal decrease in femoral neck-shaft angle (NSA) to 120° or less.[26] Femoral NSA is the angle between the lines drawn along the axis of the femoral neck and shaft. It is classified according to its etiology into congenital, acquired, or developmental.[26,27] In congenital CV, there is primary embryonic limb bud defect of the proximal femur and is commonly associated with other congenital abnormalities such as PFFD[2,26,27] (see Fig. 7A). Acquired CV is associated with skeletal abnormalities such as osteogenesis imperfecta and fibrous dysplasia (FD).[2] It is important to differentiate true from apparent CV where the NSA is decreased in the former and normal in the latter.[2] Apparent CV occurs secondary to trauma, infection, slipped capital femoral epiphysis (SCFE), and LCPD.[26] Developmental CV occurs in early childhood because of abnormal proliferation of cartilage in the medial physis resulting in dystrophic bone formation.[26]

AP radiograph is the first image modality for the assessment of CV. Normally, FH and greater trochanter ossify and become apparent on radiograph at 3 to 6 months and 4 years, respectively.[27] MR imaging is used in preoperative assessment by showing physeal changes, bone marrow edema

indicating abnormal mechanical stress, and for better evaluation of femoroacetabular impingement[2] (see Fig. 7B).

Coxa valga

Coxa valga is a deformity of the proximal femur characterized by abnormal increase in femoral NSA relative to normal standards for age. AP radiograph of the pelvis is the first imaging modality typically used (Fig. 9). It occurs because of a lack of physiologic stress to the femur caused by skeletal abnormalities or neuromuscular hip dysplasia.[2] In cases of femoral anteversion and tibial torsion, apparent coxa valga may be seen.[2] CT and MR imaging are used for preoperative assessment of femoral anteversion and tibial torsion before derotational osteotomy.[2]

Infectious Pediatric Hip Disorders

Transient synovitis and septic arthritis

TS is the most common nontraumatic hip disorder affecting pediatric patients typically between 2 and 10 years of age.[27] It is a self-limiting condition characterized by hip joint effusion and nonspecific synovial proliferation leading to limping hip pain.[18,27] TS has a male-to-female ratio of 2:1 and affects both hips in up to 25% of cases.[18] It is a diagnosis by exclusion where more severe conditions such as SA should be initially excluded.[27]

SA is mainly monoarticular and affects the hip joint in children younger than 10 years.[2] Symptoms of SA overlap with TS but patients in SA are usually acutely ill.[2] Elevated inflammatory markers such as ESR and WBC are strong predictors of infection.[2] The early diagnosis and therapeutic intervention in SA are crucial because of its devastating joint destructive nature. In cases where SA is suspected, imaging is essential for the evaluation of hip joint effusion.[26]

US is the first image modality for evaluation of hip joint effusion in TS (Fig. 10A) or SA (Fig. 11A).[18] It enables the detection of synovial thickening and joint effusion with a 95% sensitivity.[18,27] However, US does not allow to differentiate between sterile effusion of TS and purulent effusion of SA.[26] If no effusion is detected, SA is excluded because the absence of joint effusion has a 100% negative predictive value.[26] If hip joint effusion is detected and there is high clinical suspicion for SA, US-guided joint aspiration and subsequent joint fluid analysis for a definite diagnosis is recommended.[26]

Radiography is indicated in infants and in children older than 8 years where TS is less common and SA, child abuse (infants), and SFCE (older than 8 years) are more common.[18] In most patients with TS and SA, radiography is normal or demonstrates nonspecific findings such as osteoporosis, widening of the

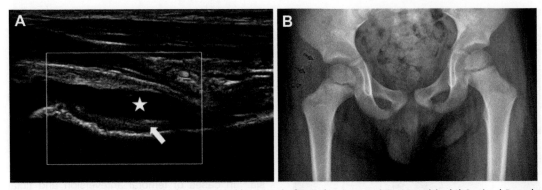

Fig. 10. A 4-year-old boy with right hip pain and low-grade fever due to transient synovitis. (*A*) Sagittal Doppler ultrasound image of right hip confirms the presence of effusion (*star*) with mild synovial thickening (*arrow*). (*B*) Frontal radiograph of the pelvis demonstrates distention of right gluteal fat pads (*arrows*) suggesting hip joint effusion.

joint space, and fat planes obliteration[2,27] (**Figs. 10B** and **11B**).

Gadolinium-enhanced MR imaging is indicated in pediatric patients with hip effusion with high inflammatory markers or TS patients experiencing clinical deterioration.[27] It allows detection of joint effusion, synovitis, and complication of SA such as abscess and avascular necrosis of femoral head (**Fig. 11**C, D).

Osteomyelitis

Osteomyelitis is a bone inflammation most commonly due to hematogenous spread of transient bacteremia.[2] It involves the most vascularized skeletal regions such as the metaphysis.[28] Osteomyelitis affects children younger than 5 years and has a male-to-female ratio of 2:1.[28]

Radiograph is the first image modality in the evaluation of osteomyelitis.[2,28] In the early stages,

radiograph can be normal (**Fig. 12A**) and in late stages, bone destruction and joint effusion can be present. Although radiograph is not sensitive for osteomyelitis, it allows to exclude other diagnoses such as trauma or tumor.[28]

Gadolinium-enhanced MR imaging is the imaging modality of choice for clinically suspected osteomyelitis affecting hip bones[28] (**Fig. 12B, C**). It allows detection of bone marrow edema and enhancement, joint effusion, and complications such as abscesses (intraosseous and soft-tissue), necrotic bone, and sinus tracks.[2]

Triple-phase RBS is used to evaluate osteomyelitis in children when radiography is normal and MR imaging is not available or contraindicated.[28] It is used in conjunction with US for better assessment of subperiosteal and soft tissue abscess and joint effusion.[28]

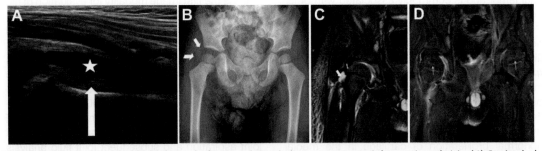

Fig. 11. A 2-year-old boy with high-grade fever and *Staphylococcus aureus* right septic arthritis. (*A*) Sagittal ultrasound of right hip shows joint effusion (*star*) with synovial thickening (*arrow*). (*B*) Frontal radiograph of the pelvis shows distention of right gluteal fat pad suggesting hip joint effusion (*arrows*). (*C*) Coronal T2-weighted fat-suppressed MR image of right hip shows joint effusion (*white arrow*), synovial thickening (*red arrow*), and subcutaneous changes (*oval*) from joint aspirate. (*D*) Coronal postcontrast T1-weighted fat-suppressed MR image of both hips shows right synovitis (*red arrow*), soft tissue enhancement with no collection (*arrowhead*), and hypoenhancement of right femoral head compared to left side (*orange arrows*). Note reactive lymph nodes of right iliac chain (*blue arrows*) in C and D.

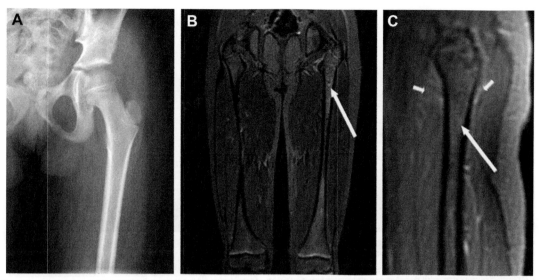

Fig. 12. An 8-year-old girl with left hip pain and fever with biopsy-proven methicillin-resistant *Staphylococcus aureus* osteomyelitis of proximal left femur. (*A*) Frontal radiograph of left hip shows no abnormality. (*B, C*) Coronal short-tau-inversion-recovery image of both femora (*B*) and sagittal postcontrast T1-weighted fat-suppressed MR image (*C*) show edema and enhancement in proximal left femoral shaft (*long arrows*) and adjacent muscles (*short arrows*) indicating acute osteomyelitis and myositis, respectively.

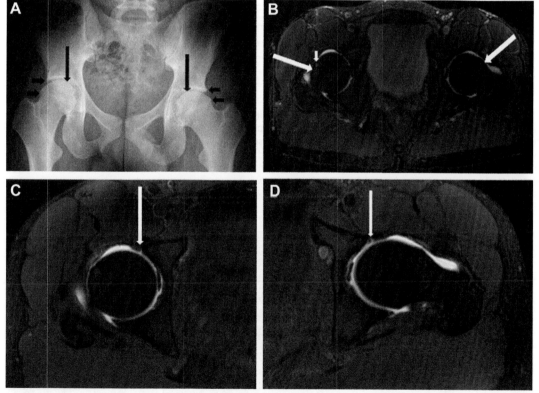

Fig. 13. A 17-year-old boy with advanced Juvenile idiopathic arthritis. (*A*) Frontal radiograph of the pelvis demonstrates bilateral hip joint narrowing (*long arrows*), marginal acetabular and femoral head (FH) osteophytes (*short arrows*). (*B*) Axial T2-weighted fat-suppressed MR image shows bony bump and marrow edema at the lateral FH-neck junction (*long arrows*), with subchondral cyst on the right (*short arrow*), suggesting CAM type of impingement. (*C, D*) Axial T1-weighted fat-suppressed MR images of right (*C*) and left (*D*) hip, respectively, show heterogeneous signal and contrast in the anterior labrum suggesting tears (*arrows*).

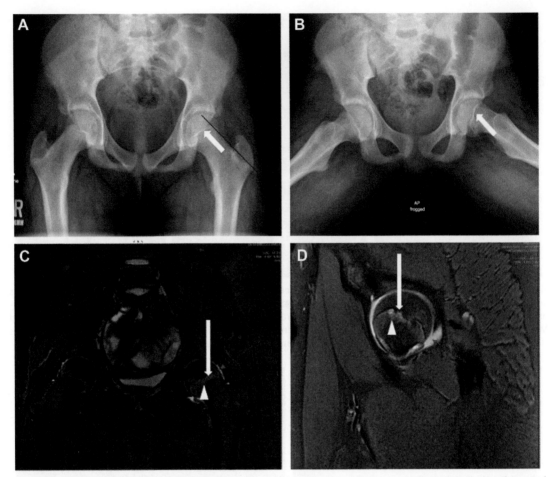

Fig. 14. A 12-year-old girl with left hip pain due to pre-slipped capital femoral epiphysis (SCFE). (*A, B*) Frontal radiographs of the pelvis in neutral (*A*) and frog-leg (*B*) positions demonstrate subtle widening of left capital femoral physis (*arrows*) with no actual slippage. Note absence of left Klein sign (*red line*). (*C, D*): Coronal T2-weighted (*C*) and sagittal proton-density (*D*) fat-suppressed MR images of left hip show widening of left femoral head (FH) physis (*white arrows*) and mild edema of adjacent metaphysis (*arrowheads*) representing pre-slippage. Note left pleural effusion (*red arrows*).

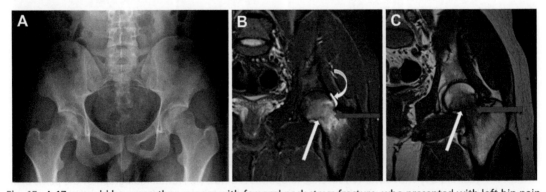

Fig. 15. A 17-year-old boy, marathon runner with femoral neck stress fracture, who presented with left hip pain. (*A*) Frontal radiograph of the pelvis shows no abnormality. (*B, C*) Coronal STIR (*C*) and coronal T1-weighted MR images of left hip show linear low signal (*white straight arrows*) of the left femoral neck consistent with stress fracture, surrounded by reactive marrow edema (*red arrows*). Note tiny left hip joint effusion (*white curved arrow*).

Inflammatory Pediatric Hip Disorders

Juvenile idiopathic arthritis

Juvenile idiopathic arthritis (JIA) is the most common cause of chronic arthritis in children.[18] It is an autoimmune noninfective inflammatory joint disease affecting children younger than 16 years with arthritis persistent for more than 6 weeks.[18,26]

Radiograph is the initial image modality in suspected cases of JIA.[2,18] In early stages, most radiographs are normal,[18] whereas late-stage radiographic findings consist of soft tissue swelling, joint

effusion, epiphyseal remodeling, and periarticular osteopenia.[18] In severe cases, radiograph may show joint space narrowing, erosions, ankyloses, and osteophytes[2] (**Fig. 13**A).

US is more sensitive than radiography for detection of joint effusion, synovitis, and synovial thickening in pediatric patients with JIA.[2,18] It is also indicated for the assessment of therapy adequacy, disease progression, and guidance during synovial fluid aspiration and intra-articular drug injection.[18]

Gadolinium-enhanced MR imaging is the best imaging modality for accurate assessment of

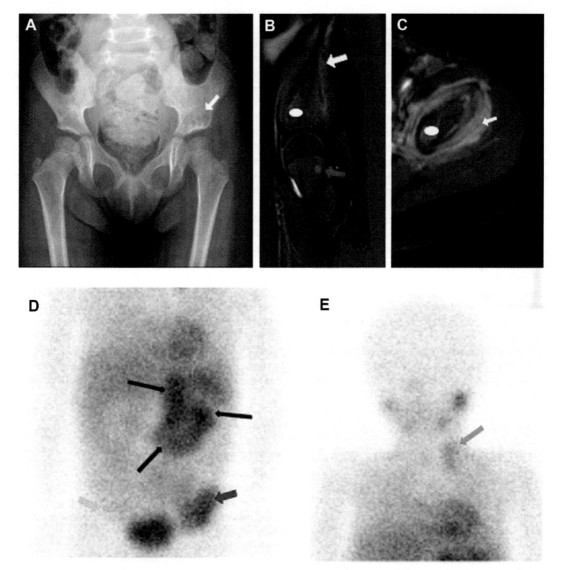

Fig. 16. A 4-year-old girl with left hip pain due to metastatic neuroblastoma. (*A*) Frontal radiograph of pelvis shows a lytic lesion in the left iliac bone (*white arrow*). (*B, C*) Sagittal T2-weighted fat-suppressed (*B*) and axial postcontrast T1-weighted fat-suppressed (*C*) MR images show destructive lesion in left acetabulum (*white oval*) with soft tissue component (*white arrows*). Note tiny metastatic lesion in the proximal left femoral metaphysis (*red arrow*). (*D, E*) Metaiodobenzylguanidine images show uptake in the primary left retroperitoneal neuroblastoma (*black arrows*) with metastasis to left lower neck (*green arrow*), left iliac bone (*red arrow*), and less seen in the right iliac bone (*yellow arrow*).

bone erosions, synovial inflammation, soft tissue, and bone marrow edema in pediatric patients with JIA.[2,18] MR imaging is superior to other modalities in the pre-erosive disease stage where it permits the early detection of subchondral bone marrow edema.[18] It is also indicated for the evaluation of therapy response and disease progression.[18] MRA helps in the assessment of complications such as femoroacetabular impingement (**Fig. 13B–D**).

Traumatic Pediatric Hip Disorders

Slipped capital femoral epiphysis

SCFE is characterized by anterosuperior slippage of FH over metaphysis.[29] It commonly affects adolescents, African Americans, and overweight children and has bilateral involvement in 20% of the cases.[27] SCFE accounts for 1 to 10 per 10,000 adolescents and has a male-to-female ratio of 2:1.4.[29]

Radiograph is the initial imaging modality for the diagnosis of SCFE. In stable disease, AP views of pelvis in neural and frog-leg positions of hips are necessary for diagnosis, whereas in unstable disease, AP and cross-table lateral views are needed.[30] Typical radiographic findings consist of irregular widening of femoral physis and loss of FH height and femoral neck anterior concavity.[29] The Klein line is an important radiographic sign in SCFE diagnosis.[29] It is a parallel line drawn from the lateral border of the femoral neck that should normally intersect with the femoral epiphysis, whereas in most cases of SCFE, it does not due to medial displacement of FH.[27,29] In preslippage stage, only widening of femoral physis is seen with absent Klein sign (**Fig. 14A, B**).

MR imaging plays a role in the early diagnosis of SCFE when radiography is equivocal, specifically in preslippage stage because it allows detection of physeal widening and periphyseal edema before slippage[27,29] (**Fig. 14C, D**). Gadolinium-enhanced MR imaging is recommended to evaluate complications such as chondrolysis and avascular necrosis of FH.[2,27] If MR imaging is contraindicated or not available, RBS is used to evaluate for complications of SCFE such as avascular necrosis. It has a 100% negative predictive value for avascular necrosis of FH.[27]

CT is used when MR imaging is not available or contraindicated. In postsurgical stage of SCFE, CT permits visualization of metalware penetration to the hip joint and successful closure of proximal femoral physis.[27]

Stress fracture

Stress fractures of the hip are uncommon in children younger than 10 years but may occur in athletes engaged in repetitive actions to the lower extremities.[2,31] Radiograph is the first imaging modality to assess stress fracture involving the hip; however, it has a low sensitivity, especially in the first 2 to 3 weeks after fracture[31] (**Fig. 15A**). Therefore, MR imaging is necessary for pediatric patients with suspected stress fracture and normal radiograph (**Fig. 15B, C**) where its sensitivity is up to 100%.[2,31] RBS has a similar sensitivity for stress fractures as MR imaging with a lower specificity,[31] usually reserved when MR imaging is not available or contraindicated.

Apophyseal injury

Apophyseal injuries are sport-induced injuries affecting adolescents due to forceful and repetitive traction of the apophysis by the corresponding attached muscular tendons.[2] The ischial tuberosity followed by the anterior inferior iliac spine is the most common injured apophysis. Radiograph is usually diagnostic in apophyseal injury where a

Table 1
Classic radiographic findings of common benign bone lesions

Benign Bone Lesions	Classic Imaging Findings
Unicameral Bone Cyst	In metaphysis of long bones or in flat bones with internal bony fragment (fallen fragment)[2,27]
Aneurysmal Bone Cyst (see **Fig. 17A–C**)	Eccentric, multiloculated radiolucent lesion (soap bubble appearance) with thin cortex in metaphysis of long bones, less commonly flat bones[2,27]
Fibrous Dysplasia	Reactive rim (rind sign) with ground-glass matrix occurring intramedullary with no outer cortex expansion and severe varus of affected proximal femur[2,27]
Multiple Osteochondromas	Clear continuity of corticomedullary portion with the parent bone (pathognomonic)[2]
Osteoid Osteoma	Subtle sclerosis with <1.5 cm central lucency

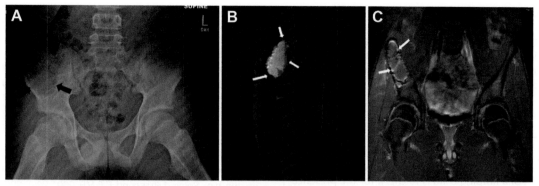

Fig. 17. A 14-year-old boy with aneurysmal bone cyst presented with right hip pain. (*A*) Frontal radiograph of the pelvis demonstrates well marginated lucent expansile and septated lesion in the right iliac wing (*black arrows*) suggestive of aneurysmal bone cyst (ABC). (*B, C*) Sagittal STIR (*B*) and coronal postcontrast T1-weighted fat-suppressed (*C*) images obtained due to progressive pain show intact cortex (*white arrows*) and absent soft tissue component excluding malignancy. Note fluid-fluid levels seen in ABC (*red arrow*).

clear displacement of the apophysis is seen.[2] This is followed by bony reaction and callus formation which could potentially be mistaken for a neoplasm.[2] MR imaging is only indicated when an apophyseal injury is suspected with normal radiograph or when atypical radiographic findings are seen. Bone marrow edema and tendon tear are common accompanying MR imaging findings at the site of injury.

Neoplastic Pediatric Hip Disorders

The 5 most common benign bone lesions of hips consist of osteochondroma, unicameral bone cyst, aneurysmal bone cyst (ABC), osteoid osteoma (OO), FD, and Langerhans cell histiocytosis.[32] They affect patients aged between 5 and 25 years and can be found incidentally after trauma.[32]

Ewing sarcoma and osteosarcoma are the 2 most common malignant pediatric bone tumors.[33] Ewing's sarcoma mainly affects the flat bones and the diaphysis of long bones in young children, whereas osteosarcoma affects the metaphysis and predominates in older children.[31,33] If multiple lytic bone lesions are detected in imaging, suspicion is raised for metastatic disease commonly from neuroblastoma, leukemia, and lymphoma[31] (Fig. 16).

Langerhans cell histiocytosis is a benign bone lesion that commonly affects hips and pelvis with variable radiographic appearance ranging from benign to malignant or mixed features.

Radiograph is the initial imaging modality.[32] In a great portion of benign conditions, radiograph is diagnostic or allows to establish a clear differential diagnosis based on the tumor location and characteristics.[32]

Radiographic findings of benign bone lesions include the following: (1) well-defined/sclerotic margins; (2) sharp transitional zone; (3) benign periosteal

reaction if any; (4) intact cortex; and (5) absence of soft tissue component.[32] Characteristic findings of common benign bone lesions are summarized in **Table 1**.

In OO, when classic features are present, CT pelvis is the main modality of choice to confirm the diagnosis.[27,34] If atypical radiographic findings, MR imaging is recommended to confirm the diagnosis and exclude other differential diagnosis.[34]

Radiographic findings of malignant bone tumors include the following: (1) ill-defined margins; (2) cortical destruction (moth-eaten or permeative pattern); (3) periosteal reaction mainly interrupted or spiculated (sunburn or onion skin appearance); and (4) soft tissue component. If there are atypical clinical or radiographic findings of a benign bone lesion (Fig. 17) or any of the malignant radiographic findings, gadolinium-enhanced MR imaging is the next imaging modality to further characterize tumors.[31] It allows accurate assessment of medullar changes, extend of the tumor, soft tissue involvement, and skip metastasis.[31] 18F-2-Fluoro-2-deoxy-D-glucose PET is used for staging malignant tumors and assess treatment response.[32] CT scan is effective in the evaluation of bone tumors. However, in pediatric patients, MR imaging is preferred because of its lack of radiation.[32]

SUMMARY

The initial assessment of pediatric hip disorders consists of a systematic approach based on patient's age, clinical history, physical examination, and laboratory findings which help in narrowing the differential diagnosis. This is further complemented by a proper selection of imaging modalities in a stepwise approach necessary to achieve a definitive diagnosis. Familiarity of the practicing radiologists and clinicians with various pediatric hip disorders and related up-to-date imaging recom-mendations and guidelines is of great importance to attain a timely and accurate diagnosis while minimizing radiation, ensure early treatment, and prevent long-term complications.

CLINICS CARE POINTS

- An important first step in imaging approach of a limping child is to check for the presence or absence of pain, trauma or repetitive sports and for signs of infection or systemic disease.

- If all these first line checkpoints are absent in a limping child, it is essential to examine the knee along with the hip joints as pediatric patients may present with a referred pain to the hip.

- Certain pediatric bone tumors such as Ewing sarcoma may clinically mimic a systemic disease and further imaging with MRI should be obtained in the absence of elevated inflammatory blood markers.

DISCLOSURE

The authors have nothing to disclose.

REFERENCES

1. Herregods N, Vanhoenacker FM, Jaremko JL, et al. Update on pediatric hip imaging. Semin Musculoskelet Radiol 2017;21(5):561-81. doi: 10.1055/s-0037-1606134.
2. Zucker EJ, Lee EY, Restrepo R, et al. Hip disorders in children. AJR Am J Roentgenol 2013;201(6):W776–96.
3. Naranje S, Kelly DM, Sawyer JR. A systematic approach to the evaluation of a limping child. Am Fam Physician 2015;92(10):908–16.
4. Nguyen JC, Dorfman SR, Rigsby CK, et al. ACR appropriateness criteria® developmental dysplasia of the hip-child. J Am Coll Radiol 2019;16(5):S94–103.
5. Barrera CA, Cohen SA, Sankar WN, et al. Imaging of developmental dysplasia of the hip: ultrasound, radiography and magnetic resonance imaging. Pediatr Radiol 2019;49(12):1652–68.
6. Croke LM. Developmental dysplasia of the hip in infants: a clinical report from the AAP on evaluation and referral. Am Fam Physician 2017;96(3):196–7.
7. Karmazyn BK, Gunderman RB, Coley BD, et al. ACR Appropriateness Criteria® on developmental dysplasia of the hip—child. J Am Coll Radiol 2009;6(8):551–7.
8. Ranawat V, Rosendahl K, Jones D. MRI after operative reduction with femoral osteotomy in developmental dysplasia of the hip. Pediatr Radiol 2009;39(2):161–3.
9. Rosenbaum DG, Servaes S, Bogner EA, et al. MR imaging in postreduction assessment of developmental dysplasia of the hip: goals and obstacles. Radiographics 2016;36(3):840–54.
10. Starr V, Ha BY. Imaging update on developmental dysplasia of the hip with the role of MRI. AJR Am J Roentgenol 2014;203(6):1324–35.
11. Blankespoor M, Ferrell K, Reuter A, et al. Developmental dysplasia of the hip in infants-a review for providers. South Dakota Med 2020;73(5):223–7.
12. Murray KA, Crim JR. Radiographic imaging for treatment and follow-up of developmental dysplasia of the hip. Semin Ultrasound CT MR 2001;22(4):306–40. doi: 10.1016/s0887-2171(01)90024-1.
13. Race C, Herring JA. Congenital dislocation of the hip: an evaluation of closed reduction. J Pediatr orthopedics 1983;3(2):166–72.
14. Biko DM, Davidson R, Pena A, et al. Proximal focal femoral deficiency: evaluation by MR imaging. Pediatr Radiol 2012;42(1):50–6.
15. Bedoya MA, Chauvin NA, Jaramillo D, et al. Common patterns of congenital lower extremity shortening: diagnosis, classification, and follow-up. Radiographics 2015; 35(4):1191–207.
16. Dillon JE, Connolly SA, Connolly LP, et al. MR imaging of congenital/developmental and acquired disorders of the pediatric hip and pelvis. Magn Reson Imaging Clin 2005;13(4):783–97.
17. Aitken GT. Proximal femoral focal deficiency. Limb Development and Deformity: Problems of Evaluation and Rehabilitation. 1969:456–76.
18. Viana SL, Ribeiro MCM, Machado BB. Joint imaging in childhood and adolescence. Springer International Publishing; 2019.
19. Herring J, Cummings D. The limb deficient child. Philadelphia: Pediatrics orthopaedics Lippincott-Raven; 1996. p. 1137–76.
20. Perry D, Skellorn P, Bruce C. The lognormal age of onset distribution in Perthes' disease: an analysis from a large well-defined cohort. Bone Joint J 2016; 98(5):710–4.
21. Dimeglio A, Canavese F. Imaging in Legg-Calvé-Perthes disease. Orthop Clin North Am 2011;42(3):297–302, v.
22. Sarwar ZU, DeFlorio R, Catanzano TM. Imaging of nontraumatic acute hip pain in children: multimodality approach with attention to the reduction of medical radiation exposure. Semin Ultrasound CT MR 2014;35(4):394-408. doi: 10.1053/j.sult.2014.05.001.
23. Hubbard AM. Imaging of pediatric hip disorders. Radiol Clin North Am 2001;39(4):721–32.
24. Dillman JR, Hernandez RJ. MRI of Legg-Calve-Perthes disease. AJR Am J Roentgenol 2009;193(5):1394–407.
25. Tsao AK, Dias LS, Conway JJ, et al. The prognostic value and significance of serial bone scintigraphy in Legg-Calvé-Perthes disease. J Pediatr Orthop 1997; 17(2):230–9.

26. Kim I-O. Radiology illustrated: pediatric radiology. Springer-Verlag Berlin Heidelberg; 2014.

27. Alshryda S, Howard JJ, Huntley JS, et al. The pediatric and adolescent hip: Essentials and evidence. Springer International Publishing; 2019.

28. Jaramillo D, Dormans JP, Delgado J, et al. Hematogenous osteomyelitis in infants and children: imaging of a changing disease. Radiology 2017;283(3):629–43.

29. Silva MS, Fernandes AR, Cardoso FN, et al. Radiography, CT, and MRI of hip and lower limb disorders in children and adolescents. Radiographics 2019;39(3):779–94.

30. Peck D. Slipped capital femoral epiphysis: diagnosis and management. Am Fam Physician 2010;82(3):258–62.

31. Jain N, Sah M, Chakraverty J, et al. Radiological approach to a child with hip pain. Clin Radiol 2013;68(11):1167–78.

32. Singla A, Geller DS. Musculoskeletal tumors. Pediatr Clin 2020;67(1):227–45.

33. Yagdiran A, Zarghooni K, Semler JO, et al. Hip Pain in Children. Dtsch Arztebl Int 2020;117(5):72.

34. French J, Epelman M, Jaramillo D, et al. Magnetic resonance imaging evaluation of osteoid osteoma: utility of the dark rim sign. Pediatr Radiol 2020;50(12):1742–50.

Pediatric Musculoskeletal Infections
Imaging Guidelines and Recommendations

Frederick E. Butt, MD[a],*, Edward Y. Lee, MD, MPH[b],
Apeksha Chaturvedi, MD[c]

KEYWORDS

- Pediatrics • Musculoskeletal • Osteomyelitis • Infection • Infectious disease • Imaging

KEY POINTS

- Pediatric musculoskeletal infections and associated complications are increasingly encountered in daily clinical practice due to epidemiologic changes over the past 2 decades.
- Conventional radiographs continue to be the first-line imaging modality of choice for evaluating pediatric musculoskeletal infections, particularly early in the course of disease, despite their low yield toward detection of musculoskeletal infections.
- Ultrasound, which is fast, noninvasive, and uses no radiation, is ideal for evaluating superficial soft tissue infections and septic arthritis. In addition, ultrasound-guided joint aspiration can both facilitate diagnosis and provide symptomatic relief.
- MR imaging, due to its superior sensitivity and specificity, is the current gold standard for diagnosis of pediatric musculoskeletal infections and associated complications.

INTRODUCTION

Pediatric musculoskeletal infections can present a diagnostic dilemma due to their often-nonspecific presentation, particularly early in the course of the disease. Missed or delayed diagnosis is frequent and can lead to potentially severe, occasionally devastating consequences in the pediatric population. Imaging is integral to the diagnostic workup of these infections, complementing history, physical examination, and laboratory testing in the pediatric population. The overarching goal of imaging evaluation is to provide an early, accurate diagnosis and minimize unwanted sequelae.

In recent years, there has been an evolution in the epidemiology of pediatric musculoskeletal infections with both the incidence and severity of disease increasing, and this has further underscored the importance of imaging evaluation for timely and accurate diagnostic workup. Therefore, it is essential for both clinicians and practicing radiologists to be aware of how to best use diagnostic imaging toward workup of pediatric musculoskeletal infections.

In this article, the unique pathophysiology of musculoskeletal infections and characteristic imaging findings in children compared with adults are reviewed. Evidence-based imaging algorithms and up-to-date recommendations regarding optimal utilization of imaging modalities toward diagnostic workup of pediatric musculoskeletal infections and, when appropriate, imaging-guided intervention, are provided.

EVIDENCE-BASED IMAGING ALGORITHM

Diagnostic workup of pediatric musculoskeletal infections involves several imaging modalities. Although conventional radiography has a low sensitivity for detection of acute osteomyelitis, especially

[a] Department of Radiology, Dartmouth-Hitchcock Medical Center, One Medical Center Drive, Lebanon, NH 03756, USA; [b] Department of Radiology, Boston Children's Hospital, Harvard Medical School, 300 Longwood Avenue, Boston, MA 02115, USA; [c] Department of Imaging Sciences, University of Rochester Medical Center, School of Medicine and Dentistry, 601 Elmwood Avenue, Rochester, NY 14642, USA
* Corresponding author.
E-mail address: Frederick.butt@hitchcock.org

radiologic.theclinics.com

early in the course of disease, radiographs should always be the first study ordered, to exclude other similarly presenting differential diagnoses. MR imaging and technetium 99m (^{99m}Tc)-MDP bone scintigraphy are both highly sensitive for the diagnosis of acute osteomyelitis. MR imaging has overtaken scintigraphy as the gold standard for diagnosis due to its lack of ionizing radiation, widespread availability, and superior delineation of extraosseous detail.

There are limited data on the exact sensitivity and specificity of imaging for diagnosis of septic joint, because imaging, by itself, cannot differentiate between sterile and infected joint fluid. Both ultrasound and conventional MR imaging are highly sensitive for detecting joint fluid. Ultrasound can guide joint aspiration, which is the gold standard for diagnosis. Dynamic contrast-enhanced MR imaging may aid distinction between a septic hip and transient synovitis.

ROLE OF IMAGING IN THE EVALUATION OF PEDIATRIC MUSCULOSKELETAL INFECTION: OSTEOMYELITIS
Epidemiology

Staphylococcus aureus has traditionally been the most common causative organism of pediatric musculoskeletal infections, especially since the advent of community immunization programs for previously common organisms such as *Haemophilus influenzae* type b (Hib). Over the past 2 decades, there has been an increase in the incidence and severity of osteomyelitis in children.[1–3] During this time, there has been a concomitant increase in the prevalence of methicillin-resistant *Staphylococcus aureus* (MRSA). Most of the cases with severe complications are secondary to an MRSA infection and are likely related to the Panton-Valentine leucocidin or PVL gene. These complications include but are not limited to multifocal infection, deep venous thrombosis, subperiosteal and intraosseous abscesses, and adjacent pyomyositis.[1,3]

Over the past 2 decades, there has been a substantial increase in the incidence of musculoskeletal infections from the facultative anaerobic gram-negative bacterium Kingella kingae, particularly in Europe and the Middle East, where it is now identified as the most common pathogen for osteomyelitis and septic arthritis in children between 6 months and 4 years of age.[4,5] This organism is highly difficult to culture. However, the increased availability of polymerase chain reaction–based assays has increased its detection. Other gram-negative organisms such as *Escherichia coli* and group B streptococci are primarily seen in neonates and young infants. *Salmonella* infection is common in patients with sickle cell disease. *Pseudomonas aeruginosa* infections are seen following puncture wounds in the feet.[6]

Osteomyelitis is considered acute if symptoms have lasted 2 weeks or less. It is most often seen in young children, with half of all pediatric cases seen in children younger than 5 years.[7,8] Male children are affected at a higher rate than female children.[9] The overall incidence of osteomyelitis in children has been increasing over the past 2 decades and now ranges between 1 and 13 per 100,000 and accounts for roughly 1% of all hospital admissions in children.[6,8,10]

Normal Anatomy and Pathophysiology

The pathogenesis of osteomyelitis in the pediatric population is unique compared with adults. Most cases of pediatric osteomyelitis occur secondary to hematogenous seeding of the metaphyseal bone marrow following an episode of transient bacteremia. Direct spread of bacteria to bone from overlying injury or infection, the predominant mechanism seen in adults, is much less common in children.

Metaphyses or metaphyseal equivalents represent the most common site of osteomyelitis in children[11] due to distinct anatomic attributes of the metaphyseal vasculature, namely the open-ended structure of the terminal metaphyseal vessels and the large number of slow-moving metaphyseal sinusoidal veins.[12] As the sluggish flow reaches the capillaries, bacteria can escape into the extravascular space via small gaps in terminal capillaries and become trapped at the junction of the metaphysis and physis. Osteomyelitis most often involves in the fast-growing long bones of the lower extremities including the femur, tibia, and fibula.[4]

Over the first 12 to 18 months of life, the metaphyseal and epiphyseal vasculature communicate directly through the growth plate, permitting direct epiphyseal seeding from a metaphyseal focus of infection (**Figs. 1** and **2**). Between 1 and 2 years of age, these transphyseal vessels begin to involute and the now avascular growth plate begins to serve as a barrier to spread of metaphyseal infection.[13]

Subacute osteomyelitis is clinically defined as infection of the bone marrow that has lasted greater than 2 weeks but less than 6 weeks (**Fig. 3**). On MR imaging, Brodie abscess, a focal region of subacute osteomyelitis is commonly characterized by the "penumbra" sign, which is a peripheral rim of vascular granulation tissue with high T1 signal surrounding the low T1 signal intensity abscess cavity (**Fig. 4**).[14,15]

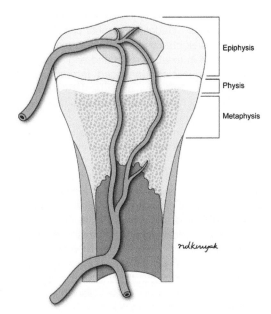

Fig. 1. Osseous vascularity during the first 18 months of life. Note transphyseal vessels that allow direct spread of metaphyseal infection to the epiphysis. (*Courtesy of* N. Kiriyak, B.F.A., Rochester, New York.)

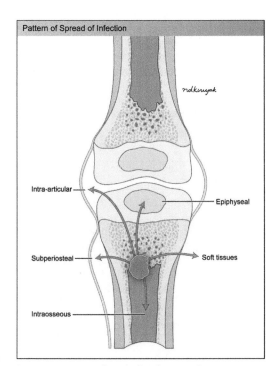

Fig. 2. Patterns of spread of acute hematogenous osteomyelitis. The infection originating in the metaphysis can spread into the epiphysis, subperiosteal space, joint, along the diaphysis of the long bone, and the surrounding soft tissues. (*Courtesy of* N. Kiriyak, B.F.A., Rochester, New York).

Chronic osteomyelitis represents infection of greater than 6 weeks duration, often with intermittent, acute exacerbations.[16,17] Chronic infection can result in necrotic bone known as sequestrum with surrounding pus and reactive new bone called an involucrum. The sequestrum can limit antibiotic efficacy by preventing penetration into the infectious cavity. A cloaca is a sinus tract extending through the involucrum, which can allow debris to drain from the necrotic bone.[5,14]

Imaging Techniques

The ultimate goal of imaging in a suspected case of osteomyelitis is to provide a prompt, accurate diagnosis in order to facilitate early and appropriate treatment and thereby decrease the likelihood of associated complications.

Radiography

Conventional radiographs are recommended as the first line of diagnostic evaluation in all cases of suspected osteomyelitis in the pediatric population. Radiographs should be obtained in conjunction with laboratory studies such as a hemogram, inflammatory markers (erythrocyte sedimentation rate [ESR] and C-reactive protein [CRP]), and blood cultures. It is important to note that the diagnostic rate of the initial conventional radiographs is less than 20% for acute osteomyelitis, with radiographic findings seen only 1 to 2 weeks after symptom onset and following loss of approximately 33% of bone mineral.[16–18] The most important role of the initial radiographs in cases of suspected acute osteomyelitis is to detect alternative causes such as trauma or malignancy, which may account for the pediatric patient's symptoms (**Box 1**).

The classic radiographic findings of acute osteomyelitis include ill-defined lytic changes with or without periosteal reaction and minimal surrounding sclerosis (**Box 2**). In subacute osteomyelitis, admission radiographs are normal in 67% to 100% of patients. When positive, bone radiographs demonstrate bone destruction, lytic lesions, and periosteal reaction/ elevation.[15]

MR imaging

In all cases with a high clinical suspicion for acute osteomyelitis, obtaining prompt MR imaging of the region of concern, regardless of the findings seen on the initial radiograph, is recommended; this is especially important in children with elevated inflammatory markers. MR imaging is the imaging modality of choice for diagnosis of acute osteomyelitis because of equivalent sensitivity to bone scintigraphy for diagnosis (97%), along with superior spatial resolution and specificity.[5,18] Performing the

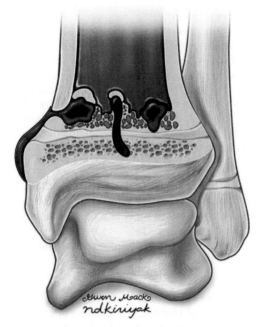

Fig. 3. Patterns of spread of Brodie abscess. (*Courtesy of* G. Mack, M.F.A., N. Kiriyak, B.F.A., Rochester, New York.)

MR imaging as soon as reasonably possible can expedite diagnosis and reduce the likelihood of complications.

MR imaging evaluation should be focused on the presumed site of infection. Non-contrast enhanced sequences include axial, coronal and sagittal T1, axial fat-suppressed T2, coronal and sagittal sh-ort-tau inversion recovery (STIR), and axial T1 with fat suppression. Gadolinium-enhanced fat suppressed T1 -weighted images should subsequently be performed in axial, coronal and sagittal planes (**Table 1**). Gadolinium-enhanced fat-suppressed T1- weighted sequences can identify epiphyseal chondritis or ischemic bone.[19] Infants and young pediatric patients (typically <5 years old) require sedation before imaging, and a multidisciplinary approach is paramount to prevent unnecessary delays in care.[20]

Acute osteomyelitis manifests as relatively decreased T1 marrow signal (when compared with the signal of adjacent muscle) and increased marrow signal on STIR or T2 sequences (**Fig. 5**). The infected bone marrow typically shows increased enhancement compared with normal bone marrow. If there is decreased or absent enhancement of portions of the infected bone marrow, there is likely a region of ischemia consistent with higher disease severity and increased complication risk (**Fig. 6**).[5]

A unique challenge in neonates and infants is their predominantly hematopoietic marrow with a low fat and high water content, which decreases sensitivity of both T1 and fluid-sensitive sequences for detection of osteomyelitis. Intravenous gadolinium-based contrast remains necessary to detect epiphyseal chondritis or ischemia (**Fig. 7**). Because of fewer localizing signs and higher incidence of multifocal infection in this age group, a whole-body MR imaging acquisition with coronal STIR sequences performed over 1 to 2 imaging stations is appropriate as an initial

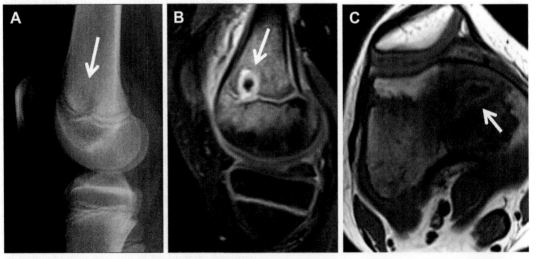

Fig. 4. An 11-year-old girl with subacute osteomyelitis and a Brodie abscess. (*A*) Lateral radiograph of the femur shows a subtle metaphyseal lucency (*arrow*) with geographic nonsclerotic margins. (*B*) Gadolinium-enhanced T1-weighted fat-suppressed MR image of the femur demonstrates a well-defined metaphyseal abscess (*arrow*) with peripheral enhancement. (*C*) Precontrast axial T1-weighted MR image obtained at the level of the distal femoral metaphysis reveals hyperintense T1-weighted signal at the rim of the abscess (*arrow*) suggesting the "penumbra" sign, characteristic of a Brodie abscess.

screening study, followed by focused MR imaging evaluation of the region of abnormality.[5]

Nuclear medicine

Before the widespread availability of MR imaging, a 3-phase bone scan using ^{99m}Tc-labeled methylene diphosphonate was the most frequent study used to confirm or exclude acute osteomyelitis. It has similar sensitivity to MR imaging, estimated to approach 97%, becomes positive within 48 hours of symptom onset, and does not require sedation.[14] Drawbacks include a high radiation dose and limited evaluation of extraosseous structures.[21] An additional challenge of scintigraphy is the difficulty of discerning metaphyseal infection due to physeal uptake of radiotracer. In addition, the predominantly cartilaginous epiphyses of infants, commonly affected in osteomyelitis, cannot be assessed with this technique.[22] For these reasons, scintigraphy is often restricted to situations where access to MR imaging is limited.

Ultrasound

Although not a routine imaging modality used for evaluation of acute osteomyelitis, ultrasound can show extraosseous findings such as adjacent soft tissue edema, subperiosteal fluid, and complications such as deep vein thrombosis in the setting of osteomyelitis.[23,24] In cases where access to MR imaging is limited, ultrasound evaluation can be performed in conjunction with scintigraphy for assessment of extraosseous structures.

Computed tomography

Computed tomography (CT) has limited benefit in the diagnosis of acute osteomyelitis because MR imaging provides superior soft tissue contrast in the pediatric population. However, CT can guide interventional procedures and surgery.[25] It is also helpful toward demonstrating osseous changes in chronic osteomyelitis such as bony sequestration, cortical destruction, and intraosseous gas.[6]

Recommended Diagnostic Workup for Suspected Osteomyelitis

As previously discussed, the clinical presentation of acute osteomyelitis and other musculoskeletal infections in the pediatric population can be highly nonspecific. In infants and toddlers, there is the added diagnostic challenge of the inability to verbalize symptoms and localize pain. Therefore, in any pediatric patient with fever and focal pain, careful consideration of initiating a workup for potential acute osteomyelitis is important. Swelling and erythema at the site of pain are helpful findings but not always present. A low threshold to initiate this workup in infant and younger pediatric patients with relatively nonspecific symptoms such as limp, refusal to bear weight, or limb pseudoparalysis is warranted.[26]

A detailed history should be obtained to clarify the duration and progression of symptoms, degree of change from baseline, and history of recent trauma. A physical examination is invaluable toward elucidating more subtle signs of bone involvement and localizing the site of pain. If physical examination suggests musculoskeletal infection, additional studies should be performed.

In general, the initial slate of studies obtained in a case of suspected acute osteomyelitis include a metabolic panel, hemogram with differential, 2 sets of blood cultures, and serum inflammatory markers including CRP, ESR, and possibly procalcitonin levels. Concurrently with these laboratory tests, focused radiographs of the site of suspected infection should be obtained in 2 orthogonal planes. If the child seems toxic on presentation, appropriate management per institutional sepsis protocol should be considered (**Fig. 8**).

ROLE OF IMAGING IN THE EVALUATION OF PEDIATRIC MUSCULOSKELETAL INFECTION: SEPTIC ARTHRITIS
Epidemiology

Septic arthritis is arthropathy secondary to intraarticular infection. This destructive arthropathy accounts for approximately 7% of all pediatric arthritis and is seen in younger patients, typically 2 to 3 years of age.[7,27] Joints of the lower extremity,

Table 1
Recommended MR imaging protocol for pediatric patients with suspected acute osteomyelitis

Sequence	Plane of Imaging
T1	Axial, coronal, sagittal
Short-tau inversion recovery (STIR)	Coronal, sagittal
T2 + [a]FS	Axial
T1 + [a]FS	Axial
T1 + [a]FS + [b]GBCA	Axial, coronal, sagittal

An optional whole-body MR imaging can be performed in cases of occult infection or multifocal osseous infection, particularly in small, nonverbal patients.

[a] FS = Fat suppression.
[b] GBCA = Gadolinium-based contrast agent.

specifically the hips and knees, are most involved. Their larger size and greater metaphyseal blood supply make them especially vulnerable to hematogenous bacterial seeding. The ankle and elbow joints are the next most commonly involved joints in the pediatric population.[3,28] Monoarticular involvement is the norm in the pediatric population with polyarticular infection seen in less than 10% of cases.[14]

As with osteomyelitis, *S aureus* including MRSA is overall the most common causative organism in septic arthritis, with *K kingae* and *Streptococcus* species making up most of the remainder.[29] Unique causative organisms include *Neisseria gonorrhoeae* in sexually active adolescents and neonates. Although there has been an increase in the incidence of osteomyelitis over the past 20 years, the incidence of septic arthritis has remained steady.[3,29]

Normal Anatomy and Pathophysiology

Hematogenous seeding of the synovium is by far the most common underlying cause of septic arthritis in the pediatric population. The synovium is highly vascularized and lacks a basement membrane allowing bacteria a pathway into the joint.[26] Rarely, direct inoculation into the joint or synovium from trauma can occur. Concomitant bone and joint infections are seen in 15% to 50% of osteoarticular infections overall and are the most common in younger pediatric patients.[30] The metaphyseal focus of infection can directly extend to the epiphysis via transphyseal vessels in younger children, and subsequently to the joint, or, when metaphyses are intraarticular, as in case of the hip, metaphyseal infection can extend directly to the joint.[31]

Imaging Techniques

Radiography

As with suspected osteomyelitis, radiographs are typically the first imaging study in case of suspected septic joint. The conventional radiograph can exclude other osseous pathology and demonstrate secondary findings of joint effusion in early cases of septic arthritis such as joint space widening and bulging of the surrounding soft tissues.[21] Joint space narrowing and joint destruction can be seen as the disease progresses.

Ultrasound

Ultrasound plays a more important role in the evaluation of septic arthritis than in acute osteomyelitis. It is fast, noninvasive, and uses no radiation. In addition, ultrasound-guided joint aspiration can both facilitate diagnosis and provide symptomatic relief.[32,33]

MR imaging

MR imaging can improve diagnostic efficacy in pediatric patients with suspected septic hip, but universal use of MR for evaluation of septic hip is currently somewhat controversial.[34,35] MR imaging is highly sensitive for detecting joint effusion and synovial thickening but cannot differentiate between sterile and septic joint effusions. Intraarticular fluid demonstrates high signal on fluid sensitive sequences and may contain internal debris.[14] An important role of MR imaging in pediatric patients with suspected or confirmed septic arthritis is to assess for adjacent osteomyelitis, which may have been the precursor to synovial and intraarticular infection, as well as detection of adjacent pyomyositis and submuscular absc-esses.[36] Dynamic contrast-enhanced MR imaging may aid distinction between septic hip and transient synovitis. Septic hip may manifest decreased perfusion and consequent hypoenhancement of the femoral head, whereas the hip affected by transient synovitis is likely to enhance normally (**Fig. 9**).[37]

Computed tomography

Similar to other cross-sectional modalities, CT can demonstrate a joint effusion, but its role is otherwise limited in the workup of septic arthritis.

Recommended Diagnostic Workup for Suspected Septic Arthritis

The presentation of septic arthritis is typically more straightforward than that of osteomyelitis in the pediatric population due to the more acute systemic manifestations of septic arthritis. Abrupt onset of fever with focal pain, erythema, and warmth at a joint is the most common presentation. If lower extremity

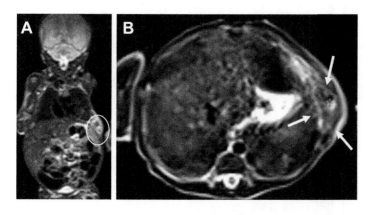

Fig. 5. A 3-week-old male neonate with osteomyelitis of the left fifth rib. During the course of his admission, patient developed methicillin-sensitive *Staphylococcus aureus* (MSSA) bacteremia. (*A*) Coronal T2-weighted MR image without fat suppression obtained as part of a whole-body MR imaging evaluation demonstrates abnormal hyperintense signal at the left lower chest (marked by oval overlay on the image). (*B*) Axial T2-weighted MR image with Dixon fat suppression obtained at the level of the abnormality shows abnormal, heterogeneous soft tissue (*arrows*) surrounding the irregular and expanded lateral aspect of the left seventh rib (*star*), compatible with osteomyelitis. No other foci of abnormality were seen through the remainder of his anatomy. Contrast agent was not administered.

joints are involved, the child may present with limp or refusal to bear weight on the affected extremity. Septic arthritis is a surgical emergency, and arthrotomy must be performed as soon as possible to prevent long-term morbidity such as degenerative arthritis, limb-length discrepancy, and ankylosis.[27]

The hip is a commonly infected joint. For pediatric patients with concern for acute bacterial infection of

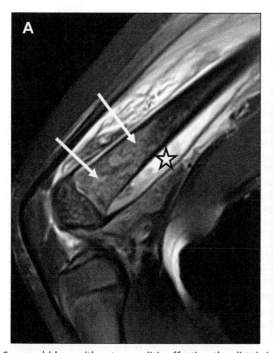
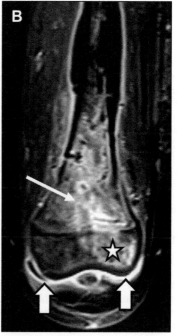

Fig. 6. A 6-year-old boy with osteomyelitis affecting the distal right femur complicated by epiphyseal and articular involvement, subperiosteal abscess, and surrounding pyomyositis. (*A*) Sagittal STIR MR image of the affected lower extremity shows abnormal, heterogeneous hyperintense signal along the distal femur metaphysis (*arrows*). Abnormal signal also extends into the anterior soft tissue planes; a subperiosteal abscess (*asterisk*) is also noted, which enhances at the rim postgadolinium. (*B*) Gadolinium-enhanced T1 MR image demonstrates enhancement of the osseous abnormality (*long arrow*), with extension into the adjacent epiphysis (*star*). There is intense synovial enhancement at the knee with knee joint fluid (*short arrows*). The patient was treated for a septic joint.

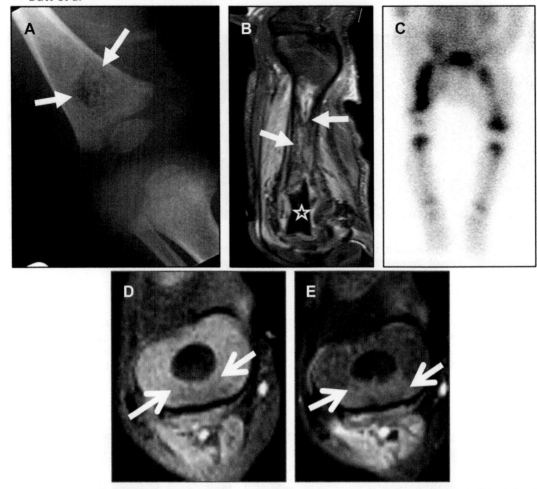

Fig. 7. A 6-month-old female infant with acute osteomyelitis of the right distal femur complicated by ischemia and epiphyseal chondritis. The patient presented to the emergency room with a red, swollen right lower extremity. (*A*) Frontal radiograph of the right knee demonstrates a poorly marginated lucent abnormality (*arrows*) within the distal femur. (*B*) Contrast-enhanced T1-weighted coronal MR image reveals abnormal patchy enhancement through most of the femoral diaphysis and the surrounding soft tissues (*arrows*). There was a well-defined region of nonenhancement within the distal femoral metadiaphysis (*star*), compatible with ischemic bone. (*C*) Tc-99m MDP bone scan corroborates the finding of bony ischemia. A photopenic defect is seen corresponding to the site of vascularity/nonenhancement at the distal femur. The remainder of the right femur shows intense radiotracer uptake compatible with bone infection. (*D*) Axial T1-weighted MR image of the distal femoral cartilage shows poorly defined hypointense signal (*arrows*) at the distal femoral cartilage. (*E*) Contrast-enhanced axial T1-weighted MR image demonstrates abnormal enhancement (*arrows*) through the distal femoral cartilage. MR imaging findings are consistent with distal femoral epiphyseal chondritis.

the hip, obtaining both radiographs of the hip as well as a targeted ultrasound of the joint to evaluate for effusion is important. If no fluid is seen in the hip joint, septic arthritis is less likely,[21,38] although recent evidence suggests that septic hip in neonates can present with scanty joint fluid and therefore a false-negative aspiration.[39] Despite a negative ultrasound, a high index of suspicion must continue to be maintained for similarly presenting periarticular infections such as adjacent osteomyelitis and/or pyogenic myositis. If symptoms persist in the setting of a negative ultrasound, MR imaging should be obtained for further evaluation (**Fig. 10**).

ROLE OF IMAGING IN THE EVALUATION OF PEDIATRIC MUSCULOSKELETAL INFECTION: SOFT TISSUE INFECTIONS

Epidemiology, Normal Anatomy, and Pathophysiology

Cellulitis, soft tissue abscesses, and pyomyositis comprise most of the pediatric soft tissue infections. Causative organisms are similar to other musculoskeletal infections with *S aureus* and *Staphylococcus pyogenes* being the most common underlying pathogens.[24,36]

Cellulitis, or infection of the superficial soft tissues, is common and, if not appropriately treated,

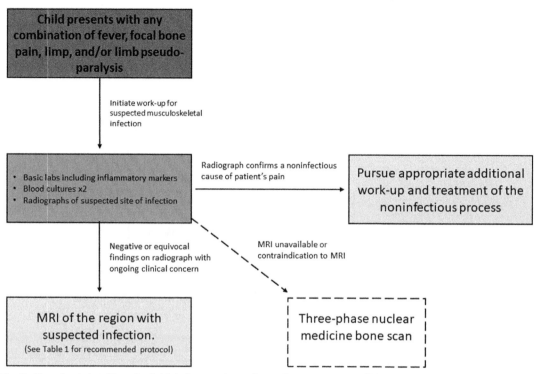

Fig. 8. Flowchart detailing the initial diagnostic workup of acute osteomyelitis in a pediatric patient.

can lead to infection of the deeper soft tissue planes. The body's attempts to contain the infection can result in abscess formation, which is a central focus of bacteria, necrotic tissue, and inflammatory debris. Extension of the infection to the skeletal muscle is termed pyomyositis, which can alternatively be a sequela of adjacent osteomyelitis or septic arthritis. The large muscles of the pelvis and lower extremities are the most often involved.

Primary skeletal muscle infection is exceedingly rare in otherwise healthy children, mostly seen in those with predisposing factors such as immunosuppression or trauma. Chronic, recurrent soft tissue infection resistant to antibiotic therapy can be secondary to a foreign body.[24]

Although rare, it is important to note that necrotizing soft tissue infections can occur in children. These infections can be rapidly fatal, with the

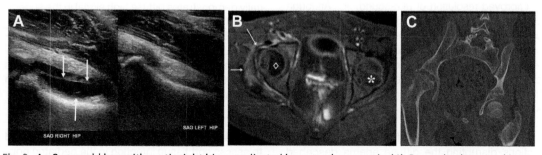

Fig. 9. An 8-year-old boy with septic right hip complicated by avascular necrosis. (*A*) Grayscale ultrasound images of the bilateral hips show abnormal fluid in the right hip joint (*arrows*). The normal left hip is provided for comparison. (*B*) Gadolinium-enhanced T1-weighted fat-suppressed MR image of the pelvis demonstrates hypoenhancement of the right femoral head (diamond) relative to the left, with surrounding synovial thickening and enhancement (*arrows*), compared with the normal left hip (*asterisk*). (*C*) Coronal CT image of the pelvis obtained several years later shows severe right hip osteoarthropathy, which arose as a result of the septic arthritis.

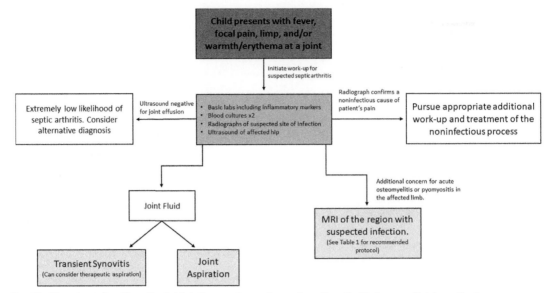

Fig. 10. Flowchart detailing the initial diagnostic workup of septic arthritis in a pediatric patient.

inciting event often innocuous. Underlying cause is usually polymicrobial.[40]

Imaging Techniques

Radiography

Conventional radiographs can demonstrate loss of fascial planes and soft tissue edema but are otherwise limited in assessing soft tissue infection. Aggressive necrotizing soft tissue infections may present with subcutaneous air, with frequency of this radiographic finding ranging between 24% and 73% as reported in different series.[40]

Ultrasound

Ultrasound is ideal for evaluating superficial soft tissue infections in the pediatric population. In younger children, the higher amount of cartilage relative to bone, lower fat, and smaller body size all contribute to improved resolution of ultrasound.[24,41] Although cellulitis is a clinical diagnosis, ultrasound is often used to exclude an associated abscess. Simple cellulitis demonstrates subcutaneous tissue thickening and hypoechoic strands interweaving through hyperechoic subcutaneous fat. As the infection progresses, there is increased disarray of tissues with pus accumulation and eventual abscess formation.[42]

Abscesses typically manifest as focal fluid collections disrupting the diffuse edema described earlier. The internal liquefied, necrotic components of an abscess can vary in echogenicity, appearing iso- or hyperechoic to adjacent inflammation.[43] Additional findings include lack of Doppler flow internally with surrounding hyperemia.[43,44] Abs-

cesses can be aspirated under ultrasound guidance with direct needle visualization through the duration of the procedure.

Imaging findings of pyomyositis progress in a similar manner to more superficial soft tissue infections. Early phlegmonous infection shows muscular edema as ill-defined hypoechoic regions with distorted muscular planes. The later suppurative phase shows findings more typical of abscess.[45,46] The presence of dirty shadowing suggests intramuscular gas, suggesting infection with an anaerobic bacterium.

MR imaging

MR imaging can be a useful adjunct to ultrasound in the workup of a suspected soft tissue infection. If the lesion is too deep to be adequately characterized by ultrasound, MR imaging should be considered, especially if an abscess is suspected. Cellulitis typically demonstrates diffuse high signal in the superficial soft tissues on fluid sensitive sequences. Abscesses in the superficial soft tissues or in the muscle are often accompanied by low signal on T1-weighted and high signal on T2-weighted images with a rim of surrounding contrast enhancement on postgadolinium sequences.[14]

Computed tomography

Because of ionizing radiation, CT is rarely used to assess soft tissue infection in the pediatric population. MR imaging can better depict soft tissue changes without the use of radiation. CT should only be considered if MR imaging is not available and there is concern for deep soft tissue infection that cannot be visualized by ultrasound.

Recommended Diagnostic Workup for Suspected Soft Tissue Infection

Cellulitis is diagnosed clinically, and imaging is not required. However, if there is concern for an abscess, imaging should be considered. Ultrasound of the area of concern is the recommended initial imaging modality of choice. Ultrasound is preferred over MR imaging due to ease of use, low cost, and no need for sedation. If an abscess is not visualized and pediatric patient's symptoms either persist or worsen, ultrasound can be repeated because the classic ultrasound findings of abscess can be slow to develop. MR imaging should be considered if there is high suspicion for a deep soft tissue infection that cannot be visualized by ultrasound.

SUMMARY

The potentially devastating consequences of pediatric musculoskeletal infections necessitate a high index of clinical suspicion and prompt diagnostic workup and proper treatment. Recent changes in epidemiology of acute musculoskeletal infections have led to more severe sequelae, further amplifying diagnostic urgency.

Imaging is central to diagnostic workup. Conventional radiographs are the first line of diagnostic evaluation, with negative radiographs common during the early course of the disease. Ultrasound can assess for soft tissue infections and joint effusions but cannot conclusively distinguish between sterile and septic effusions. Joint aspiration for definitive diagnosis should be performed if there is concern for septic arthritis. CT has a markedly limited role in assessment of pediatric musculoskeletal infections. Bone scintigraphy, previously central to diagnosis of pediatric musculoskeletal infections, has now mostly been replaced by MR imaging. Optimal pediatric patient management for musculoskeletal infections can be achieved by close multidisciplinary collaboration with imaging playing a central role, and this can lead to timely, accurate diagnosis and prevent potential complications.

CLINICS CARE POINTS

- Initial radiographs are very often negative for findings of acute osteomyelitis early in the disease process. A high index of suspicion must be maintained in the setting of negative radiographs.
- MR imaging is the imaging study of choice for evaluating for acute osteomyelitis.

- Ultrasound is an ideal, cost-effective way to evaluate for joint effusion in patients with septic arthritis.
- Imaging alone cannot differentiate between sterile and infected joint effusion. If there is concern for a septic joint, joint aspiration should be performed expeditiously to prevent treatment delays.
- Infections of the bone, joint, and muscle can often occur simultaneously, and MR imaging is useful to assess the extent of infection.
- CT plays in an extremely limited role in the evaluation of suspected musculoskeletal infection in the pediatric population.

ACKNOWLEDGMENTS

The authors wish to acknowledge Nadezhda Kiriyak and Gwen Mack from Graphics, Imaging Sciences, University of Rochester Medical Center for contributing original artwork to this article.

DISCLOSURE

The authors have nothing to disclose.

REFERENCES

1. Goergens ED, McEvoy A, Watson M, et al. Acute osteomyelitis and septic arthritis in children. J Paediatr Child Health 2005;41(1–2):59–62.
2. Browne L, Guillerman P, Orth R, et al. Community-acquired staphylococcal musculoskeletal infection in infants and young children: necessity of contrast-enhanced MRI for the diagnosis of growth cartilage involvement. AJR Am J Roentgenol 2012; 198:194
3. Gafur OA, Copley LAB, Hollmig ST, et al. The impact of the current epidemiology of pediatric musculoskeletal infection on evaluation and treatment guidelines. J Pediatr Orthop 2008;28(7):777–85.
4. Peltola H, Pääkkönen M. Acute osteomyelitis in children. N Engl J Med 2014;370(4):352–60.
5. Jaramillo D, Dormans JP, Delgado J, et al. Hematogenous osteomyelitis in infants and children: imaging of a changing disease. Radiology 2017;283(3): 629–43.
6. Dartnell J, Ramachandran M, Katchburian M. Haematogenous acute and subacute paediatric osteomyelitis: a systematic review of the literature. J Bone Joint Surg Br 2012;94:584.
7. Dolitsky R, DePaola K, Fernicola J, et al. Pediatric musculoskeletal infections. Pediatr Clin North Am 2020;67(1):59–69.
8. Riise Ø, Kirkhus E, Handeland K. Childhood osteomyelitis: incidence and differentiation from other

acute onset musculoskeletal features in a population-based study. BMC Pediatr 2008;8:45.

9. Grammatico-Guillon L, Vermesse ZM, Baron S, et al. Paediatric bone and joint infections are more common in boys and toddlers: a national epidemiology study. Acta Paediatr 2013;102(3):e120–5.

10. Yeo A, Ramachandran M. Acute haematogenous osteomyelitis in children. BMJ 2014;348(20 3):g66.

11. Trueta J. The three types of acute haematogenous osteomyelitis. J Bone Joint Surg Br 1959;41-B(4): 671–80.

12. Stephen RF, Benson MKD, Nade S. Misconceptions about childhood acute osteomyelitis. J Child Orthop 2012;6(5):353–6.

13. Ogden JA. Pediatric osteomyelitis and septic arthritis: the pathology of neonatal disease. Yale J Biol Med 1979;52(5):423–48.

14. Ranson M. Imaging of pediatric musculoskeletal infection. Semin Musculoskelet Radiol 2009;13(03): 277–99.

15. González-López JL, Soleto-Martín FJ, Cubillo-Martín A, et al. Subacute osteomyelitis in children. J Pediatr Orthop B 2001;10(2):101–4.

16. Weiland A, Moore J, Daniel R. The efficacy of free tissue transfer in the treatment of osteomyelitis. J Bone Joint Surg 1984;66(2):181–93.

17. Termaat MF, Raijmakers PGHM, Scholten HJ, et al. The accuracy of diagnostic imaging for the assessment of chronic osteomyelitis: a systematic review and meta-analysis. J Bone Joint Surg Am 2005; 87(11):2464–71.

18. Mandell GA. Imaging in the diagnosis of musculoskeletal infections in children. Curr Probl Pediatr 1996;26(7):218–37.

19. Averill LW, Hernandez A, Gonzalez L, et al. Diagnosis of osteomyelitis in children: utility of fat-suppressed contrast-enhanced MRI. AJR Am J Roentgenol 2009;192(5):1232–8.

20. Mueller AJ, Kwon JK, Steiner JW, et al. Improved Magnetic Resonance Imaging Utilization for Children with Musculoskeletal Infection. J Bone Joint Surg 2015;97(22):1869–76.

21. Jaramillo D, Treves ST, Kasser JR, et al. Osteomyelitis and septic arthritis in children: appropriate use of imaging to guide treatment. AJR Am J Roentgenol 1995;165(2):399–403.

22. Karmazyn B. Imaging approach to acute hematogenous osteomyelitis in children: an update. Semin Ultrasound CT MR 2010;31(2):100–6.

23. Karmazyn B. Ultrasound of pediatric musculoskeletal disease: from head to toe. Semin Ultrasound CT MRI 2011;32(2):142–50.

24. Robben SGF. Ultrasonography of musculoskeletal infections in children. Eur Radiol 2004;14(4):L65–77.

25. Pineda C, Vargas A, Rodríguez AV. Imaging of osteomyelitis: current concepts. Infect Dis Clin North Am 2006;20(4):789–825.

26. Frank G, Mahoney HM, Eppes SC. Musculoskeletal infections in children. Pediatr Clin North Am 2005; 52(4):1083–106.

27. Offiah AC. Acute osteomyelitis, septic arthritis and discitis: Differences between neonates and older children. Eur J Radiol 2006;60(2):221–32.

28. Arnold JC, Bradley JS. Osteoarticular infections in children. Infect Dis Clin North Am 2015;29(3): 557–74.

29. Sucato D, Schwend R, Gillespie R. Septic arthritis of the hip in children. J Am Acad Orthop Surg 1997;5: 249.

30. Chen W-L, Chang W-N, Chen Y-S, et al. Acute community-acquired osteoarticular infections in children: high incidence of concomitant bone and joint involvement. J Microbiol Immunol Infect 2010; 43(4):332–8.

31. Jackson M, Burry V, Olson L. Pyogenic arthritis associated with adjacent osteomyelitis. Pediatr Infect Dis J 1992;11:9.

32. Mooney JF, Murphy RF. Septic arthritis of the pediatric hip: update on diagnosis and treatment. Curr Opin Pediatr 2019;31(1):79–85.

33. Givon U, Liberman B, Schindler A, et al. Treatment of septic arthritis of the hip joint by repeated ultrasound-guided aspirations. J Pediatr Orthop 2004;24(3):266–70.

34. Gottschalk HP, Moor MA, Muhamad AR, et al. Improving diagnostic efficiency: analysis of pelvic MRI versus emergency hip aspiration for suspected hip sepsis. J Pediatr Orthop 2014;34(3):300–6.

35. Refakis CA, Arkader A, Baldwin KD, et al. Predicting periarticular infection in children with septic arthritis of the hip: regionally derived criteria may not apply to all populations. J Pediatr Orthop 2019;39(5): 268–74.

36. Mignemi ME, Menge TJ, Cole HA, et al. Epidemiology, diagnosis, and treatment of pericapsular pyomyositis of the hip in children. J Pediatr Orthop 2014;34(3):316–25.

37. Kim EY, Kwack K-S, Cho JH, et al. Usefulness of dynamic contrast-enhanced MRI in differentiating between septic arthritis and transient synovitis in the hip joint. AJR Am J Roentgenol 2012;198(2):428–33.

38. Zawin J, Hoffer F, Rand F. Joint effusion in children with an irritable hip: ultrasound diagnosis and aspiration. Radiology 1993;187:459.

39. Lee SH, Park JH, Lee JH, et al. False-negative joint aspiration of septic arthritis of the hip in neonates. J Pediatr Orthop B 2020. https://doi.org/10.1097/BPB.0000000000000814.

40. Fontes RA, Ogilvie CM, Miclau T. Necrotizing soft-tissue infections. J Am Acad Orthop Surg 2000; 8(3):151–8.

41. Shahid M, Holton C, O'Riordan S, et al. Sonography of musculoskeletal infection in children. Ultrasound 2020;28(2):103–17.

42. Chao HC, Lin SJ, Huang YC, et al. Sonographic evaluation of cellulitis in children. J Ultrasound Med 2000;19(11):743–9.

43. Loyer EM, DuBrow RA, David CL, et al. Imaging of superficial soft-tissue infections: sonographic findings in cases of cellulitis and abscess. AJR Am J Roentgenol 1996;166(1):149–52.

44. Struk DW, Munk PL, Lee MJ, et al. Imaging of soft tissue infections. Radiol Clin North Am 2001;39(2):277–303.

45. Chou H, Teo HEL, Dubey N, et al. Tropical pyomyositis and necrotizing fasciitis. Semin Musculoskelet Radiol 2011;15(05):489–505.

46. Chau CLF, Griffith JF. Musculoskeletal infections: ultrasound appearances. Clin Radiol 2005;60(2):149–59.

Pediatric Vascular Malformations
Imaging Guidelines and Recommendations

Jonathan D. Samet, MD[a],*, Ricardo Restrepo, MD[b], Shankar Rajeswaran, MD[a], Edward Y. Lee, MD, MPH[c], Jared R. Green, MD[d]

KEYWORDS
- Vascular malformation • Vascular anomaly
- ISSVA (International Society for the Study of Vascular Anomalies)

KEY POINTS
- Ultrasound and MR imaging are the mainstay for imaging diagnosis of vascular malformations in infants and children.
- Vascular malformations should be characterized as low flow or high flow to direct management.
- Radiologic reports should employ terminology of the International Society for the Study of Vascular Anomalies classification to effectively communicate findings with multidisciplinary vascular anomaly subspecialists.

INTRODUCTION

Vascular anomalies encompass a wide-range of entities differing in clinical presentation, natural history, imaging findings, and management. Vascular malformations, a subset of vascular anomalies, are congenital and grow proportional to the patient. Vascular malformations are diagnosed most commonly in the first 2 decades of life and occur in approximately 0.5% of the population.[1,2]

Mulliken and Glowacki[3] devised a cell-oriented classification of vascular anomalies in 1982, delineating entities based on pathophysiology, namely endothelial cell characteristics.[3,4] Vascular tumors, such as hemangiomas, are true neoplasms that exhibit endothelial proliferation and hyperplasia.[4] On the other hand, vascular malformations do not exhibit endothelial proliferation; rather, they the result from errors in vascular morphogenesis. Vascular malformations are categorized by predominant vessel type, including capillary, venous, lymphatic, arterial, and combinations thereof.[5] The most widely accepted classification of vascular anomalies was created by the multispecialty International Society for the Study of Vascular Anomalies (ISSVA) in 1996 and was last revised in 2018.[6] The ISSVA classification provides a standardized nomenclature, which takes into account clinical presentation, lesion histology, natural history, imaging findings, and management. Radiologists should utilize accurate ISSVA terminology when evaluating vascular malformations, because the use of improper or nonuniform terminology may lead to diagnostic delay and preclude appropriate clinical management.[7]

Clinical history and physical examination often can lead to a correct diagnosis for a vascular malformation, although imaging remains essential for characterizing clinically indeterminate lesions and establishing the extent of disease as well as planning and monitoring treatment.[8,9] Radiologists may recommend additional imaging in cases of

[a] Ann and Robert H. Lurie Children's Hospital of Chicago, Northwestern University Feinberg School of Medicine, 225 East Chicago Avenue Box 9, Chicago, IL 60611, USA; [b] Department of Interventional Radiology and Body Imaging, Nicklaus Children's Hospital, 3100 SW 62nd Avenue, Miami, FL 33155, USA; [c] Department of Radiology, Boston Children's Hospital, Harvard Medical School, 300 Longwood Avenue, Boston, MA 02115, USA; [d] Joe DiMaggio Children's Hospital, Envision Radiology associates of Hollywood, 500 N Hiatus Road, Suite 200, Pembroke Pines, FL 33026, USA
* Corresponding author.
E-mail address: JSamet@luriechildrens.org

Radiol Clin N Am 60 (2022) 179–192
https://doi.org/10.1016/j.rcl.2021.08.011

suspected syndromic association or multiorgan involvement.[5] The purpose of this article is to review evidence-based imaging guidelines and recommendations for the evaluation of pediatric vascular malformations.

EVIDENCE-BASED IMAGING ALGORITHM

There is a relative paucity of rigorous scientific evidence concerning imaging of vascular malformations. This may in part be due to limited adherence to ISSVA terminology in clinical practice, which has been shown to hamper management.[10] In a study of more than 5000 referrals to a dedicated center of excellence for vascular lesions, 65% of referrals were vascular malformations and 35% were tumors, yet up to 50% of these referrals carried with incorrect referral diagnosis.[8] Multidisciplinary vascular anomaly clinics have been shown to overcome to these hurdles and improve treatment success.[10–13] Vascular anomaly centers of excellence have been shown crucial for accurate evaluation and treatment of these conditions.[14,15] Additionally, value-based care achieved through multidisciplinary vascular anomaly clinics has been shown to be financially advantageous to patients and the health care system at large.[16]

Ultrasound (US) and MR imaging are the mainstay modalities in vascular malformation imaging work-up and often are complementary in establishing a diagnosis and treatment plan.[17–19] Distinction between high-flow and low-flow lesions is essential to guide management.[18,19] In general, low-flow lesions that require treatment can be treated percutaneously with sclerotherapy, whereas high-flow lesions often require intravascular embolization.[18] Dynamic US images and maneuvers and key MR imaging features, discussed later, can help distinguish types of low-flow lesions.[5,18,19]

PRACTICAL IMAGING APPROACH TO PEDIATRIC VASCULAR MALFORMATIONS
Ultrasound

US should be the initial examination performed in the work-up of a suspected vascular malformation, because it often can make a correct diagnosis, especially in superficial and focal lesions (Fig. 1).[5,20,21] Superficial lesions may be entirely characterized with US, whereas deeper or more extensive lesions may be more difficult to assess. UA is widely available, is inexpensive, is noninvasive, and does not require sedation, which is an important consideration in pediatric patients.[5]

Grayscale
Presence of a solid hypervascular mass is not consistent with the US appearance of vascular malformations and therefore an important distinction for the initial evaluation. The presence of a solid mass virtually excludes an arteriovenous malformation (AVM) and should prompt suspicion of a neoplasm.[22] Cystic or heterogenous lesions are common appearances for lymphatic malformations (LMs) and venous malformations (VMs). VMs and LMs both can have anechoic spaces with intervening septations. If thrombosed or after intralesional hemorrhage, a malformation may demonstrate features, such as fluid-fluid levels or masslike solid appearance.

Spectral Doppler
Spectral Doppler US is an essential component of the initial imaging evaluation and is obtained relatively easily, especially in superficial lesions.[5] Doppler is needed to distinguish high-flow and low-flow lesions, a critical part of the US interpretation. High-flow lesions, such as AVMs, demonstrate arterial waveforms, although septations within a low-flow malformation may contain vessels that demonstrate arterial or venous waveforms and should not be confused with AVMs. Low-flow lesions include VMs and LMs, discussed later.

Dynamic maneuvers
Compressibility, a feature suggestive of VMs and to a lesser extent LMs, can be assessed and documented on cine images easily. If a VM undergoes thrombosis, it may not compress, however. Maneuvers, such as tourniquet application for lesions located in the extremities and Trendelenburg for head and neck lesion, can demonstrate lesional engorgement suggestive of VM.

MR Imaging

MR imaging plays a pivotal role in the imaging evaluation of vascular malformations owing to excellent contrast resolution and ability to depict a lesion's relationship to adjacent anatomic structures.[4] MR imaging, better than US, allows depiction of the relationship of the lesion with adjacent critical structures, in particular nerves, which is important when intervention is contemplated.[18] The full extent of a lesion, including focal, multifocal, or diffuse, can be assessed accurately with MR imaging.[18] In a study comparing the utility of MR imaging versus US in head and neck vascular malformations, delineation of lesion extent was superior with MR imaging (54% of cases) compared with US (44% of cases).[23] A disadvantage of MR imaging compared with US is the need for sedation in younger or uncooperative patients, because MR imaging examinations are lengthy and may require intravenous insertion for contrast administration.

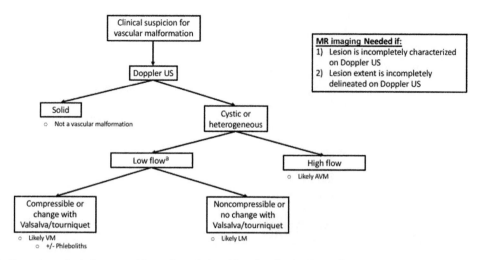

Fig. 1. Flow chart depicting an evidence based algorithm for the workup of a suspected vascular malformation. [a]Low-flow malformations may show arterial or venous flow in vascularized septations or crossing vessels. US, ultrasound; MR, magnetic resonance; AVM, arteriovenous malformation; VM, venous malformation; LM, lymphatic malformation.

On routine MR imaging sequences, high-flow lesion, such as AVMs, may have tortuous signal flow voids indicative of fast flow.[18] Intravenous contrast with dynamic, multiphase magnetic resonance angiogram (MRA) can subcategorize vascular malformations into low-flow and high-flow lesions.[4,24,25] The feeding arteries and draining veins of high-flow lesions often are well depicted on time-resolved maximum intensity projection (MIP) reconstructions.[18] Low-flow lesions, such as VMs, and LMs, typically are hypointense on T1-weighted images and hyperintense (fluid signal) on T2-weighted images and may contain internal septations.

Radiography

Radiographs often are performed in the initial evaluation of extremity pain or mass. Although soft tissue lesions often are occult on radiographs, important information sometimes can be gleaned regarding the nature of a vascular malformation. Phleboliths appear as small rounded calcifications and are characteristic of VMs. Studies have shown, however, that phleboliths are seen on radiographs in only 15% to 25% of cases (**Fig. 2**), although can be seen in 80% of cases with high-resolution US[23] Phleboliths that are present argue against LMs or high-flow lesions, such as AVMs. Radiographs also may give insight into the presence of intraosseous involvement. Intraosseous involvement occurs in up to 18% of AVMs and is important to recognize because it can lead to orthopedic complications.[26] Radiographic findings of AVM intraosseous extension include lucent serpiginous lesions involving the bony cortex and medullary space. Radiographs also may be useful in the evaluation of limb length discrepancy and hemihypertrophy, which may occur in the setting of complex vascular malformation syndromes.

Computed Tomography

Computed tomography (CT) often is avoided in pediatric patients due to associated radiation burden.[27] For example, in the evaluation of suspected VMs and AVMs, multiple phases are required to assess the lesion accurately, which increase the overall radiation dose. The relatively lower-contrast resolution of CT compared with MR imaging makes CT less helpful in the characterization of vascular malformations. CT can be used when MR imaging is not available, in cases less amenable to MR imaging evaluation, such as those with lung involvement, and in pediatric patients requiring cross-sectional imaging who are not able to undergo general anesthesia for MR imaging. If used, however, CT requires the administration of intravenous contrast. CT with its 3-dimensional capabilities can depict the degree of intraosseous involvement and deformity critical in the preoperative planning, particularly with AVMs.[26] On noncontrast CT, VMs usually are low attenuation and enhance gradually after intravenous contrast. Depending on the timing and presence of contrast, VM appearance on postcontrast imaging may range from hypodense

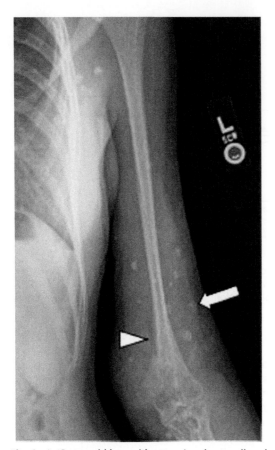

Fig. 2. A 13-year-old boy with extensive chest wall and upper extremity venous malformation (VM). Frontal radiograph of the left humerus demonstrates numerous phleboliths (*arrow*). Left humerus distal metaphysis periosteal reaction (*arrowhead*) is present at the site of a healing pathologic fracture related to intraosseous extension of the VM.

to hyperdense.[28] Phleboliths easily are detected on CT due to the presence of calcium.[28]

Interventional Radiology

Invasive imaging, including arteriography and venography, is used primarily in the treatment of vascular malformations, although may be required to fully characterize AVMs and other high-flow lesions.[29]

SPECTRUM OF PEDIATRIC VASCULAR MALFORMATIONS

With appropriate adherence to ISSVA terminology in daily radiology practice, the most commonly encountered vascular malformations fall under the simple category, in particular LMs and VMs, with AVMs and arteriovenous fistulas (AVFs) seen less frequently. The first step when it comes to

imaging is to distinguish low-flow and high-flow vascular malformations, because the treatment of these lesions is vastly different. LMs and VMs are low-flow lesions, and AVMs/AVFs are high-flow lesions. Vascular malformations associated with other anomalies are less common but often produce characteristic imaging appearances. Capillary malformations (CMs) often are diagnosed clinically, and MR imaging usually is not necessary. Combined malformations include varying combinations of LM, VM, CM, and AVM.

Low-flow Vascular Malformations

Venous malformations

VMs are the most common vascular malformations (67% overall), encountered in the head/neck (40% of cases), extremities (40%), and trunk (20%).[4] VMs have 2 distinct morphologic forms that are reflected on imaging, including spongiform and dysplastic types. Dysplastic types frequently have a collection of ectatic veins, often spanning multiple tissue planes and compartments.[5] Intramuscular VMs can have a delayed presentation, leading to higher morbidity; given these disparate appearances, diagnosis of VM not always is straightforward.[21]

US typically shows a hypoechoic lesion, sometimes with internal anechoic channels. Up to 78% of VMs demonstrate presence of venous waveforms on Doppler US, with up to 16% showing no substantial flow detected.[21] Arterial flow may be present within VM septations or normal vessels crossing through the VM and should not be confused with the arterial flow of an AVM.[21] Phleboliths have been reported to be seen in 80% of cases with high-resolution US, previously reported in 16% to 22% on older US studies.[21,23]

Applying compression is essential to distinguish from other malformations or tumors, because VMs without intralesional thrombosis demonstrate compressibility (Fig. 3). With Valsalva or Trendelenburg maneuvers or the application of a tourniquet, VMs often engorge or fill on color Doppler (Fig. 4).

If additional imaging is required to characterize a lesion or delineate its extent further, MR imaging usually is the complementary modality of choice to evaluate VMs, especially those in deeper locations or extensive lesions. Classically, VMs are T2 hyperintense and slightly hyperintense to muscle on T1-weighted imaging. Spongiform type has lobulated margins. Internally, it may have thrombi or phleboliths, which are T2 hypointense. Fluid-fluid levels can be seen due to blood flow stagnation and isolation from the systemic circulation, especially in the spongiform subtype. Contrast enhancement of VM is variable and erratic from

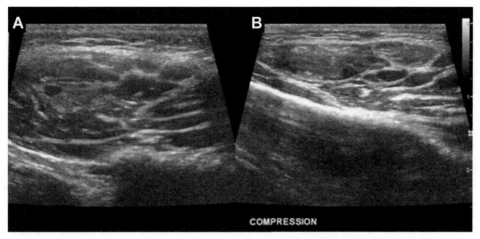

Fig. 3. A 15-year-old girl with lower leg intramuscular venous malformation (VM). (A) Grayscale US image shows an intramuscular circumscribed hypoechoic lesion with thin septations and no soft tissue component. (B) Grayscale US image during US-guided compression demonstrates compressibility of the lesion.

minimal and spotty to fairly homogeneous and on time-resolved MRA, VMs enhance only on delayed or very delayed phases.[18] Dynamic images show gradual filling of the lesion with contrast over time (Fig. 5).[18]

Lymphatic malformations

LMs are the second most common vascular malformation after VMs and are seen most commonly in the neck (80%) and axillary region (20%) and are uncommon in the extremities.[4] LMs are located most commonly within the subcutaneous tissues, although often are trans-spatial[1]; 65% are seen at birth and 80% by 1 year.[2] LMs can be microcystic macrocystic or a combination thereof. Macrocystic lesions have larger multiloculated cystic spaces, typically greater than 1 cm.[1] Microcystic LMs are ill-defined and cysts measure less than 1 cm, typically 2 mm or smaller.[4,5] LMs may become clinically apparent only with swelling in the setting of internal bleeding–related minor trauma or infection (Fig. 6).[1,18]

On US, the cystic spaces of LMs typically are anechoic in their unstimulated state (Fig. 7), although microcystic LMs can appear as sheets of hyperechoic tissue with loss of normal tissue planes (Fig. 8). Unlike VMs, LMs are not very compressible. LMs should not contain a substantial vascular component, although may show minimal peripheral or septal flow on Doppler US.

With MR imaging, LMs are substantially hyperintense on T2 although signal intensity may become

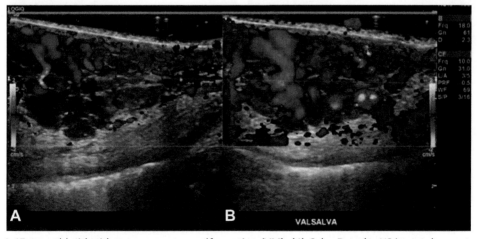

Fig. 4. A 17-year-old girl with tongue venous malformation (VM). (A) Color Doppler US image demonstrates internal low-level color flow within the VM at rest. (B) Color Doppler US image shows substantially increased internal color flow within the VM during Valsalva maneuver.

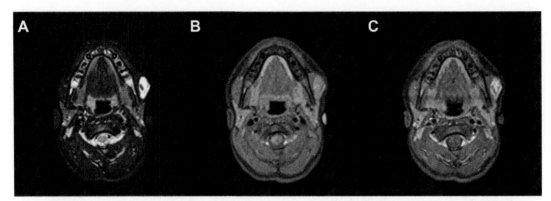

Fig. 5. A 9-year-old boy with left facial venous malformation (VM). (*A*) Axial T2-weighted fat-suppressed MR image demonstrates hypointense lesion located within the left masseter muscle, with low-signal phlebolith versus clot present. (*B*) Axial T1-weighted, fat-suppressed, precontrast MR image shows the lesion is slightly hyperintense to muscle. (*C*) Axial T1-weighted, fat-suppressed postcontrast MR image demonstrates inhomogeneous enhancement of the lesion.

heterogeneous in the setting of intralesional hemorrhage. Macrocystic LMs have well-defined margins whereas the microcystic ones can have infiltrative borders and appear solid. With contrast-enhanced MR imaging, macrocystic LMs should dem-onstrate only rim and septal enhancement (Fig. 9); the presence of a homogenous enhancing component should raise consideration for alternate diagnoses. With microcystic LMs, the enhancement may be homogenous mimicking a solid neoplasm.

High-flow Vascular Malformations

Vascular malformations that contain arterial components or bypass the capillary bed are termed high-flow lesions, accounting for 10% of extremity malformations.[18] AVMs and AVFs are high-flow lesions that must be distinguished from low-flow lesions due to substantial treatment differences. On Doppler US, high-flow lesions, such as AVMs, have an arterial waveform with spectral broadening and arterialized venous waveform. Time-resolved MRA detects arterial flow in the early phases of lesional enhancement.[4,18] If only delayed-phase imaging is performed, this hemodynamic information is lost. AVMs have arterial inflow, vascular nidus, and early drainage into dilated veins. In AVFs, there is a direct connection between arteries and veins. AVMs are present at birth but

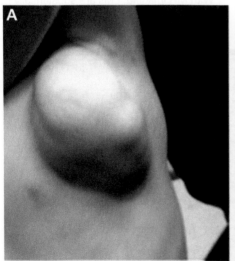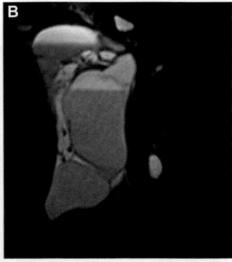

Fig. 6. A 2-year-old girl with sudden expansion of a previously occult left chest wall lesion. (*A*) Clinical photograph shows a multilobulated lesion arising in the axillary region, with no overlying skin discoloration. (*B*) Axial T2-weighted fat-suppressed MR image of the left axilla demonstrates multiple macrocystic and microcystic spaces with fluid-fluid levels, consistent with lymphatic malformation.

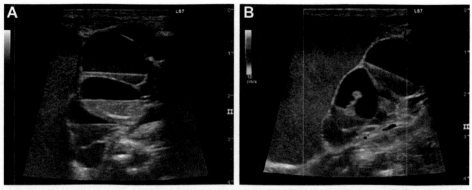

Fig. 7. A 3-year-old girl with chest wall lymphatic malformation (LM). (*A*) Transverse grayscale US image demonstrates multiple macrocysts of varying sizes within the LM, some of which show fluid-fluid levels. (*B*) Transverse color Doppler US image demonstrates absence of flow within the cystic spaces, although flow is present within a vessel adjacent to the LM.

may not become symptomatic until later.[4,5] AVFs can be congenital or posttraumatic, such as those due to prior venous line access.[30]

On grayscale US, AVMs' and AVFs' lack of a mass lesion[4,5] is a feature that helps distinguish them from other vascular anomalies, such as hemangiomas. On color and spectral Doppler, there is increased vascularity and arterial waveforms (**Fig. 10**) with high diastolic flow.[5] Arterialized venous waveforms are a clue to the diagnosis.[5] On routine precontrast MR imaging sequences, high-flow lesions may show tangles of flow voids, representing the abnormal arteries and/or veins of the malformation. Time-resolved MRA shows arterial inflow in the early phases, best visualized on the MIPs (**Fig. 11**). In AVFs especially, there is early shunting into dilated veins.[18,24,31]

Vascular Malformations Associated with Other Anomalies

Vascular malformations can be diffuse, complex, and associated with syndromes or other anomalies. Close collaboration with multidisciplinary teams, including dermatology, interventional radiology, diagnostic radiology, and orthopedics, is key to arriving at the correct diagnosis and best management.[32] Five well-known syndromes associated with vascular malformation, including Klippel-Trénaunay syndrome, Parkes Weber syndrome, Maffucci syndrome, blue rubber bleb nevus (Bean) syndrome, generalized lymphatic anomaly (GLA), and Gorham-Stout disease (GSD), are discussed.

Klippel-Trénaunay syndrome

Klippel-Trénaunay syndrome is an overgrowth syndrome with extensive low flow combined vascular malformation, including capillary, venous, and lymphatic components.[5] The lower extremities are involved most commonly. The unilateral limb is involved in 85% and bilateral in 12.5%.[2] Limb length discrepancy is reported in 66%.[33] There is a pathognomonic draining marginal vein in the subcutaneous fat of the lateral lower leg and thigh (**Fig. 12**).

Parkes Weber syndrome

Parkes Weber syndrome consists of AVFs, CM, and limb overgrowth. It is a high-flow lesion with substantial AVFs, a main distinguishing feature.[34] This arteriovenous shunting may lead to high-output cardiac failure.[35] It involves the lower limbs in 77% of cases.[2]

Maffucci syndrome

Enchondromatosis plus vascular lesions is the hallmark of Maffucci syndrome, distinguishing it from enchondromatosis alone as seen in Ollier disease. The vascular lesions can be low-flow lesions, such as VMs, or high-flow lesions, such as spindle cell hemangiomas (**Fig. 13**).[6] Phleboliths in the soft tissues are within VMs in this entity. Malignant transformation is a feared complication, reported in 20% to 30%.[2]

Blue rubber bleb nevus (Bean) syndrome

Blue rubber bleb nevus (Bean) syndrome is characterized by numerous VMs, particularly in the skin and gastrointestinal system but also in the musculoskeletal system. The lesions can result in soft tissue and osseous extremity deformities.[36] On MR imaging, the VMs are multiple but retain their characteristic appearance, as in solitary disease. Gastrointestinal hemorrhage is a primary concern; therefore, prompt diagnosis is essential.[2]

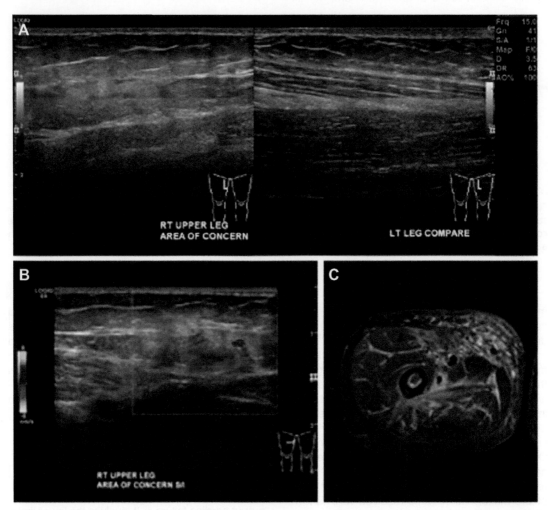

Fig. 8. An 11-year-old girl with right thigh microcystic lymphatic malformation (LM). (*A*) Longitudinal grayscale US image (*left*) of the involved area demonstrates diffuse, trans-spatial hyperechoic appearance of the subcutaneous and deep soft tissues, with loss of normal tissue planes; comparison image (*right*) of the left thigh demonstrates preservation of the normal tissue planes and architecture. (*B*) Transverse color Doppler US image of the involved area shows no evidence of hyperemia or abnormal vascular flow otherwise. (*C*) Axial T2-weighted, fat-suppressed MR image of the right thigh demonstrates the trans-spatial nature of the hyperintense microcystic LM and better delineates lesion extent.

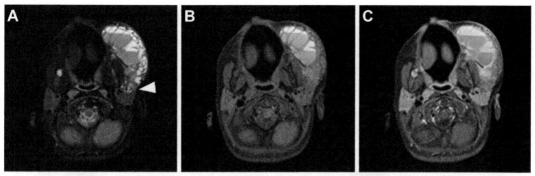

Fig. 9. A 3-year-old girl with a facial lymphatic malformation (LM). (A) Axial T2-weighted, fat-suppressed MR image demonstrates mixed macrocystic and microcystic LM, with trans-spatial extension into the left parotid gland (arrowhead). (B) Axial T1-weighted, fat-suppressed MR image shows mixed isointense to hyperintense contents of the cysts, with numerous fluid levels present. (C) Axial T1-weighted, fat-suppressed, postcontrast MR image demonstrates septal enhancement, with no MR imaging evidence of a solid enhancing component.

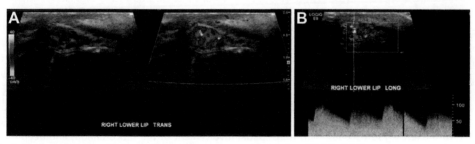

Fig. 10. A 12-year-old boy with lower lip arteriovenous malformation (AVM). (A) Transverse grayscale US demonstrates a hypoechoic nidus of vessels with no soft tissue mass, with color Doppler imaging showing multidirectional avid internal vascularity. (B) Longitudinal spectral Doppler US image within the AVM nidus demonstrates pulsatile low-resistance waveforms.

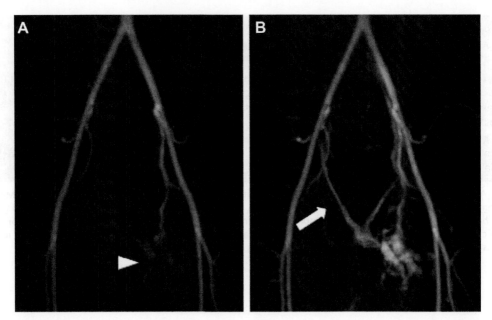

Fig. 11. A 10-year-old boy with pelvic arteriovenous malformation (AVM). (*A*) Coronal MIP, dynamic, time-resolved contrast-enhanced MRA image in the early arterial phase demonstrates enhancement of the nidus (*arrowhead*) via the left internal iliac artery. (*B*) Subsequent arterial-phase MRA image shows early drainage of the AVM via the bilateral internal iliac veins (*arrow*), without opacification of the systemic veins otherwise.

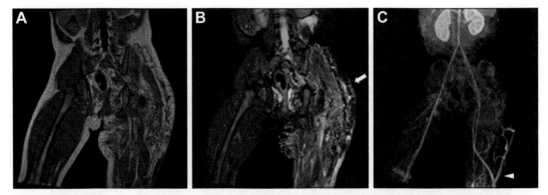

Fig. 12. A 3-year-old girl with Klippel-Trénaunay syndrome. (*A*) Coronal T1-weighted MR image demonstrates overgrowth of the left leg soft tissues, with trans-spatial involvement of the subcutaneous and deep intramuscular planes with mixed capillary, venous, and lymphatic malformation (LM) components. (*B*) Coronal T2-weighted, fat-suppressed MR image shows extent of the hyperintense vascular malformation (*arrow*). (*C*) Coronal MIP, dynamic time-resolved, contrast-enhanced MRA image demonstrates numerous ectatic abnormal veins, including the marginal vein of Servelle (*arrowhead*).

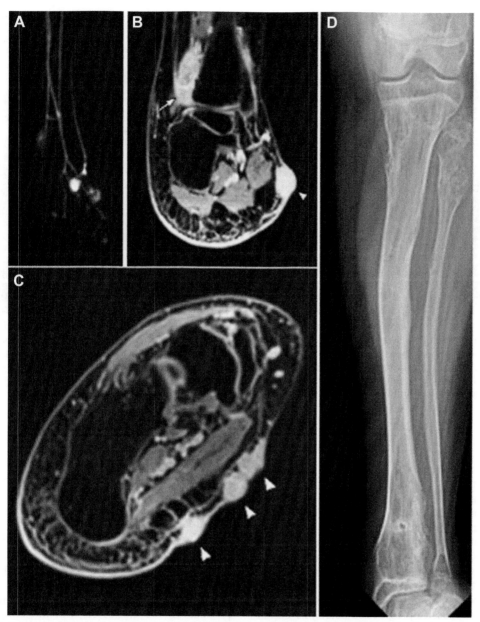

Fig. 13. A 19-year-old girl with Maffucci syndrome. (*A*) Coronal MIP image from time-resolved MRA demonstrates 3 high-flow soft tissue lesions of the right foot and ankle, compatible with hemangiomas in the setting of Maffucci syndrome. (*B*) Delayed postcontrast, T1-weighted, fat-suppressed, coronal MR image showing multiple hypervascular soft tissues masses along the medial foot (*arrowhead*), and within the syndesmosis (*arrow*). (*C*) Delayed postcontrast, T1-weighted, fat-suppressed, axial MR image shows multiple hypervascular soft tissues masses (*arrowheads*) along the medial foot and within the syndesmosis. (*D*) Frontal radiograph of the other leg, with numerous irregular shaped lucent lesions of the proximal and distal tibia and fibula, compatible with enchondromatosis.

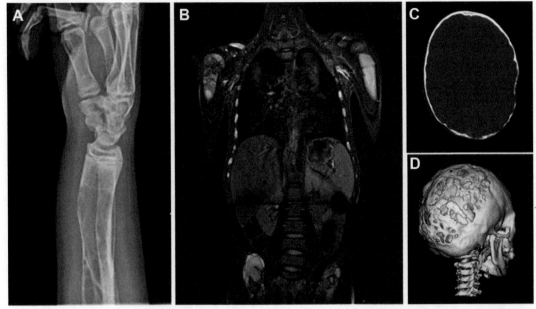

Fig. 14. A 14-year-old boy with Gorham-Stout disease (GSD). (*A*) Lateral radiograph of the right wrist demonstrates intramedullary lucent, expansile lesions with cortical erosions and no periostitis. (*B*) Coronal short tau inversion recovery composite MR image shows numerous hyperintense cystic lesions of the axial and appendicular skeleton, with no visceral or soft tissue involvement. (*C*) Axial contrast-enhanced bone algorithm head CT image demonstrates multiple lytic lesions of the calvarium. (*D*) A 3-dimensional volume-rendered reconstruction CT image of the calvarium best delineates lytic lesion extent.

Gorham-Stout disease and generalized lymphatic anomaly

Gorham-Stout disease (GSD), vanishing bone disease, is a rare disorder with progressive osteolysis. Generalized lymphatic anomaly (GLA), cystic lymphangiomatosis, is an extensive multisystem LM that may affect solid organs, soft tissue, and bone. GLA and GSD have overlapping imaging features, but there are distinguishing features[37] (**Fig. 14**).

Although both can have osseous involvement, GSD has massive progressive osteolysis that involves the cortex and medullary space, often extensive. In GLA, there are multiple lytic lesions but they are confined to the medullary space. Visceral organ involvement, in particular liver and splenic lesions, is greater in GLA.[37]

SUMMARY

Vascular malformations can be focal or diffuse and associated with other syndromes. Diagnosis and classification are complicated and continuously evolving, therefore requiring subspecialist evaluation based on an evidence-based practical approach and multidisciplinary collaboration.

CLINICS CARE POINTS

- Imaging work-up of pediatric vascular malformations should begin with US and then followed by MR imaging for further characterization, as needed.

- Vascular malformations should be characterized mainly as low flow or high flow.

- Vascular malformation extent in different tissues can be elucidated with MR imaging, including subcutaneous, muscular, articular, neural, and osseous.

- Vascular malformations associated with syndromes should be diagnosed and managed in conjunction with a multidisciplinary team.

DISCLOSURE

No disclosures.

REFERENCES

1. White CL, Olivieri B, Restrepo R, et al. Low-flow vascular malformation pitfalls: from clinical examination

to practical imaging evaluation—part 1, lymphatic malformation mimickers. AJR Am J Roentgenol 2016; 206(5):940–51.

2. Redondo P, Aguado L, Martínez-Cuesta A. Diagnosis and management of extensive vascular malformations of the lower limb: part I. Clinical diagnosis. J Am Acad Dermatol 2011;65(5):893–906.

3. Mulliken JB, Glowacki J. Hemangiomas and vascular malformations in infants and children: a classification based on endothelial characteristics. Plast Reconstr Surg 1982;69(3):412–22.

4. Flors L, Leiva-Salinas C, Maged IM, et al. MR imaging of soft-tissue vascular malformations: diagnosis, classification, and therapy follow-up. Radiographics 2011;31(5):1321–40.

5. Dubois J, Alison M. Vascular anomalies: what a radiologist needs to know. Pediatr Radiol 2010;40(6): 895–905.

6. 3-30-2021 ICoVAISftSoVAAaiocA.

7. ISSVA Classification of Vascular Anomalies ©2018 International Society for the Study of Vascular Anomalies. Available at: issva.org/classification.

8. Greene AK, Liu AS, Mulliken JB, et al. Vascular anomalies in 5621 patients: guidelines for referral. J Pediatr Surg 2011;46(9):1784–9.

9. Mulligan P, Prajapati H, Martin L, et al. Vascular anomalies: classification, imaging characteristics and implications for interventional radiology treatment approaches. Br J Radiol 2014;87(1035): 20130392.

10. Mathes EF, Haggstrom AN, Dowd C, et al. Clinical characteristics and management of vascular anomalies: findings of a multidisciplinary vascular anomalies clinic. Arch Dermatol 2004;140(8): 979–83.

11. Lee B-B, Bergan JJ. Advanced management of congenital vascular malformations: a multidisciplinary approach. Cardiovasc Surg 2002;10(6): 523–33.

12. Dubois J, Garel L. Imaging and therapeutic approach of hemangiomas and vascular malformations in the pediatric age group. Pediatr Radiol 1999;29(12):879–93.

13. Rochon PJ. Vascular anomalies: importance of multidisciplinary approach to vascular malformation management. Semin intervent radiol 2017;34(3): 301–2.

14. Rockson SG. Lymphatic Centers of Excellence: A New Reality, Long Overdue. Lymphat Res Biol 2021; 19(1):1–2. https://doi.org/10.1089/lrb.2021.29100.sr.

15. Nassiri N, Thomas J, Cirillo-Penn NC. Evaluation and management of peripheral venous and lymphatic malformations. J Vasc Surg Venous Lymphatic Disord 2016;4(2):257–65.

16. Straughan AJ, Mudd PA, Silva AL, et al. Cost analysis of a multidisciplinary vascular anomaly clinic. Ann Otol Rhinol Laryngol 2019;128(5):401–5.

17. Hussein A, Malguria N. Imaging of vascular malformations. Radiol Clin 2020;58(4):815–30.

18. Fayad L, Hazirolan T, Bluemke D, et al. Vascular malformations in the extremities: emphasis on MR imaging features that guide treatment options. Skeletal Radiol 2006;35(3):127–37.

19. Flors L, Leiva-Salinas C, Norton PT, et al. Ten frequently asked questions about MRI evaluation of soft-tissue vascular anomalies. AJR Am J Roentgenol 2013;201(4):W554–62.

20. Reis J III, Koo KS, Monroe EJ, et al. Ultrasound evaluation of pediatric slow-flow vascular malformations: practical diagnostic reporting to guide interventional management. AJR Am J Roentgenol 2021;216(2): 494–506.

21. Olivieri B, White CL, Restrepo R, et al. Low-flow vascular malformation pitfalls: from clinical examination to practical imaging evaluation—part 2, venous malformation mimickers. AJR Am J Roentgenol 2016;206(5):952–62.

22. Paltiel HJ, Burrows PE, Kozakewich HP, et al. Soft-tissue vascular anomalies: utility of US for diagnosis. Radiology 2000;214(3):747–54.

23. Ahuja A, Richards P, Wong K, et al. Accuracy of high-resolution sonography compared with magnetic resonance imaging in the diagnosis of head and neck venous vascular malformations. Clin Radiol 2003;58(11):869–75.

24. Hammer S, Uller W, Manger F, et al. Time-resolved magnetic resonance angiography (MRA) at 3.0 Tesla for evaluation of hemodynamic characteristics of vascular malformations: description of distinct subgroups. Eur Radiol 2017;27(1):296–305.

25. Green JR, Resnick SA, Restrepo R, et al. Spectrum of imaging manifestations of vascular malformations and tumors beyond childhood: what general radiologists need to know. Radiol Clin North Am 2020; 58(3):583–601.

26. Do YS, Park KB. Vascular anomalies: special consideration for intraosseous arteriovenous malformations. Semin intervent radiol 2017;34(03):272–9.

27. Obara P, McCool J, Kalva SP, et al. ACR appropriateness criteria® clinically suspected vascular malformation of the extremities. J Am Coll Radiol 2019;16(11):S340–7.

28. Legiehn GM, Heran MK. Venous malformations: classification, development, diagnosis, and interventional radiologic management. Radiol Clin North Am 2008;46(3):545–97.

29. Hawkins CM, Chewning RH. Diagnosis and management of extracranial vascular malformations in children: arteriovenous malformations, venous malformations, and lymphatic malformations. Semin Roentgenol 2019;54(4):337–48.

30. Teichgräber U, Gebauer B, Benter T, et al. Central venous access catheters: radiological management of complications. Cardiovasc Intervent Radiol 2003; 26(4):321–33.

31. Merrow AC, Gupta A, Patel MN, et al. 2014 revised classification of vascular lesions from the international society for the study of vascular anomalies: radiologic-pathologic update. Radiographics 2016; 36(5):1494–516.

32. Donnelly LF, Adams DM, Bisset GS III. Vascular malformations and hemangiomas: a practical approach in a multidisciplinary clinic. AJR Am J Roentgenol 2000;174(3):597–608.

33. Redondo P, Aguado L, Martínez-Cuesta A. Diagnosis and management of extensive vascular malformations of the lower limb: part II. Systemic repercussions, diagnosis, and treatment. J Am Acad Dermatol 2011;65(5):909–23.

34. Ziyeh S, Spreer J, Rössler J, et al. Parkes Weber or Klippel-Trenaunay syndrome? Non-invasive diagnosis with MR projection angiography. Eur Radiol 2004;14(11):2025–9.

35. Nozaki T, Nosaka S, Miyazaki O, et al. Syndromes associated with vascular tumors and malformations: a pictorial review. Radiographics 2013;33(1): 175–95.

36. Kassarjian A, Fishman SJ, Fox VL, et al. Imaging characteristics of blue rubber bleb nevus syndrome. AJR Am J Roentgenol 2003;181(4):1041–8.

37. Lala S, Mulliken JB, Alomari AI, et al. Gorham-Stout disease and generalized lymphatic anomaly—clinical, radiologic, and histologic differentiation. Skeletal Radiol 2013;42(7):917–24.

Moving?

Make sure your subscription moves with you!

To notify us of your new address, find your **Clinics Account Number** (located on your mailing label above your name), and contact customer service at:

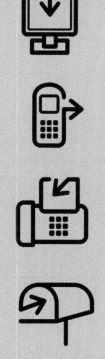

Email: journalscustomerservice-usa@elsevier.com

800-654-2452 (subscribers in the U.S. & Canada)
314-447-8871 (subscribers outside of the U.S. & Canada)

Fax number: 314-447-8029

Elsevier Health Sciences Division
Subscription Customer Service
3251 Riverport Lane
Maryland Heights, MO 63043

ELSEVIER

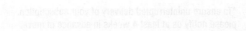

Printed and bound by CPI Group (UK) Ltd, Croydon, CR0 4YY

08/05/2025

01864704-0019